W9-BIM-725

Lithium in Medical Practice

Lithium in Medical Practice

Proceedings of the
First British Lithium Congress
University of Lancaster, England. 15-19 July 1977

Edited by
F. Neil Johnson, PhD
Senior Lecturer in Psychology, University of Lancaster, England
and
Susan Johnson, PhD
Department of Psychology, University of Lancaster, England

University Park Press
Baltimore

Published in USA and Canada by
University Park Press,
233, East Redwood Street,
Baltimore, Maryland 21202

Published in UK by
MTP Press Limited
St. Leonard's House
Lancaster, Lancs.

Library of Congress Cataloging in Publication Data

British Lithium Congress, 1st, University of Lancaster, 1977.
Lithium in medical practice.

Includes bibliographical references and index.
1. Lithium—Therapeutic use—Congresses.
2. Lithium—Physiological effect—Congresses.
I. Johnson, F. N. II. Johnson, Susan. III. Title.

RC483.B74 1977 615'.2'381 77-18031
ISBN 0-8391-1210-6

Printed in Great Britain

To all those research workers, clinicians and patients who have played their part in establishing the place of lithium in modern medical practice.

List of Contributors

S. Andrews	Royal Park Psychiatric Hospital, Melbourne, Australia
P. C. Baastrup	Department of Psychiatry, Glostrup Hospital, Glostrup, Denmark
J. Bailey	Medical Research Council Neuropsychiatry Laboratory, West Park Hospital, Epsom, Surrey, England
E. H. Bennie	Leverndale Hospital, Glasgow, Scotland
P. A. Bond	St. John's Hospital, Stone, Aylesbury, Buckinghamshire, England
N. J. Birch	Department of Biochemistry, University of Leeds, Leeds, England
J. F. J. Cade	655 Orrong Road, Toorak, Victoria, Australia
R. Chalmers	Leverndale Hospital, Glasgow, Scotland
E. Chiu	Royal Park Psychiatric Hospital, Melbourne, Australia
C. Christiansen	Department of Clinical Chemistry, Glostrup Hospital, Glostrup, Denmark
K. J. Collard	Department of Physiology, University College, Cardiff, Wales
A. Coppen	Medical Research Council Neuropsychiatry Laboratory, West Park Hospital, Epsom, Surrey, England
H. Dam	Psychochemistry Institute, Copenhagen, Denmark
J. T. Dancey	Department of Medicine, Montreal General Hospital, McGill University, Montreal, Canada
D. A. T. Dick	Department of Anatomy, University of Dundee, Dundee, Scotland
E. G. Dick	Department of Anatomy, University of Dundee, Dundee, Scotland
P. R. Eastwood	Medical Research Council Unit for Metabolic Studies in Psychiatry, Middlewood Hospital, Sheffield, England

F. Eisenried	Psychiatric Clinic, University of Munich, Munich, West Germany
L. Fenoglio	Clinica delle Malattie Nervose e Mentali, University of Pavia, Pavia, Italy
A. Geisler	Department of Pharmacology, University of Copenhagen, Copenhagen, Denmark
A. I. M. Glen	Medical Research Council Brain Metabolism Unit, Thomas Clouston Clinic, Edinburgh, Scotland
J. D. Gommersall	Whiteley Wood Clinic, University Department of Psychiatry, Sheffield, England
W. Greil	Psychiatric Clinic, University of Munich, Munich, West Germany
N. Hariharasubramanian	Department of Physiology, Madurai Medical College, Madurai, India
P. E. Harrison-Read	Department of Pharmacology, Medical College of St. Bartholomew's Hospital, London, England
J. Ph. Hes	Department of Psychiatry, Ichilov Government Municipal Hospital, Tel Aviv, Israel
D. S. Hewick	Department of Pharmacology and Therapeutics, Ninewells Hospital, Dundee, Scotland
D. F. Horrobin	Clinical Research Institute, Montreal, Canada
M. F. Hussain	St. Augustine's Hospital, Canterbury, Kent, England
J. M. Hsu	Veterans Administration Center, Bay Pines, Florida, USA
F. A. Jenner	Medical Research Council Unit for Metabolic Studies in Psychiatry, University Department of Psychiatry, Middlewood Hospital, Sheffield, England
T. C. Jerram	Regional Metabolic Research Unit, High Royds Hospital, Menston, West Yorkshire, England
F. N. Johnson	Department of Psychology, University of Lancaster, Lancaster, England
S. Johnson	Department of Psychology, University of Lancaster, Lancaster, England
M. Karmazyn	Clinical Research Institute, Montreal, Canada

R. J. Kerry	Woodside Psychiatric Unit, Middlewood Hospital, Sheffield, England
R. Klysner	Department of Physiology, University of Copenhagen, Copenhagen, Denmark
J. H. Lazarus	Department of Medicine, University Hospital of Wales, Cardiff, Wales
C. R. Lee	Medical Research Council Unit for Metabolic Studies in Psychiatry, Middlewood Hospital, Sheffield, England
B. Lena	District General Hospital, Eastbourne, East Sussex, England
R. McDonald	High Royds Hospital, Menston, West Yorkshire, England
T. M. McMillan	Department of Pharmacology, University College, London, England
R. Maggs	District General Hospital, Eastbourne, East Sussex, England
M. S. Manku	Clinical Research Institute, Montreal, Canada
K. Martin	Department of Pharmacology, University of Cambridge, Cambridge, England
E. T. Mellerup	Psychochemistry Institute, Copenhagen, Denmark
J. Merry	West Park Hospital, Epsom, Surrey, England
J. P. Mtabaji	Department of Physiology, University of Newcastle-upon-Tyne, Newcastle-upon-Tyne, England
G. J. Naylor	Department of Psychiatry, University of Dundee, Dundee, Scotland
S. Parvathi Devi	Department of Physiology, Madurai Medical College, Madurai, India
C. Paschalis	Medical Research Council Unit for Metabolic Studies in Psychiatry, Middlewood Hospital, Sheffield, England
J. Perez-Cruet	Department of Psychiatry, Missouri Institute of Psychiatry, St. Louis, Missouri, USA
P. Plenge	Psychochemistry Institute, Copenhagen, Denmark
O. J. Rafaelsen	Psychochemistry Institute, Copenhagen, Denmark
C. M. Reynolds	West Park Hospital, Epsom, Surrey, England
A. A. Rider	Department of Biochemistry and Behavioral Sciences, Johns Hopkins University, Baltimore, Maryland, USA

M. Schou	Institute of Psychiatry, Aarhus University, Aarhus, Denmark
D. M. Shaw	Department of Psychological Medicine, Welsh National School of Medicine, Cardiff, Wales
V. Srinivasan	Department of Physiology, Madurai Medical College, Madurai, India
H. Steinberg	Department of Pharmacology, University College, London, England
S. J. Surtees	District General Hospital, Eastbourne, East Sussex, England
P. Thams	Department of Physiology, University of Copenhagen, Copenhagen, Denmark
P. Tosca	Clinica delle Malattie Nervose e Mentali, University of Pavia, Pavia, Italy
I. Transbøl	Department of Internal Medicine, Hvidovre Hospital, Hvidovre, Denmark
S. P. Tyrer	Department of Psychiatry, McMaster University, Hamilton, Ontario, Canada
P. Vendsborg	Psychochemistry Institute, Copenhagen, Denmark
A. Venkoba Rao	Department of Psychiatry, Madurai Medical College, Madurai, India
J. Waite	Department of Psychiatry, Missouri Institute of Psychiatry, St. Louis, Missouri, USA
G. Wildschiødtz	Psychochemistry Institute, Copenhagen, Denmark
E. P. Worrall	Department of Psychological Medicine, Southern General Hospital, Glasgow, Scotland
O. Wraae	Department of Psychiatry, University Hospital, Odense, Denmark
F. Zerbi	Clinica delle Malattie Nervose e Mentali, University of Pavia, Pavia, Italy

Preface

This book contains the full proceedings of the First British Lithium Congress. The title given to this unique occasion bears closer inspection. For the first time ever, a whole scientific conference, spanning several days, was devoted to the subject of lithium and its biological effects: in this sense the conference was truly a "first". It was a British occasion only insofar as it was held on British soil; the speakers and those who attended to listen and to discuss, came not only from England, Scotland and Wales but also from many other lands — from the USA, Canada, Chile and Panama in the New World; from Germany, France, Italy, Denmark, Sweden and the Netherlands in Europe; from Israel and Egypt in the Middle East; from India and Japan in the Old World; from Australia on the other side of the globe, from Iceland, and from our nearest neighbour, Ireland. Lithium was the bond holding together this cultural mix; it was the purpose for which so many experts had congressed in the University of Lancaster for five days in July, 1977.

In that relatively brief period, virtually all aspects of lithium research and lithium therapy were aired, discussed, and argued about. The latest research findings were made public and new cooperative research endeavours established.

From an exciting and stimulating meeting comes a book which we hope will be worthy of those same adjectives. Whilst the book has, so far as its overall organisation into sections is concerned, been cast in a form similar to that of its immediate predecessor, *Lithium Research and Therapy,* it is, in fact, quite a different kind of work and is intended not so much to replace as to supplement the earlier volume. *Lithium Research and Therapy* was explicitly a review text, defining the status of all facets of research on lithium up to 1975: *Lithium in Medical Practice* attempts to update some of the particularly important areas reviewed in the former book (such as the use of lithium in treating conditions other than the affective disorders, and the potentially highly significant effects of lithium on renal functioning), but it does more than this. It reflects in a powerful way the dynamism of ongoing research endeavour in this rapidly expanding field in a manner which was not possible in a volume dedicated to a review of established knowledge. What *Lithium Research and Therapy* said, in effect, was "this is where we have reached so far", but *Lithium in Medical Practice* says "these are the frontiers, the problems, the broad conceptual issues, the directions in which future research may lead us."

In order to build into this book some of the feeling of the drive and energy which were so evident during the Congress, we have to some extent reorganised the order of presentation. The Congress consisted of five major symposia, each having a long review paper and several shorter research papers. The review paper was intended to set the scene, both in historical terms and in the light of the most recent findings, for the subsequent research papers; the latter not only presented data from new (and in many cases, ongoing) experimental research, but outlined the special kinds of problems facing research workers in this area and the ways in which such problems might be overcome. Additionally, a large number of free communications were accepted for presentation at the Congress, and these covered such an astonishingly large variety of topics, evidencing again the vitality and importance from a general biological standpoint of work in this area, that we have included all of them in this book.

In grouping the papers together under the section headings used in this book, we have chosen not to take into account the original designation of the papers as review papers, research papers or free communications. Consequently, long reviews rub shoulders with short expositions of tightly defined research problems, and with discussions of a more speculative nature. But that is as it should be; research is like that. It is not a tidily organised business, but a mixture of established knowledge and exciting speculation, of problems solved and unsolved, of accepted precept and violently contested assertion.

We hope that *Lithium in Medical Practice* will allow those who were unable to attend the First British Lithium Congress to share in the enthusiasm which the meeting engendered, and that it will stimulate others to engage in this most promising field of psychiatric research.

Neil and Susan Johnson,
Lancaster, 1977

Acknowledgements

In an undertaking such as the First British Lithium Congress a great many people become involved — not to say embroiled — in one way or another, and it is not possible to acknowledge each by name: we nevertheless sincerely thank them all. A few, however, have made such major contributions that we are more than pleased to express our gratitude to them in these pages. Mrs. Julie West, Miss Sheila Young and Mrs. Frances Sharples proved to be invaluable in running the Congress Secretariat, and Frances Sharples also typed all the Abstracts which were bound and presented to each delegate and speaker. Paul Johnson, Julie Sockett, Catherine Midgley, Andrew Tolmie and Christine Simpson helped to ensure the smooth running of the Congress. All these, individually and collectively, showed a commitment to the Congress and a personal loyalty to the Organising Secretary which can never be adequately acknowledged.

The final insurance of the success of the Congress and, ultimately, of this book, was the way in which all the speakers put so much thought and energy into their presentations which were of a uniformly high quality. The standard of the papers was reflected in the discussions which followed each session, and it is a great pity that, for reasons both of time and publishing costs, it has not been possible to include edited excerpts from the discussions in this book.

Finally, we must thank all the delegates to the Congress for being so pleasant and courteous to the organisers: it made our lives much easier.

Contents

Part I:
The Historical Context of Lithium Research

Introduction

It is probably true to say that lithium research is today one of the most active areas of investigation in biological psychiatry. In the early nineteen fifties one could number the lithium research workers on one hand—certainly on two. Now, it would be an extremely difficult task to provide a definitive list of all those who are devoting a major portion of their research effort to investigating the effects of lithium on the whole gamut of biochemical, physiological and psychological processes. The story of the discovery of the therapeutic actions of lithium is one which has been told before, and there is no doubt that it will be retold many times in the future. It is a story of a man—John Cade, an Australian—who had the clinical acumen, coupled with an insight into the biological bases of psychopathological states, to launch a timely investigation into the biochemical concomitants of manic depression, and who then had the vision to recognise the biological significance of an unexpected result in his research. But the acumen, the insight and the vision would have been wasted if John Cade had not also had the courage (and it took courage) to press home his advantage into the sphere of practical medicine. In Chapter 1, John Cade tells his own story in a typically blunt and straightforward style. When the history of 20th century medicine comes to be written, the year 1949, the name of John Cade, and the story which he tells, will figure prominently and may indeed gain their true recognition as marking the transition from custodial treatment procedures to rational therapeutic techniques in the control of major psychopathological conditions.

1

Lithium — Past, Present and Future

J. F. J. CADE

INTRODUCTION

In reviewing the history of lithium in medicine an appropriate starting point would have been an account of medieval spas, wells and springs, detailing their alleged medicinal and curative properties, especially of so-called mental illness and then to correlate these alleged benefits with subsequently determined mineral content, with particular reference to lithium salts. I spent a fruitless day researching this topic in the National Library in Melbourne. There are so many variables, conjectures and unsubstantiated statements that it quickly became apparent that it was a fruitless exercise.

However, I was more fortunate in discovering in the library of the Medical Society of Victoria, Sir John Floyer's *History of Cold Bathing* (5th edition 1722 — London) wherein he gives a vivid description of the successful treatment of a case of mania, or at least of acute psychotic excitement. I produce the case report verbatim in Figure 1.1.

Certainly this was over 250 years ago but let us not forget that only slightly less extreme forms of hydrotherapy were practised in cases of great excitement or confusion until quite recently. Less than 25 years ago I visited in Britain a famous psychiatric establishment which still boasted a magnificent hydrotherapy department — fine jets, coarse jets, cold jets, warm jets, low pressure jets, high pressure jets, blanket baths hot and cold, and several other refinements. I rejoice to say that its therapeutic popularity had waned and that patients and staff all jumped together into a spacious heated indoor swimming pool — much more civilized and even

This Man was ſo raving *mad*, that he was bound in *Fetters*; having firſt tryed all Evacutions, uſual in ſuch Caſes, together with Opiats in great Quantity, but to no purpoſe, I, at length, plung'd him *ex improviſo*, into a great Veſſel of *cold Water*, and at the ſame time throwing on him, with great Violence, ten or twelve Pails full of cold Water on his *Head*; but that not ſucceeding, the next day having the Conveniency of a Fall of Water, about half a Mile off, I caus'd him to be plac'd in a Cart, and ſtript from his Clothes; and, being blindfold, that the *Surprize* might be the greater, let fall on a ſudden a great Fall or Ruſh of Water about 20 Foot high, and continued him under it as long as his Strength would well permit: This ſucceeded ſo well, that after his Return home, he fell into a *deep Sleep* for the Space of 29 hours, and awaken'd in a quiet and ſerene State of *Mind* as ever, and ſo continues to this day, it being now about Twelve Months ſince; but in ſome *hypochondriac* and *paralytic* Caſes, I have not ſound it to ſucceed ſo well.

Figure 1.1 Case report from Sir John Floyer's *History of Cold Bathing* (1722)

more therapeutically effective. Indeed, it is the only sensible place to conduct a group therapy session, with the possible exception of the bar at the village pub.

You may well ask, at this stage, what this has to do with lithium. It is relevant in so far as the treatment of recurrent psychotic excitement is concerned: it was the picture up till relatively recently but the advent of the modern psychotropic drugs, including lithium, has changed everything.

Lithium (the metal) was discovered in 1817 by Johan August Arfwedson in analysing the mineral petalite. It constitutes about 20 parts per million of the igneous rocks of the earth's crust, so it is sparsely but widely distributed.

Lithium salts were first introduced into medicine in the 1850s by the English physician Garrod in his book *Gout and Rheumatic Gout* (1), following the demonstration that lithium urate was the most soluble of the urates.

By 1876 the *British Pharmaconoeia* was listing only two preparations of containing carbonate of lithia 10 grains to 1 pint of water, the dose being given as up to ½ pint. Unfortunately it omitted to mention how often such a dose should be taken, still less what it was used for. Exactly the same entry appears in the 1885 edition.

However, Lauder Brunton, in his *Textbook of Pharmacology, Therapeutics and Materia Medica* (1891) expands the list of lithium salts to include the benzoate, salicylate and bromide, quoting from the *United States Pharmacopoeia,* in which they were included. Additionally he gives a rationale for the use of lithium which reads as follows:-

> "The urate of lithium being much more soluble than those of either potassium or sodium, lithia is often employed in preference to these others in gout. It is given internally in order to aid in the elimination of uric acid by the kidneys, to prevent the gouty paroxysm, and to lessen the acidity of the urine, to prevent deposit of uric acid gravel or calculi in the kidneys or bladder, and also to aid in their solution when already formed. It is applied locally to parts affected with gouty inflammation in order to aid in the solution and absorption of the urate of sodium in the tissues. For this purpose it may be applied to stiff joints and chalk-stones whether covered by skin or laid bare by ulceration. A solution of lithia, five grains to the ounce is kept constantly applied to the part for several weeks together."
>
> As for lithium salicylate "It is used as a remedy in gout and rheumatism and is intended to unite the properties of salicylic acid and lithium. It is less irritant to the stomach than salicylic acid." The recommended dose was 20-40 grains or 1.3-2.6 g but there was no mention of frequency of dosage.
>
> Of bromide of lithium, Lauder Brunton goes on:
>
> "It is said by some to have a stronger hypnotic action than the other bromides but by others to be less effective than the potassium salt. It may be preferable to the potassium salt in the irritability of gouty subjects."

The benzoate, he says "has been used as a remedy for gout and uric acid".

By 1898 the *British Pharmacopoeia* was still only listing three preparations — the carbonate, the citrate and the effervescent citrate. They were obviously not highly regarded but Martindale in the 1908 edition of the *Extra Pharmacopoeia* waxes more enthusiastic. He lists the benzoate, the bromide "of great use in Bright's disease" as well as epilepsy, the carbonate which is "diuretic and increases the alkalinity of the blood", the citrate both ordinary and effervescent, the glycerophosphate, the guaiacate "for chronic gout and rheumatism", the hippurate, the iodide which is claimed to be "an anti-arthritic and has been employed in syphilis by kataphoresis", the salicylate both ordinary and effervescent and the tartrate, the last being "of special use in gouty cases with gum affections".

However, by 1941 Martindale is becoming more realistic about the use of lithium salts, pointing out that their introduction into medicine was due to a misconception.

> "Lithium urate being relatively soluble, the lithium salts were introduced as solvents for uric acid, but since the soluble urate cannot exist in the body or the urine in the presence of sodium or potassium ions there is no rational foundation for the use of these salts. When given they should be freely diluted."

In this edition the bromide no longer appears and seems to have been replaced by the chloride, of which more anon.

By 1952 Martindale is playing lithium in a very minor key indeed. The various salts are not listed under the heading of lithium but under the headings of the appropriate and supposedly active anions. Of the carbonate, the following advice is given:-

> "Usually administered in copious draughts as lithia water, preferably on an empty stomach."

It was mildly esteemed as a diuretic, which is interesting in view of its subsequent history in the treatment of manic-depressive illness and the occasional diabetes insipidus-like syndrome that develops.

So the introduction of the lithium ion into medicine was all the result of an elementary mistake. It was perfectly useless for the conditions for which it was prescribed although of course the various anions to which it was united had some therapeutic value. But worse was to follow. From useless it became dangerous. By the late 1940s lithium chloride was being used — in many cases in quite an uncontrolled way — as a salt substitute for flavouring low-sodium diets in patients suffering from oedema due to congestive cardiac failure. In short, it was being used in the wrong way in quite the last kind of patient for whom one would think of prescribing it, and under the worst possible physiological condition, i.e. that of sodium depletion. Fatal intoxication, not surprisingly, was being reported.

The *Journal of the American Medical Association* in its issue of 12 March 1949 tolled the death knell for lithium in medicine, or so it seemed. The first two papers in that issue are devoted to accounts of lithium poisoning from the use of salt substitutes. The first, by Corcoran *et al.* (2) makes a very percipient observation.

> "That the cause of the intoxication was lithium ion and not sodium depletion as such, seems evident from a study of these cases . . . nevertheless, the data indicate that sodium depletion, incident to

treatment with low sodium diets, increases the susceptibility to intoxication from orally ingested lithium salts.''

In the second paper, by Hanlon *et al.* (3) it is stated:-

> ''Recently a 25% solution of lithium chloride which has a taste similar to table salt has been made commercially available. Although there are, in the older literature, scattered records suggesting that ingestion of inorganic lithium salts may cause weakness, tremors and blurring of vision, the solution has been marketed by the distributors with the assurance that it is perfectly safe . . . . Our acquaintance with lithium began in the last two months of 1948 . . . . In the preliminary phase of the report the possibility of serious toxicity from the drug was brought to our attention by the cases presented in this report.''

Both these papers give excellent descriptions of severe and fatal lithium intoxication.

In the same issue of the *JAMA* there is another case report (4) concerning lithium chloride poisoning, this time with complete recovery, and a letter to the Editor on the same topic.

So in March 1949 lithium was effectively excommunicated as a therapeutic substance, at least in the USA.

But strangely enough its pharmacological rehabilitation was commenced in that very same year when a relatively short paper (5) claiming a specific anti-manic effect of the lithium ion appeared in the *Medical Journal of Australia* on 3rd September. That the process was a slow one, extending over more than 20 years was due to a variety of factors. The claim was made by an unknown psychiatrist, with no research experience, working alone in a small chronic mental hospital using primitive techniques and negligible equipment. Additionally, it was published in a journal which had a relatively small circulation outside Australia. This, combined with recent bitter experience with lithium in the States almost threatened the claim with extinction apart from some local interest in Australia and amongst a few psychiatrists in the United Kingdom. It was fortunate indeed that the paper came to the attention of Mogens Schou in Denmark quite early and he enthusiastically followed it up. He has done more than anyone to validate and extend my original observations.

People inevitably ask why lithium should have been tried in the treatment and prophylaxis of affective illness and especially, in the first place, of manic episodes. It is, of course, a perfectly valid question. Why not try potable pearl, or crocodile dung or unicorn horn? I was asked by a reporter some years ago — I thought rather unkindly — whether I had discovered it whilst shaving one morning.

It is naturally the profoundest mystery unless one is aware of the preceding and intermediate steps. Then it can be seen, with such hindsight, to have been the almost inevitable result of experimental work I was engaged in, in an attempt to elucidate the aetiology of manic-depressive illness.

First, of course, was the formulation of an hypothesis. What was the essential nature of manic-depressive illness? Psychopathological explanations seemed to me to be singularly unconvincing, and completely useless when it came to treatment or prevention of attacks. Perhaps it was partly because I was first trained as a physician that I was attracted to a medical model as an explanatory hypothesis. Certainly manic and melancholic patients appeared to me to be sick people in the medical sense. But what medical conditions appeared to provide some sort of analogy?

Manic patients behave in many ways as if they were intoxicated — noisy, restless, disinhibited and flamboyant. Could it be that they were in fact intoxicated, perhaps by a normal product of metabolism circulating in excess? Then melancholia could be explained as the corresponding deprivative condition. The parallel between manic-depressive illness and thyrotoxicosis/myxoedema seemed an attractive proposition and a promising jumping off point. The first dilemma was to decide in which direction to jump. I suppose an obvious thought was that if mania were indeed due to some metabolic substance circulating in excess, some of it might be excreted in the urine and be demonstrable therein. The problem at this stage was that, even supposing such a substance existed, one knew nothing whatever about its properties and therefore had no clear idea how to demonstrate it. The only solution seemed to be to devise an extraordinarily crude differential toxicity test and discover whether any differentials emerged. And crude it was. It involved simply the intraperitoneal injection into guinea pigs of a concentrated sample of urine (the early morning specimen passed after abstinence from fluid for 12-14 hr) in varying amounts from manics, melancholics, schizophrenics and normal controls.

It quickly became evident that the urine from some manic patients was far more toxic than that from any of the other groups. The urine from some manic patients would kill the animals in doses as low as 0.25 ml per 30 g body weight, whereas the most toxic specimen from others was not lethal in doses lower than 0.75 ml per 30 g body weight. All that had been demonstrated so far was that any concentrated urine in sufficient quantity would kill a guinea pig, but that urine from a manic patient often killed much more readily.

Now the mode of death is the same in all cases, manic and non-manic, suggesting that the same toxic agent is at work. After a latent period of 12-28 min, in which the animal appears perfectly well, apart from occasional distress of a few minutes following the injection, it becomes tremulous and ataxic, and in a few minutes quadriplegic, the hind legs being the first affected. It remains fully conscious and often squeals when picked up at this stage. Myoclonic twitching precedes a severe tonic convulsion, and from then on the animal remains unconscious in status epilepticus of tonic type with convulsive gasping until its death a few or many minutes later. An occasional animal recovers.

In an attempt to identify the actual toxic agent in the urine the principal end products of nitrogenous metabolism were first investigated. It was not very surprising to find that urea was the guilty substance. In a 4% aqueous solution its lethal dose for guinea pigs was 1.0-1.25 ml per 30 g of body weight, a relatively enormous dose, roughly equivalent to 100 g in a 70 kg man. The mode of death is exactly the same as with urine. It is an interesting point that there appear to be no intermediate effects. The animal either develops no symptoms whatever following the injection or it dies.

Uric acid 0.1% solution in normal saline, and creatinine 0.1% solution in normal saline, appeared to have no toxic effects at all when injected intraperitoneally in guinea pigs in maximum doses. It is impossible to inject more than about 2 ml of fluid per 30 g of body weight into the peritoneal cavity of a guinea pig.

So, although the actual toxic agent was identified this was only a first step. The next was to identify the quantitative modifiers that made specimens of urine from some manics so much more toxic than any specimens from other sources. It was not simply that these more toxic urines contained a higher concentration of urea. As the lethal dose of a 4% aqueous solution of urea is about 1 ml per 30 g body weight, one would have to postulate an impossible concentration of 8-16% urea in these specimens. In fact quantitative estimations showed that urine from manic patients did not differ significantly from that of non-manics or controls in urea content.

Were uric acid or creatinine the quantitative modifiers? Uric acid has, if anything, a slight effect in enhancing the toxicity of urea, but the most surprising observation was the remarkable protective action of creatinine. The minimal lethal dose of an aqueous solution of 0.025% creatinine and 4% urea is double that of a 4% solution of urea only. The same degree of protection is afforded by a fairly wide range of creatinine concentrations; 0.025% gives as much protection as 0.2% and more than counter-balances the mildly enhancing toxic effect of uric acid.

Creatinine is also strongly protective against the convulsive and lethal effects of "Cardiazol" (pentamethylenetetrazol).

It now appeared important to estimate more accurately, if possible, how much uric acid increased the toxicity of urea. The practical difficulty was the comparative insolubility of uric acid in water, so the most soluble urate was chosen — the lithium salt. And that is how lithium came into the story.

When an aqueous solution of 8% urea, saturated with lithium urate, was injected, the toxicity was far less than expected. It appeared as though the lithium ion may have been exerting a protective effect.

Substitution of the carbonate for the urate was equally effective in preventing the convulsant death produced by toxic doses of urea.

To determine whether lithium salts by themselves had any discernible effects on guinea pigs, animals were injected intraperitoneally with large doses of 0.5% aqueous solution of lithium carbonate. A noteworthy result was that after a latent period of about 2 hr the animals, although fully conscious, became extremely lethargic and unresponsive for 1-2 hr before once again becoming normally timid and active. Those who have experimented with guinea pigs know to what extent a ready startle reaction is part of their make-up. It was thus even more startling to the experimenter to find that after the injection of a solution of lithium carbonate they could be turned on their backs and that, instead of their usual frantic righting reflex behaviour, they merely lay there and gazed placidly back at him.

It may seem a long way from lethargy and tranquillity in guinea pigs to the control of manic excitement but as the emphasis in these investigations from the very beginning had been upon mania, its possible aetiology and (hopefully) its management, the association of ideas is readily understandable.

Since, as recounted earlier, lithium salts had been in use in medical practice since the middle of the nineteenth century, there seemed no ethical contraindications to using them in mania, especially as single and repeated doses of lithium citrate and lithium carbonate in the doses contemplated produced no discernible ill effects on the experimenter himself.

Originally two alternative salts were used — the citrate because of its solubility but increasingly the carbonate because this salt seemed considerably less likely to produce alimentary disturbance. The original therapeutic dose decided on fortuitously proved to be the usual optimum, that is 1200 mg of the citrate or 600 mg of the carbonate thrice daily.

It may be of interest to record once again the case report of the very first manic patient ever deliberately and successfully treated with lithium salts. This was a little wizened man of 51 who had been in a state of chronic manic excitement for 5 years. He was amiably restless, dirty, destructive, mischievous and interfering. He had enjoyed pre-eminent nuisance value in a back ward for all those years and bid fair to remain there for the rest of his life. He commenced treatment with lithium citrate 1200 mg thrice daily on 29 March 1948. On the fourth day, the optimistic therapist thought he saw some change for the better but acknowledged that it could have been his expectant imagination (it was April Fool's Day!). The nursing staff were non-committal but loyal. However, by the 5th day it was clear that he was in fact more settled, tidier, less disinhibited and less distractible. From then on there was steady improvement so that in 3 weeks he was enjoying the unaccustomed and quite unexpected amenities of a convalescent ward. As he had been ill so long and confined to a closed chronic ward he found normal surroundings and liberty of movement strange at first. Owing to this, as well as housing difficulties and the necessity of determining a satisfactory maintenance dose, he was kept under observation for a further 2 months.

He remained perfectly well and left hospital on 9 July 1948, on indefinite leave, with instructions to take a maintenance dose of lithium carbonate 300 mg twice daily.

The carbonate had been substituted for the citrate as he had become intolerant of the latter, complaining of severe nausea. He was soon back working happily at his old job.

It was with a sense of the most abject disappointment that I readmitted him to hospital 6 months later as manic as ever but took some consolation from his brother who informed me that Bill had become overconfident about having been well for so many months, had become lackadaisical about taking his medication and had finally ceased taking it about 6 weeks before. Since then he had become steadily more irritable and erratic. His lithium carbonate was at once recommenced and in 2 weeks he had again returned to normal. A month later he was recorded as completely well and ready to return to home and work.

And so lithium, after its dubious beginning in medicine and its disastrous apparent finale, was launched again — precariously, it is true — as a powerful psychotropic drug in affective illness.

I will review only briefly progress since 1949: later chapters in this book will cover the various aspects in great detail.

There has been, in the first place, an extension of the clinical indications for the use of lithium. My original claim was simply that it was therapeutic and prophylactic in chronic and recurrent mania and that it seemed to have some use as a non-specific tranquillizer in the disturbed schizophrenic without, however, affecting the fundamental schizophrenic process. In my extremely limited experience at the time I could not discern that it had any therapeutic value as an anti-depressant in the few chronic depressives in whom it was tried.

Since then various workers, foremost amongst whom have been Schou and Baastrup (6) in Denmark, have shown in a series of papers that it is powerfully prophylactic against depressive swings in both bipolar and unipolar depressive illness.

In some cases of schizo-affective illness and so-called chronic schizophrenia lithium may prove dramatically effective. In such cases it is usually given as "end-of-the-line" medication, more in desperation than expectation. Those in the latter category who do respond have frequently had manic or hypomanic features documented from time to time in their bulky clinical histories. I have been sufficiently impressed of latter years by this admittedly uncommon phenomenon to urge colleagues working in large hospitals with clinical responsibility for considerable numbers of chronic schizophrenics to carefully review such patients' medical files and, where they find affective episodes recorded, to essay a clinical trial with lithium. I point out that it will only take two weeks or so to determine whether they are responders or non-responders, warning too that they will have many failures but the occasional brilliant success.

Lithium may prove an essential therapeutic weapon in the total management of young people with character or personality disorders in whom there is clear evidence of cyclothymia, as one of my younger colleagues (7), and others since, have pointed out. In these young people their sociopathic behaviour is to a large extent merely a symptom of their cyclothymia which they themselves recognize once their mood swings have been stabilized.

I will not do more than mention the use of lithium in what are as yet only relatively thinly explored areas — explosive aggressive prisoners, childhood hyperkinesis, hyperthyroidism and Huntington's chorea. Schou, in Chapter 2, covers such topics in detail.

Secondly, there is now documentation of various side-effects of which I was initially unaware, and I refer especially to fine digital tremor, the polydypsia/polyuria syndrome and the depression of thyroid function, the last of which has been extensively studied.

Thirdly, there have been notable advances in clinical practice and management, topics covered in the later chapters of this book.

Looking back, I am amazed by the crudity of my early practice, however effective the results. The rules were simple. Patients, relatives and nursing staff were all thoroughly briefed about toxic symptoms. The instructions were peremptory — prompt and complete cessation of lithium on the first appearance of such symptoms and immediate medical review. What almost invariably happened was that such symptoms completely abated after 2-3 days and dosage was resumed at a lower level.

There was no thought of monitoring treatment with measurement of serum lithium levels. Indeed at that time laboratory facilities were such that it was impossible anyhow.

I was not aware then of the necessity of ensuring adequate sodium status of patients and the possible perils of sodium depletion but we did have a rule of thumb as some sort of insurance policy against the dangers of intoxication — and that was one rest day a week, arbitrarily on Sundays.

By comparison present day management is highly sophisticated, with the proliferation of properly organized lithium clinics (just as it became necessary years ago to organize diabetic clinics and more recently "Modecate" clinics). Only in this way can adequate follow up, dosage schedules, clinical status and blood levels be properly monitored.

It might not be amiss at this point to discuss the prescribing of lithium. The decision should not be taken lightly as in most cases it is a life sentence as it often is with insulin in diabetes.

When should it be prescribed? For a first affective swing in early adult life — never. Psychiatrists these days know little about the natural history of untreated affective illness. The patient may not have another affective episode of treatable proportions for 20 years, so to prescribe lithium on this first occasion may be to prescribe it unnecessarily for all that time. If the patient has two affective swings in 1 year, perhaps in opposite directions, and associated with a positive family history, it should certainly be seriously considered. With three episodes in 2 years, there is no doubt it should be given.

It can be strongly argued that this decision in the vast majority of cases should be taken by a psychiatrist, on the grounds that if a person is sufficiently incapacitated to require lithium he is ill enough to have been referred for a psychiatric opinion. As lithium is in many cases only thought of in affective illness of sufficient severity to warrant hospitalization, treatment is preferably commenced on an inpatient basis. This ensures that the therapeutic response can be more accurately assessed, satisfactory maintenance dosage determined, side and toxic effects and associated precautions discussed with the patient and relatives and blood levels frequently monitored with minimal inconvenience. As well, of course, the patient is introduced to the milieu and philosophy of the lithium clinic which will later be responsible for long term follow-up.

What has been the impact of lithium in the treatment of affective illness and the practice of psychiatry? The most dramatic tribute to its effectiveness is given by Fieve (8)

> "Our group of over 200 manic-depressive patients had been subjected to a total of approximately 5000 shock treatments and many courses of anti-depressant drugs before coming under lithium control of the illness. (Over a period of 1-40 years). During a 1-10 year period on lithium they have had a total of only 25 shock treatments. . . . We have for the first time in the history of psychiatry a simple drug that controls a complex major mental illness."

In conclusion may I quote once again from that August publication the *British Pharmacopoeia.* Lithium salts had completely disappeared as therapeutic substances by 1932 and had not been reinstated as late as the 1968 edition. I rejoice to say however that the phoenix has arisen from its ashes and that lithium carbonate reappears in the 1973 edition. Under 'Action and Use', the *BP* states succinctly "Used in the prophylaxis and treatment of manic depressive disorders".

References

1. Garrod, A.B. (1859). *Gout and Rheumatic Cout.* (London: Walton and Maberly)
2. Corcoran, A.C., Taylor, R.D. and Page, I.H. (1949). *J. Am. Med. Assoc.,* **139**, 685
3. Hanlon, L.W., Romaine, M., Gilroy, F.J. and Dietrick, J.E. (1949). *J. Am. Med. Assoc.,* **139**, 688
4. Stern, R.L. (1949). Severe lithium chloride poisoning with complete recovery. *J. Am. Med. Assoc.,,* **139**, 710
5. Cade, J.F.J. (1949). *Med. J. Aust.,* **2**, 349
6. Baastrup, P.C., Poulson, J.C., Schou, M., Thomsen, K. and Amidsen, A. (1970). *Lancet,* **ii**, 326
7. Serry, M. (1969). *Aust. N.Z. J. Psychiat.,* **3**, 390

Part II:
Clinical Uses

Introduction

When lithium therapy was still in its early stages of development (in the nineteen fifties, particularly) there was considerable excitement at the prospect of discovering a medication specific to a single psychopathological entity. Had it been the case that lithium was effective against recurrent endogenous affective disorders and against no other form of psychiatric disorder, the chances of uncovering a physiological/biochemical lesion responsible for producing mood disorders, would undoubtedly have been greatly enhanced. This possibility is, however, rapidly fading as it becomes increasingly clear that lithium may be effective against a variety of other conditions. Professor Schou, in an admirably comprehensive review (Chapter 2), lists all the uses which have been, and are being, suggested for lithium. There seems, at present, no single simple common denominator linking these various lithium-responsive states, but should such a factor be eventually elucidated it would provide a potentially fruitful new approach to the classification of psychiatric disorders, and might possibly also give a clue to new ways of treating psychopathological states.

Dr Bennie, in Chapter 3, examines the use of lithium in the treatment of acute depressive illness, an issue which frequently arouses controversy.

Sometimes lithium is used as a "last resort" treatment when all else has failed, and may, under such circumstances, prove to be surprisingly effective: in this context, Dr Hussain and Dr Gomersall report the use of lithium to treat schizo-affective disorders which had proved refractory to other forms of therapy (Chapter 4).

Considerable interest has been aroused in the past two or three years in the possibility of using lithium to treat various forms of drug abuse and addiction. Lithium treatment of alcoholism is covered by Dr Merry and his colleagues in Chapter 5, whilst in the following chapter Professor Steinberg gives an interesting account of animal behaviour studies which are currently in progress in this area. It is encouraging that there is the interplay between clinical usage and laboratory study which is evidenced by Chapters 5 and 6.

Work on animals and human volunteer subjects suggested that lithium might have anti-aggressive potential, and Dr Worrall looks at recent developments in this area (Chapter 7).

Part 2 ends with Chapter 8, by Dr Lena and his colleagues considering the case for the use of lithium in children and adolescents. There is — and quite rightly so — a reluctance amongst psychiatrists to employ pharmaceutical methods to control childhood psychopathology, but it is nevertheless important that the matter should receive careful scrutiny.

In the next few years we may expect to see further widening in the scope of therapeutic usage of lithium. No doubt some early enthusiasms will, with hindsight, be seen to have been misplaced, but it is important to recognise that a precise specification of the therapeutic profile of lithium is as important in elucidating its mode of action as are the biochemical and physiological investigations outlined in the rest of this book.

2

The Range of Clinical Uses of Lithium

M. SCHOU

INTRODUCTION

Examination of the range of clinical uses of lithium may serve two purposes:

1. One may try to find out whether there are other diseases than manic-depressive disorder in which lithium exerts therapeutic or prophylactic action. If this is so, accumulated knowledge about the safe and efficient handling of lithium treatment could be utilized for the benefit of new groups of patients.

2. Through determining the therapeutic profile of lithium one may get a clue to its mode of action. Common features among diseases or syndromes that respond to lithium could give an indication of the particular biochemical or physiological or psychological mechanisms that are influenced by lithium treatment. Let me exemplify by asking three questions: Does lithium act specifically on manic-depressive illness? Does lithium have an effect on all diseases that are characterised by an abnormal mood or by mood changes? Does lithium exert a stabilizing action on periodic diseases in general?

These and similar questions may be worth examining, and I shall go through the various lithium uses systematically. Special attention will be paid to reports that have appeared since I reviewed the field three years ago (1). The presentation is only a survey; detailed reports about particular uses of lithium are presented by others. The terms "indication" and "use" refer to experimental indications and suggested uses. There are only two established and well documented indications for lithium today: the therapeutic use in mania and the prophylactic use in recurrent manic-depressive disorder of bipolar and monopolar type.

SUGGESTED PSYCHIATRIC USES

Mania

The therapeutic use in mania, initiated in Cade's seminal study (2), is well established (3).

Depression

Lithium seems to exert some therapeutic action in some patients with endogenous (primary, vital) depression, but the treatment can hardly compete with antidepressant drugs and electroconvulsive treatment (4). Observations by Bennie (5) indicate that lithium may be of therapeutic value when antidepressant drugs and ECT have failed.

Recurrent affective disorder, bipolar and monopolar

The prophylactic action of lithium in recurrent affective disorders, for some time the subject of considerable debate, is now well established (6). Lithium attenuates or prevents recurrences in the monopolar as well as in the bipolar type.

Schizophrenia, periodic catatonia

Some anecdotal reports but no systematic studies indicate that lithium given as the only treatment may be of benefit in schizophrenia. Small *et al.* (7) compared the effects of lithium plus a neuroleptic with those of placebo plus a neuroleptic in a double-blind study involving 22 chronically ill schizophrenics. Treatment results were significantly better when neuroleptics were combined with lithium than when they were given together with placebo. The improvements involved a number of the clinical measures tested and all subtypes of schizophrenia.

Gjessing (8) and Pétursson (9) each gave lithium to one patient with periodic catatonia. In Gjessing's patient intervals were prolonged from 3 to 6 weeks, but there was no shortening of psychotic episodes. In the patient reported by Pétursson lithium treatment led to dramatic improvement with total disappearance of symptoms; the improvement lasted for many years.

Recurrent schizo-affective disorder

The prophylactic effect of lithium in this ill-defined condition seems indisputable but is less pronounced than in typical affective disorder (10-13). Combination with neuroleptic drugs may offer advantages.

Pathological emotional instability in children and adolescents

Lithium maintenance treatment seems to exert a stabilizing action in children with rapid changes of mood and activity (14-25). Later case reports by Lena and O'Brien (26) and Kelly *et al.* (27) tell the same story. Adolescents with "emotionally unstable character disorder" may also, when given lithium treatment, reach a condition that is more satisfying to themselves and to others, as indicated by a double-blind study carried out by Rifkin *et al.* (28).

Not much has happened in this field in recent years. It would be interesting to learn about the later fate of the patients given lithium treatment. How long did they stay on lithium? What happened when they were taken off lithium? Is is possible today to characterize the children and teenagers who may benefit from lithium maintenance treatment?

Observations published until now indicate that lithium is well tolerated by children and that few side effects are seen, but any long-term administration of drugs to the growing organism should obviously be undertaken with caution.

It may be worth emphasising that lithium is without effect on the hyperkinetic syndrome in psychotic children (29,30).

Pathological impulsive aggressiveness

Aggressiveness is sometimes a prominent feature of mania, which subsides when the mania is treated with lithium. Lithium has furthermore been shown to counteract animal aggressive behaviour such as pain-elicited aggression, mouse killing in rats, isolation-induced aggression in mice, drug-induced aggression in rats, and hypothalamically induced aggression in cats (31). These observations have led to lithium treatment trials with aggressive prisoners, mostly those in whom aggressiveness has been recurrent and sudden. None of the studies included manic-depressive prisoners. Some of the prisoners were diagnosed as having schizophrenic features, but most were non-psychotic.

Tupin *et al.* (32) and Morrison *et al.* (33) in non-blind studies on groups of 27 and 23 prison or hospital inmates found significant decreases in combative behaviour as compared with the subjects' behaviour prior to lithium administration. The subjects themselves reported that lithium gave them an increased capacity to reflect on the consequences of a rash action, increased capacity to control angry feelings when evoked, diminished intensity of anger, and generally a more reflective mood.

The most systematic and penetrating studies on lithium and aggression have been carried out by Sheard and his associates (34-39). Starting with animal experiments they went on to investigate the antiaggressive action of lithium in prison inmates in non-blind, single-blind and double-blind trials.

Their subjects were not manic-depressive and not psychotic; they were characterized by a history of chronic assaultive behaviour or chronic impulsive antisocial behaviour. Patient groups ranged from 12 in the non-blind and single-blind studies to 66 in the double-blind study. All the trials showed a significant reduction of aggressiveness during lithium treatment whether compared with the subjects' previous behaviour or with the behaviour of matched controls given no lithium. Marini and Sheard (39), on the basis of the literature and their own studies, conclude that the antiaggressive effect of lithium is not due to toxicity or side effects, to subjective or objective weakness, to reduced reaction time, coordination or motor performance, to frank cognitive deficits, to hypothyroidism, to reduction of serum testosterone, to placebo effects, or to underlying manic-depressive illness. They point out that although the studies clearly show the existence of strongly lithium responsive aggressive subjects, the observations do not yet provide a clear definition of these subjects.

Further observations of antiaggressive effects of lithium include case reports of satisfactory treatment response in a female child batterer (40), a patient with postpsychotic antisocial aggressive behaviour (41), and a patient with "diabolical behaviour", conversion symptoms, and diffuse violence and cruelty (42). Shader *et al.* (43), who reported lithium dampening of aggression in a nonpsychotic subject, felt that lithium treatment had added a delay factor in their patient, who previously went automatically from stimulus to response.

Whereas in the studies mentioned so far it is reasonably certain that the patients did not suffer from manic-depressive disorder, such certainty is not possible in studies on mental defective persons with aggressive behaviour. Dostal and Zvolsky (44, 45) treated 14 adolescents with severe mental retardation, Cooper and Fowlie (46) one self-mutilating subnormal girl in her early twenties, Worrall *et al.* (47) 8 patients with mental deficiency with ages ranging from 33 to 57 years, and Lion *et al.* (48) a 27-year-old mentally retarded man with temper outbursts. In all the studies there was marked reduction of self-mutilation and aggressiveness towards others, but in some instances side effects prevented continuation of the treatment.

Pathological hypersexuality

Among prison inmates given lithium for aggressiveness Sheard (31) noted a dampening of sexual responsiveness in three subjects, two with a history of promiscuous homosexual behaviour who stopped taking lithium presumably because they did not like the suppression of sexuality, and a third who was a recurrent rapist with compulsive masturbation and in whom lithium treatment led to naturally infrequent masturbation without rape phantasies. Sheard does not actually suggest pathological hypersexualism as an indication for lithium treatment, but the observations are interesting.

Transvestism

Ward (49) described a patient who suffered from transvestism as well as from recurrent manic-depressive disorder. The patient would wear female clothes during hypomanic or manic episodes. Lithium treatment led to disappearance of the affective episodes, and the transvestism also disappeared. The author emphasised that there is no evidence to support the use of lithium in transvestite patients without manic-depressive disorder.

Premenstrual tension syndrome

The premenstrual tension syndrome is a periodical complaint, thought to involve electrolyte disturbances. It therefore invites therapeutic trials with lithium. Sletten and Gershon (50) treated eight patients and Fries (51) and Rosman (52) each one patient with good results. In contrast to this, double-blind studies carried out by Mattsson and von Schoultz (53, 54) with 18 patients and by Singer *et al.* (55) with 14 patients showed lithium to be no better than placebo. Gershon (personal communication 1977) has observations which indicate that lithium treatment is of value in a subgroup of patients in whom mood and behaviour are severely affected premenstrually.

Alcoholism with and without depression

Most psychiatrists with experience of lithium treatment have seen manic-depressive patients who drink during manic or depressed episodes and who, when their condition has been stabilized through lithium maintenance treatment, get their alcohol consumption under control. Is this purely due to an action of lithium on the manic-depressive disorder, or does lithium have a more specific effect on the cerebral processes underlying alcoholism?

Under appropriate experimental conditions lithium treated rats drink less than control rats (56, 57), but observations in animals cannot be extrapolated to human alcoholics. Fries (51) found lithium possibly useful in one out of 17 cases of alcoholism. More systematic studies were carried out by Kline, Wren and their associates (58, 59) who started more than 70 patients in a lithium-placebo double-blind trial. Only 30 patients completed the trial. In these patients lithium seemed to have influenced the drinking habits so that the patients had fewer disabling drinking episodes than they had before lithium and also than the patients given placebo. The patients suffered from chronic alcoholism associated with nonpsychotic depression, but the reports do not characterize the depression further, nor do they indicate whether the depression had a recurrent course.

The study carried out by Merry *et al.* (60) had a somewhat similar design. The patients were treated double-blind with lithium or placebo. Some of the patients were depressed, i.e. had a Beck inventory score of 15 or higher, others were not. Also in this study there was a marked drop-out rate, with 71 patients starting the trial and only 38 finishing it. Among 16 depressed patients lithium was significantly superior to placebo as regards number of days incapacitated by drink and percentage of time on trial incapacitated. Among 22 patients who were not depressed, there was no difference between lithium and placebo. Whereas Merry *et al.* (60) were cautiously optimistic about the use of lithium in depressive alcoholics, Young and Keeler (61) were more sceptical. Their 15 patients with alcoholism and depression all suffered relapse within one year, alcoholic symptoms usually appearing earlier than affective. It is conceivable that a sub-group of alcoholic patients may benefit from lithium maintenance treatment, but one wonders whether it will differ from the manic-depressives who drink when they are manic or depressed.

Revusky and his group (62-64) suggest, on the basis of rat data, that lithium could be used as a sickness producing agent and hence employed for chemical aversion therapy of alcoholism. They have presented no human data. To produce strong nausea, lithium must be given in doses that are close to the toxic level; the proposal by Revusky should presumably be viewed with some scepticism.

Lithium treatment of alcohol withdrawal symptoms has been suggested by Sellers *et al.* (65, 66). They found with 18 chronic alcoholics that in mild alcoholic withdrawal lithium treatment diminished subjective symptoms of withdrawal and normalized performance on a motor tracking task. Since lithium does not reach steady-state levels until after several days, the authors suggest that patients might start lithium while drinking. They do not recommend lithium for severe withdrawal, and they emphasise that the comparative efficacy and safety of lithium and benzodiazepines in ameliorating alcohol withdrawal symptoms yet have to be determined. Also as regards this proposal one is tempted to express reservations due to the possible toxic action of lithium in patients with deranged fluid and electrolyte metabolism.

Drug addiction

Experiments on animals and humans have shown that lithium antagonizes certain effects of amphetamine, morphine, and cocaine (67-76).

There are few therapeutic trials in drug addiction. Nahunek *et al.* (77)

gave lithium to 23 drug dependent subjects and after 28 weeks found clinical improvement and lowered drug usage in 15. As the authors point out, the results are difficult to analyse due to the small number of patients in the study, to interfering abstinence symptoms, and to the lack of placebo controls. Altamura (78) administered lithium to 20 opiate addicts, but only nine patients took the medication for more than a few weeks. In our own hospital we tried giving lithium to young morphine addicts but found them so unreliable as regards intake of lithium, of food and of opiates that a meaningful study could not be completed. No convincing evidence indicates that lithium is a useful agent in the treatment of drug addiction.

Acute anxiety

Lackroy and van Praag (79) studied 35 mentally healthy subjects who were to undergo myelography. Double-blind comparison of lithium and placebo provided no evidence that lithium is able to alleviate acute anxiety.

Obsessive-compulsive neurosis

Baastrup (80) saw relief of obsessive features in some patients with monopolar affective disorder who were given prophylactic lithium treatment. Forssman and Wålinder (81) noted improvement during lithium treatment in obsessive patients who did not seem to suffer from affective disorder but who had a periodic course. Van Putten and Sanders (82) found lithium superior to placebo in a patient with severe intractable obsessive neurosis.

These positive reports are contrasted by the failure by Gottfries (83) to obtain a lithium effect in five patients with phobic disorders and by the double-blind placebo-controlled studies by Geisler and Schou (84, 85) and Hessö and Thorell (86), who in groups of 6 to 8 patients, respectively, with obsessive-compulsive neurosis found lithium as ineffective as placebo.

Anorexia nervosa

Working on the hypothesis that mania and anorexia nervosa share a number of features Barcai (87) gave lithium treatment to two patients who had suffered from anorexia nervosa for many years and had failed to respond to other treatments. Both patients gained weight (12 kg and 9 kg) during the treatment and the weight gain was maintained during therapy for a year. The author found his hypothesis supported but correctly drew attention to the fact that many patients not suffering from anorexia nervosa gain weight during lithium treatment. The author suggests that lithium should be tried in anorexia nervosa but only in adults. It should perhaps be added that since anorexia nervosa patients often have low and variable intakes of food and fluid, they should be under particularly careful supervision during such treatment.

Affective psychoses in organic brain syndromes

Lithium is apt to produce toxic reactions when given to patients suffering from organic brain damage. Nevertheless it has been shown to exert therapeutic action in some patients with affective psychoses that were secondary to neurological disease: hypomania developing after a cerebral vascular accident (88), depressions accompanying neurological disease, possibly multiple sclerosis (89), and mania developing in multiple sclerosis (90). Beneficial effects of lithium have also been seen in four patients with psychotic reactions precipitated by intake of LSD (91).

It is not clear whether in some of these patients pre-existing manic-depressive disorder may have been precipitated by the neurological disease or by treatment with ACTH. None of the studies included controls; non-specific effects of the treatment and spontaneous recoveries cannot be excluded.

Psychosomatic disorders

It has been suggested that some psychosomatic disorders may be atypical depressions; lithium treatment has therefore been tried. Favourable results have been reported in patients suffering from colitis, asthma, various types of pain, paraesthesias, and painful shoulder syndrome (92-96). It should be remembered, however, that patients with psychosomatic complaints are often placebo responders. Double-blind trials must therefore be considered indispensable for reliable assessment of treatment effects. Such studies have yet to be carried out with lithium.

Failure of other treatments

This ill-defined indication for lithium treatment should hardly be taken at face value. Van Putten (97) gave lithium to a group of patients with chronic and incapacitating mental illness, who had failed to respond to other treatments. None of the patients seemed to suffer from manic-depressive disorder. Lithium was given double-blind in a cross-over design with placebo. Of the 39 patients started on lithium, 15 improved, 9 dramatically so. Retrospective diagnosis revealed that the patients who improved suffered from non-remitting manic-depressive illness, psychotic excitement, or character disorder. It seems that manic-depressive disorder, especially in its chronic form, may present itself under unusual and not easily recognisable pictures, and that lithium treatment occasionally may give benefit in cases with uncertain diagnosis. Van Putten suggests that the best candidates for a trial of lithium appear to be those patients in whom such mood states as irritability, anger, excitement, and impulsive aggressivity are core problems.

SUGGESTED NONPSYCHIATRIC USES

Movement disorders

Certain disorders of movement may be caused by disturbances in brain amine metabolism. Lithium affects brain amines; it has consequently been tried therapeutically in various movement disorders.

Improvement of abnormal movements or reduction in anger and irritability was observed in patients with Huntington's chorea given lithium treatment (98-105). Lithium was without effect in studies reported by Aminoff and Marshall (106), Carman *et al.* (107), Leonard *et al.* (108, 109) and Vestergaard *et al.* (110). Andén *et al.* (111) saw aggravation of hyperkinesias in a patient given lithium concurrently with baclofen.

There may be several reasons for the discrepancy of observations in lithium treated Huntington patients. The patient groups may have differed as regards type and intensity of the disease, the rating scales may have differed in sensitivity, the lithium treatment may have been carried out with different intensity, and drugs given concurrently with lithium may have influenced the results. The reports do not permit any clear choice among these possibilities, but it is noteworthy that the studies with positive results were all carried out non-blind, whereas the negative studies used a double-blind design with placebo controls. Psychological factors and observer bias may have been responsible for the positive findings.

The situation is unclear as regards lithium treatment of neuroleptic-induced tardive dyskinesia. In four non-blind studies lithium was found to decrease the dyskinetic movements (98, 105, 112, 113). In two placebo controlled studies (114, 115) lithium induced a slight reduction of dyskinesias and suppressed psychomotor agitation and aggression. On the other hand, Simpson *et al.* (116), who also used placebo controls, found no change in the patients' dyskinetic symptoms.

Lithium treatment of spasmodic torticollis led to improvement in one case reported by Couper-Smartt (117) and in one of two cases published by Foerster and Regli (105). McCaul and Stern (118) had mixed results of treatment with lithium plus haloperidol in nine patients with chronic refractory spasmodic torticollis, one patient with torsion dystonia and one patient with bilateral choreoathetosis.

Levodopa-induced hyperkinesias in Parkinsonism were relieved by lithium in two patients treated by Dalén and Steg (119). Van Woert and

Ambani (120) saw only slight reduction of dyskinesias in two of their four patients. McCaul and Stern (121) treated 16 patients with lithium and apart from some relief of painful muscle spasms and cramps did not obtain results indicating that lithium may be helpful in the management of Parkinsonism.

Lithium was administered by Messiha *et al.* (122) to two patients with Gilles de la Tourette's syndrome; in both cases tics, involuntary sounds, and coprolalia responded to the treatment.

It may be relevant to the topic of movement disorders to mention that lithium treatment itself may lead to the development of extrapyramidal symptoms. In one study (123) cogwheel rigidity was found in more than half of the patients. In another study (124) it was found in only few cases. Bien (125) saw cogwheel rigidity in a patient with impending lithium intoxication. Johnels *et al.* (126) observed development of Parkinsonism in two lithium treated patients. The role played by concurrently administered drugs (neuroleptics, antidepressants) in these studies is not clear.

Meniere's disease

Meniere's disease occurs periodically and is thought to be based on disturbances of the fluid and electrolyte balance in the inner ear. This led Thomsen *et al.* (127) to give lithium to 30 Meniere patients in an open trial, and they obtained promising results. Lutz (128) also observed relief from Meniere's disease in a patient given lithium for recurrent manic-depressive disorder.

However, Thomsen and his associates later checked their results in a double-blind cross-over trial with 21 patients given 6 months of lithium and 6 months of placebo treatment (129). Under these circumstances no difference could be demonstrated between the two treatments. The evidence accordingly does not favour a prophylactic effect of lithium in Meniere's disease.

Migraine and cluster headache

Of 44 patients given lithium treatment for headache, migraine and hemicrania no less than 39 reported the therapy to be thoroughly effective (95). The patients apparently did not suffer from manic-depressive disorder. No control group or placebo medication was employed in this study.

Ekbom (130, 131) gave lithium treatment to five patients with chronic migrainous neuralgia (cluster headache). There was a slight improvement in two patients with periodic symptoms, marked improvement in three patients with chronic symptoms. Relief set in very quickly. Discontinuation of lithium treatment led to aggravation of the headache, and a second treatment resulted once more in definitive improvement. There was placebo control for one patient. None of the patients in this series seems to have suffered from manic-depressive disorder. Lithium treatment was continued successfully for 18-36 months in three patients.

Selecting patients according to Ekbom's suggestions Kudrow (132) gave lithium to 32 patients with chronic cluster headache. Four dropped out due to side effects. Marked and continued improvement occurred in 27 out of the remaining 28, and the improvement was maintained throughout 32 weeks of therapeutic trial.

Lauritsen (133) found that 16 of 73 manic-depressive patients suffered from periodic headaches. Lithium maintenance treatment failed to alter the frequency or severity of the migraine attacks.

The therapeutic and prophylactic effects of lithium in various forms of headache clearly require further investigation in systematic trials.

Periodic hypersomnia

Periodic hypersomnia, sometimes combined with hyperphagia, is designated the Kleine-Levin-Critchley syndrome. The periodic course of this condition has led to therapeutic trials with lithium. Jeffries and Lefebvre (134) treated a 16-year-old girl who in addition to the syndrome had evidence of endogenous depression. Lithium administration led to improvement of the condition, and the authors suggest that the Kleine-Levin-Critchley syndrome may be related to manic-depressive disorder. Ogura *et al.* (135) treated a 17-year-old male who was moderately depressed during the somnolent periods. Lithium treatment was able to prevent the occurence of new periods of somnolence, but it has no effect when administered during a somnolent period. A prophylactic action but no therapeutic effect is a pattern which resembles that seen with lithium administration to patients with endogenous depressions. Abe (136) found that lithium effectively prevented hypersomniac episodes in a 15-year-old male. This patient did not seem to suffer from affective disorder. When lithium was discontinued, there was a relapse of hypersomniac periods.

Treatment results with three patients cannot provide strong evidence, but the results were obtained by different groups of authors and they seem to invite further investigations on the effect of lithium in periodic hypersomnia.

Periodic hypokalaemic paralysis

This condition occurs periodically and is caused by electrolyte disturbance. Ottosson and Persson (137) gave prolonged lithium therapy to a patient with the disease; the treatment did not alter the frequency, duration or severity of the paralytic attacks.

Cyclical vomiting

A mentally defective patient with mood swings often vomited when she was depressed. Other treatments had proved ineffective; lithium was then administered for two years. There was a significant fall in the frequency of manias and depressions and also in the periods of vomiting (138). The authors assume that lithium corrected a hypothalamic defect in this patient. They suggest trying lithium treatment on resistant cases of cyclical vomiting in children.

Inappropriate secretion of antidiuretic hormone

Among the side effects of lithium treatment is polyuria caused by a lowering of the renal response to ADH. Lithium would therefore seem a rational treatment for the syndrome of inappropriate ADH secretion. The studies carried out until now do not, however, give a clear picture of its efficacy. Forrest *et al.* (139), on the one hand, found no change of urine volume, urine osmolality or serum sodium concentration in three patients given lithium. White and Fetner (140), Jacobs (141) and Baker *et al.* (142), on the other hand, each treated one patient with inappropriate ADH secretion and saw prompt water diuresis, normalization of urine osmolality and correction of serum sodium. The changes occurred within a few days and could be maintained for many months. Baker *et al.* (142) recommend lithium treatment for patients who cannot comply with long-term fluid restriction.

Hyperthyroidism, thyroid cancer

Among several actions exerted by lithium on the thyroid gland, inhibition of hormone release is prominent. In patients given lithium treatment this occasionally leads to development of goitre or myxoedema. Endocrinologists have taken advantage of this side effect and administered lithium to patients with hyperthyroidism or metabolizing thyroid cancer.

In the studies on hyperthyroidism lithium has sometimes been given alone, sometimes in combination with thiocarbamides or radioactive iodine. A number of therapeutic trials have shown lithium treatment to counteract hyperthyroidism (143-151), but opinions differ as to its practical value. Some authors feel that lithium, given alone or together with other therapies, is useful for the treatment of thyrotoxicosis; others feel that it may be useful but should be given only for a short time, since after the initial striking effect there may be accumulation of iodine in the gland with risk of later aggravation. Some have found lithium largely without side effects and recommend it as a safe treatment; others have seen side effects that detract from its value. The place of lithium in the treatment of hyperthyroidism is still uncertain.

A few reports deal with lithium treatment of metabolizing thyroid cancer. In this condition lithium is used together with radioactive iodine. Due to its inhibition of hormone release from the gland, lithium reduces the disappearance rate of the radioactive iodine and therefore increases the ratio of gland irradiation to body irradiation (152, 153).

Granulocytopenia

Granulocytopenia is a serious condition, and the few therapies available are not always effective. Lithium administration is accompanied by granulocytosis, and treatment with lithium has consequently been tried in granulocytopenic states. Many of the reports deal with only few patients.

Among the patients with Felty's syndrome given lithium treatment, positive effects were obtained in one case by Rampon *et al.* (154), one case by Pointud *et al.* (155), all of eight patients treated by Kurnick *et al.* (155), and all of ten patients treated by Gupta *et al.* (157, 158). The rise in leukocyte count occurred within a week after start of treatment, was sustained throughout the treatment period, and disappeared when lithium was discontinued. Kaplan (159) saw no effect of lithium treatment in two patients with Felty's syndrome.

Barrett *et al.* (160, 161) obtained good effects of lithium treatment in two patients with aplastic anaemia, temporary in one and sustained in the other. Greco *et al.* (162) found that lithium treatment counteracted granulocytopenia induced by cancer chemotherapy in 25 patients.

It is not clear what place lithium administration may have in the long-term treatment of granulocytopenic states, but the results obtained up to now seem encouraging.

DISCUSSION

The therapeutic trials with lithium were initiated for a number of reasons: because the disease in question was thought to resemble manic-depressive illness with respect to mood abnormality or periodicity; because one assumed the existence of common chemical pathology with affective disorders; or because side effects observed during lithium treatment of manic-depressive patients indicated that lithium might exert a therapeutically useful action on particular biological processes.

The clinical evidence concerning a therapeutic or prophylactic action of lithium in the various diseases varies considerably in weight and reliability. It ranges from casuistic reports about treatment of a single or a few patients to extensive controlled trials involving large numbers of patients treated over long periods of time. Table 2.1 lists the lithium uses where an effect of lithium or the lack of an effect has been proved with a reasonable degree of certainty. It should be noted that proved effect of lithium does not necessarily mean that lithium treatment is clinically better than or equal to other treatment modalities.

Table 2.1. Uses where effect or lack of effect of lithium has been proved

Effect proved	Lack of effect proved
Mania	Acute anxiety
Recurrent affective disorder, bipolar type	Obsessive-compulsive neurosis
Recurrent affective disorder, monopolar type	Meniere's disease
Pathological impulsive aggressiveness	
Hyperthyroidism	
Granulocytopenia	

There is good reason to use lithium for the treatment of mania, alone for manias of mild or moderate intensity, combined initially with a neuroleptic of rapid action for violent mania. Lithium prophylaxis in recurrent endogenous affective disorders is presumably the most valuable use of the drug. Lithium is clearly superior to other treatments in the bipolar cases; in the monopolar ones the relative merits of lithium maintenance treatment and continuation treatment with tricyclic antidepressants are still under investigation. One cannot yet define clearly the pathologically aggressive patient who may benefit from lithium treatment; nevertheless therapeutic trials with lithium seem indicated for both clinical and investigatory reasons. The clinical value of lithium treatment of hyperthyroidism relative to the value of other treatments is still sub judice. In states of granulocytopenia, lithium therapy seems worth trying, especially when treatment with steroids has failed.

We asked ourselves three questions in the introduction. They can be answered now, and the answers are all negative. First, lithium is not specific for manic-depressive illness. Not only does it counteract impulsive aggressiveness and presumably other psychopathological conditions; it also acts on somatic diseases that have nothing to do with manic-depressive disorder. Secondly, lithium is not a general mood normalizer; it fails to counteract acute anxiety and does not relieve the obsessive-compulsive patients. And thirdly, lithium does not cure all disturbances with an episodic course; Meniere's disease and periodic hypokalaemic paralysis, for example, are not affected.

Our survey has accordingly served to refute hypotheses that were too comprehensive, too crude. Now let us try to formulate something that is slightly more specific by asking what it is that characterizes conditions which respond to lithium. We may include in our considerations conditions where there is some evidence of a lithium effect even if the evidence is not yet conclusive. We should perhaps also, in the present context, disregard such conditions as inappropriate ADH-secretion, thyrotoxicosis, and granulocytopenia, and concentrate on diseases or syndromes which involve psychopathology.

It is at present not easy to distinguish psychopathological features that are common to such a variety of conditions as recurrent affective disorders, emotional instability in children and adolescents, pathological impulsive aggressiveness, alcoholism with mood changes and drinking bouts, periodic hypersomnia, and possibly premenstrual tension with pronounced mental changes. The only thing that seems reasonably clear is that inclusion of all these conditions under the diagnostic label "manic-depressive illness" would stretch this beyond recognition and clinical reason. We must content ourselves with the fact that a number of psychopathological conditions respond or appear to respond to lithium treatment but that common psychopathological features have not yet been identified.

There is, however, another feature that seems to be common to all the responsive conditions, namely a course that is episodic or cyclical or periodic or recurrent, a course with intervals which are free, or nearly free, of symptoms. It is of course possible that this common feature of recurrences and intervals is due to preferential selection of such diseases for therapeutic trials with lithium, but it should at least be noted that no psychiatric disease has yet been found which is responsive to lithium and which does not take a recurrent course.

This seems to be where we stand today. A clearer picture may emerge from further studies on the range of clinical lithium uses.

References

1. Schou, M. (1976). In: A. Villeneuve (ed.) *Lithium in Psychiatry. A Synopsis,* pp. 49-77. (Québec: Presses Univ. Laval)
2. Cade, J. F. J. (1949). *Med. J. Aust.,* **36**, 349
3. Peet, M. (1975). In: F. N. Johnson (ed.) *Lithium Research and Therapy,* pp. 25-41. (London, New York and San Francisco: Academic Press)
4. Mendels, J. (1975). In: F. N. Johnson (ed.) *Lithium Research and Therapy* pp. 43-62. (London, New York and San Francisco: Academic Press)
5. Bennie, E. H. (1975). *Lancet,* **i**, 216
6. Schou, M (1976). In: D. M. Gallant and G. M. Simpson (eds.) *Depression: Behavioral, Biochemical, Diagnostic and Treatment Concepts,* pp. 309-334 (New York: Spectrum)
7. Small, J. G., Kellams, J. J., Milstein, V. and Moore, J. (1975). *Am. J. Psychiat.,* **132**, 1315
8. Gjessing, L. R. (1967). *Acta Psychiat. Scand.,* **43**, 372

9. Pétursson, H. (1976). *Acta Psychiat. Scand.*, **54**, 248
10. Angst, J., Weis, P., Grof, P., Baastrup, P. C. and Schou, M. (1970). *Br. J. Psychiat.*, **116**, 604
11. Egli, H. (1971). *Schweiz. Med. Wochenschr.*, **101**, 157
12. Quitkin, F. M., Rifkin, A. and Klein, D. F. (1973). In: S. Gershon and B. Shopsin (eds.) *Lithium. Its Role in Psychiatric Research and Treatment,* pp. 295-315. (New York and London: Plenum)
13. Perris, C. (1976). *Pharmakopsychiat.*, **9**, 149
14. Frommer, E. A. (1968). In: A. Coppen and A. Walk (eds.) *Recent Developments in Affective Disorders,* pp. 117-136. (London: Headley)
15. Annell, A.-L. (1969). *Acta Psychiat. Scand.*, suppl. **207**, 19
16. Annell, A.-L. (1969). *Acta Paedopsychiat.*, **36**, 292
17. Uddenberg, G. (1969). *Acta Psychiat. Scand.*, suppl. **207**, 31
18. Dyson, W. L. and Barcai, A. (1970). *Curr. Ther. Res.*, **12**, 286
19. Feinstein, S. C. and Wolpert, E. A. (1972). *Psychiat. Enf.*, **15**, 133
20. Frommer, E. A. (1972). *Diagnosis and Treatment in Clinical Child Psychiatry.* (London: William Heinemann)
21. Gram, L. F. and Rafaelsen, O. J. (1972). *Acta Psychiat. Scand.*, **48**, 253
22. Schou, M. (1972). In: A.-L. Annell (ed.) *Depressive States in Childhood and Adolescence.* (Stockholm: Almqvist and Wiksell)
23. Výborová, L. and Náhunek, K. (1972). *Activ. Nerv. Sup. (Praha)*, **15**, 104
24. Feinstein, S. C. (1973). *Early Child Devel. Care,* **3**, 1
25. Feinstein, S. C. and Wolpert, E. A. (1973). *J. Am. Acad. Child Psychiat.*, **12**, 123
26. Lena, B. and O'Brien, E. M. D. (1975). *Lancet,* **i**, 1307
27. Kelly, J. T., Koch, M. and Buegel, D. (1976). *Dis. Nerve. Syst.*, **37**, 90
28. Rifkin, A., Quitkin, F., Carrillo, C., Blumberg, A. G. and Klein, D. F. (1972). *Arch. Gen. Psychiat.*, **27**, 519
29. Whitehead, P. L. and Clark, L. D. (1970). *Am. J. Pscyhiat.*, **127**, 824
30. Greenhill, L. L., Rieder, R. O., Wender, P. H., Buchsbaum, M. and Zahn, T. P. (1973). *Arch. Gen. Psychiat.*, **28**, 636
31. Sheard, M. H. (1975). *J. Nerv. Ment. Dis.*, **160**, 108
32. Tupin, J. P., Smith, D. B., Clanon, T. L., Kim, L. I., Nugent, A. and Groupe, A. (1973). *Comprehens. Psychiat.*, **14**, 311
33. Morrison, S. D., Erwin, C. W., Gianturco, D. T. and Gerber, C. J. (1973). *Dis. Nerv. Syst.*, **34**, 186
34. Sheard, M. H. (1970). *Nature (London)*, **228**, 284
35. Sheard, M. H. (1971). *Nature (London)*, **230**, 113
36. Sheard, M. H. (1973). *Agressologie,* **14**, 327
37. Sheard, M. H. (1974). *J. Psychiat. Res.*, **10**, 151
38. Sheard, M. H., Marini, J. L., Bridges, C. I. and Wagner, E. (1976). *Am. J: Psychiat.*, **133**, 1409
39. Marini, J. L. and Sheard, M. H. (1977). *Acta Psychiat. Scand.*, **55**, 269
40. Kerr, W. C. (1976). *Med. J. Aust.*, **2**, 414
41. Liebowitz, J. H., Rudy, V., Gershon, E. S. and Gillis, A. (1976). *Comprehens. Psychiat.*, **17**, 655
42. Putten, T. van and Alban, J. (1977). *J. Nerv. Ment. Dis.*, **164**, 218
43. Shader, R. I., Jackson, A. H. and Dodes, L. M. (1974). *Psychopharmacologia (Berl.).*, **40**, 17
44. Dostal, T. and Zvokský, P. (1970). *Int. Pharmacopsychiat.*, **5**, 203
45. Dostal, T. (1972). In: A.-L. Annell (ed.) *Depressive States in Childhood and Adolescence,* pp. 491-498. (Stockholm: Almqvist and Wiksell)
46. Cooper, A. F. and Fowlie, H. C. (1973). *Br. J. Psychiat.*, **122**, 370

47. Worrall, E. P., Moody, J. P. and Naylor, G. J. (1976). *Br. J. Psychiat.,* **126**, 464
48. Lion, J. R., Hill, J. and Madden, D. J. (1975). *Dis. Nerv. Syst.,* **36**, 97
49. Ward, N. G. (1975). *J. Nerv. Ment. Dis.,* **161**, 204
50. Sletten, I. W. and Gershon, S. (1966). *Comprehens. Psychiat.,* **7**, 197
51. Fries, H. (1969). *Acta Psychiat. Scand.,* suppl. **207**, 41
52. Rosman, C. (1969). *Acta Psychiat. Scand.,* suppl. **207**, 89
53. Mattsson, B. and von Schoultz, B. (1973). *Nord. Psykiat. T.,* **27**, 406
54. Mattsson, B. and von Schoultz, B. (1974). *Acta Psychiat. Scand.,* suppl. **255**, 75
55. Singer, K., Cheng, R. and Schou, M. (1974). *Br. J. Psychiat.,* **124**, 50
56. Ho, A. K. S. and Kissin, B. (1976). In: D. H. Ford and C. H. Clouet (eds.) *Tissue Response to Addictive Drugs,* pp. 447-459. (New York. Spectrum)
57. Truitt, E. B. and Vaughen, C. M. (1976). *Fed. Proc.,* **35**, 814
58. Kline, N. S., Wren, J. C., Cooper, T. B., Varga, E. and Canal, O. (1974). *Am. J. Med. Sci.,* **268**, 15
59. Wren, J. C., Kline, N. S., Cooper, T. B., Varga, E. and Canal, O. (1974). *Clin. Med.,* **81**, 33
60. Merry, J., Reynolds, C. M., Bailey, J. and Coppen, A. (1976). *Lancet,* **ii**, 481
61. Young, L. D. and Keeler, M. H. (1977). *Lancet.* **i**, 144
62. Revusky, S. (1973). *J. Behav. Ther. Exp. Psychiat.,* **4**, 15
63. Revusky, S. and Taukulis, H. (1975). *Behav, Res. Ther.,* **13**, 163
64. Revusky, S., Parker, L. A., Coombes, J. and Coombes, S. (1976). *Behav. Res. Ther.,* **14**, 189
65. Sellers, E. M., Cooper, S. D., Sen, A. K. and Zilm, D. H. (1974). *Clin. Pharmacol. Ther.,* **15**, 218
66. Sellers, E. M., Cooper, S. D., Zilm, D. H. and Shanks, C. (1976). *Clin. Pharmacol. Ther.,* **20**, 199
83. Gottfries, C. G. (1968). *Acta Psychiat. Scand.,* suppl. **203**, 157
84. Geisler, A. and Schou, M. (1970). *Nord. Psykiat. T.,* **23**, 493
85. Geisler, A. and Schou, M. (1973). *Foreign Psychiat.,* **2**, 90
86. Hessö, R. and Thorell, L.-H. (1970). *Nord Psykiat. T.,* **23**, 496
87. Barcai, A. (1977). *Acta Psychiat. Scand.,* **55**, 97
88. Rosenbaum, A. H. and Barry, M. J. (1975). *Am. J. Psychiat.,* **132**, 1072
89. Mehta, D. B. (1976). *Am. J. Psychiat.,* **133**, 236
90. Kemp, K., Lion, J. R. and Magram, G. (1977). *Dis. Nerv. Syst.,* **38**, 210
91. Horowitz, H. A. (1975). *Dis. Nerv. Syst.,* **36**, 159
92. López-Ibor Alino, J. J. and López-Ibor Alino, J. M. (1970). *Int. Pharmacopsychiat.,* 5, 187
93. Straker, M. (1970). *Can. Psychiat. Assoc. J.,* **15**, 21
94. Zisook, S. (1972). *J. Am. Med. Assoc.,* **219**, 755
95. Nieper, H.-A. (1973). *Agressologie,* **14**, 407
96. Tyber, M. A. (1974). *Can. Med. Assoc. J.,* **111**, 137
97. Putten, T. van (1976). *Curr. Psychiat. Ther.,* **16**, 155
98. Dalén, P. (1973). *Lancet,* **i**, 107
99. Manyam, N. V. B. and Bravo-Fernandez, E. (1973). *Lancet,* **i**. 1010
100. Mattsson, B. (1973). *Lancet,* **i**, 718
101. Mattsson, B. and Persson, S.-A. (1973). *Lancet,* **ii**, 684
102. Schenk, G. and Leijnse-Ybema, H. J. (1974). *Lancet,* **i**, 364
103. Rorbaek-Jacobsen, I. (1975). *Nord. Psykiat. T.,* **29**, 109
104. Vestergaard, P. (1975). *Nord Psykiat. T.,* **29**, 41
105. Foerster, K. and Regli, F. (1977). *Nervenarzt,* **48**, 228
106. Aminoff, M. J. and Marshall, J. (1974). *Lancet,* **i**, 107

107. Carman, J. S., Shoulson, I. and Chase, T. N. (1974). *Lancet,* **i**, 811
108. Leonard, D. P., Kidson, M. A., Shannon, P. J. and Brown, J. (1974). *Lancet,* **ii**, 1208
109. Leonard, D. P., Kidson, M. A., Brown, J. G. E., Shannon, P. J. and Taryan, S. (1975). *Aust. N.Z. J. Psychiat.,* **9**, 115
110. Vestergaard, P., Baastrup, P. C. and Petersson, H. (1977). *Acta Psychiat. Scand.* (in the press)
111 .Andén, N.-E., Dalén, P. and Johansson, B. (1973). *Lancet,* **ii**, 93
112. Simpson, G. M. (1973). *Br. J. Psychiat.,* **122**, 618
113. Reda, F. A., Escobar, J. I. and Scanlan, J. M. (1975). *Am. J. Psychiat.,* **132**, 560
114. Prange, A. J., Wilson, I. C., Morris, C. E. and Hall, C. D. (1973). *Psychopharmacol. Bull.,* **9**, No. 1, 36
115. Gerlach, J., Thorsen, K. and Munkvad, I. (1975). *Pharmakopsychiat.,* **8**, 51
116. Simpson, G. M., Branchey, M. H., Lee. J. H., Voitashevsky, A. and Zoubok, B. (1976). *Pharmakopsychiat.,* **9**, 76
117. Couper-Smartt, J. (1973). *Lancet,* **ii**, 741
118. McCaul, J. A. and Stern, G. M. (1974). *Lancet,* **i**, 1058
119. Dalén, P. and Steg, G. (1973). *Lancet,* **i**, 936
120 .Woert, M. H. van and Ambani, L. M. (1973). *Lancet,* **ii**, 1390
121. McCaul, J. A. and Stern. G. M. (1974). *Lancet,* **i**, 1117
122. Messiha, F. S., Erickson, H. M. and Goggin, J. E. (1976). *Res. Commun. Chem. Pathol. Pharmacol.,* **15**, 609
123. Shopsin, B. and Gershon, S. (1975). *Am. J. Psychiat.,* **132**, 536
124. Branchey, M. H., Charles, J. and Simpson, G. M. (1976). *Am. J. Psychiat.,* **133**, 444
125. Bien, R. D. (1976). *Am. J. Psychiat.,* **133**, 1093
126. Johnels, B., Wallin, L. and Walinder, J. (1976). *Br. Med. J.,* **3**, 642
127. Thomsen, J., Bech, P., Geisler, A., Jorgensen, M. B., Rafaelsen, O. J., Terkildsen, K., Udsen, J. and Zilstorff, K. (1974). *Acta Oto-laryng (Stockh.),* **78**, 59
128. Lutz, E. G. (1974). *J. Med. Soc. N.J.,* **71**, 502
129. Thomsen, J., Bech, P., Geisler, A., Prytz, S., Rafaelsen, O. J., Vendsborg, P. and Zilstorff, K. (1976). *Acta Oto-laryng. (Stockh.)* **82**, 294
130. Ekbom, K. (1974). *Opusc. Med (Stockh.),* **19**, 148
131. Ekbom, K. (1977). *Headache,* **17**, 39
132. Kudrow, L. (1977). *Headache,* **17**, 15
133. Lauritsen, B. J. (1977). *Nord. Psykiat. T.,* **31**, 110
134. Jeffries, J. J. and Lefebvre, A. (1973). *Can. Psychiat. Assoc. J.,* **18**, 439
135. Ogura, C., Okuma, T., Nakazawa, K. and Kishimoto, A. (1976). *Arch. Neurol.,* **33**, 143
136. Abe, K. (1977). *Br. J. Psychiat.,* **130**, 312
137. Ottosson, J.-O. and Persson, G. (1971). *Acta Psychiat. Scand.,* suppl. **221**, 39
138. Reid, A. H. and Leonard, A. (1977). *Br. J. Psychiat.,* **130**, 316
139. Forrest, J. N., Cox, M., Hong, C., Morrison, G. and Singer, I. (1976). *Kidney Int.,* **10**, 498
140. White, M. G. and Fetner, C. D. (1975). *N. Engl. J. Med.,* **292**, 390
141. Jacobs, R. S. (1976). *Am. J. Hosp. Pharm.,* **33**, 1127
142. Baker, R. S., Hurley, R, M. and Feldman, W. (1977). *J. Pediat.,* **90**, 480
143. Spaulding, S. W., Burrow, G. N., Bermudez, F. and Himmelhoch, J. M. (1972). *J. Clin. Endocrinol.,* **35**, 905
144. Temple, R., Berman, M., Robbins, J. and Wolff, J. (1972). *J. Clin. Invest.,* **51**, 2746
145. Gerdes, H., Littmann, K.-P., Joseph, K. and Mahlstedt, J. (1973). *Deutsch. Med. Wochenschr.,* **98**, 1551
146. Lazarus, J. H., Richards, A. R., Addison, G. M. and Owen, G. M. (1974). *Lancet,* **ii**, 1160
147. Bell, R. L. (1976). *J. Tenn. Med. Assoc.,* **69**, 31

148. Kristensen, O., Andersen, A. H. and Pallisgaard, G. (1976). *Lancet,* **i**, 603
149. Turner, J. G., Brownlie, B. E. W., Sadler, W. A. and Jensen, C. H. (1976). *Acta. Endocrinol.,* **83**, 86
150. Turner, J. G., Brownlie, B. E. W. and Rogers, T. G. H. (1976). *Lancet,* **i**, 614
151. Turner, J. G. and Brownlie, B. E. W. (1976). *Lancet,* **ii**, 904
152. Brière, J., Pousset, G., Darsy, P. and Guinet, P. (1974). *Ann. Endocrinol. (Paris).,* **35**, 281
153. Gershengorn, M. C., Izumi, M. and Robbins, J. (1976). *J. Clin, Endocrinol. Metab.,* **42**, 105
154. Rampon, S., Bussiere, J.-L., Sauvezie, B., Missioux, D., Lopitaux, R. and Prive, L. (1976). *N. Presse Méd.,* **5**, 1756
155. Pointud, P., Clerc, D., Allard, C., Manigand, G. and Deparis, M. (1976). *Sem. Hôp. Paris,* **52**, 1719
156. Kurnick, J. E., Gupta, R. C. and Robinson, W. A. (1975). *Clin. Res.,* **23**, 486 A
157. Gupta, R. C., Robinson, W. A. and Smyth, C. J. (1975). *Arthr. Rheum.,* **18**, 179
158. Gupta, R. C., Robinson, W. A. and Kurnick, J. E. (1976). *Am. J. Med.,* **61**, 29
159. Kaplan, R. A. (1976). *Ann. Intern. Med.,* **84**, 342
160. Barrett, A. J., Longhurst, P. A., Newton, K. A. and Humble, J. G. (1976). *Exp. Hematol.,* **4**, (suppl.), 42
161. Barrett, A. J. (1977). *Lancet,* **i**, 202
162. Greco, F. A., Brereton, H. D. and Pomeroy, T. (1976). *Proc. Am. Assoc. Cancer Res.,* **17**, 250

3

Lithium in the Management of Acute Depressive Illness

E. H. BENNIE

INTRODUCTION

Depressive illness has been shown to be responsive to ECT (1), to tricyclic antidepressant drugs and to L-tryptophan (2). However, some patients remain refractory and lithium has been shown to benefit some of these patients (3, 4). It is important that lithium's antidepressant action be evaluated as the drug has been found to succeed in situations where established therapies have failed (5). Mendels (6) has stated that while the use of lithium for the treatment of depression remains controversial, with controlled trials yielding conflicting results (7, 8) there may be evidence supporting the view that lithium is an effective antidepressant in a sub-group of patients. Fourteen clinical studies demonstrating that depressive illness has responded to lithium have been summarized in Table 3.1

Table 3.1. A summary of 14 studies on the effectiveness of lithium in acute depressive illness

Type of study	Uncontrolled studies	Controlled studies
Number of patients	189	128
Number of patients responding to lithium	110	51 (77)
Percentage of patients improved	52	40 (60)
Number of studies	9	5

* Figures in parentheses: patients showing some response

Approximately 50% of patients given lithium in both open and controlled studies improved significantly. Coppen (9) has shown that lithium is superior to Maprotiline in the prevention of depressive relapse. This chapter reports the results of successful lithium treatment in depressive illness which has not responded to tricyclic drugs.

SUBJECTS AND METHODS

The patients reported are the ones who responded to lithium. They received lithium in the course of their ordinary clinical treatment. Lithium was added to the treatment regime of patients who were diagnosed as suffering from recurrent affective psychosis depressed phase. The criteria for the prescribing of lithium for the patient's illness were as follows:—

1. At least two previous episodes of affective illness
2. The current episode had not responded to tricyclic drugs.

The presence of at least four of the following eight points assisted in the decision to give the patient lithium.

1. History of bipolar affective disorder
2. Obsessional personality
3. Somatic symptomatology
4. Symptoms of retardation and agitation
5. Chronic depression
6. Psychotic symptomatology
7. Difficult, demanding or hostile behaviour
8. Family history of affective illness.

Thirty patients have been given lithium for acute depressive illness during the period 1971 to 1976. Lithium was given in the form of lithium carbonate in tablets of 400 mg. The patients were started with a low dose of lithium and this was gradually increased until symptoms subsided or the patient's serum levels were 1 mmol/1. The lithium was prescribed on a once daily dose schedule using the sustained release preparation Priadel.

The study was completely retrospective in the first twelve patients. In the eighteen subsequent illnesses a deliberate attempt was made to treat depression with lithium.

Table 3.2. Basic clinical data

Number of patients	30
Men	12
Women	18
Out-patients	13
In-patients	17
Age range (years)	29-74
Average age (years)	53

Previous therapy was not always discontinued when lithium was commenced and it was found that lithium was given along with tricyclic antidepressant drugs on nine occasions, together with phenothiazine drugs on ten occasions, with ECT on one occasion and as a sole therapy on ten occasions.

RESULTS

Table 3.3: Diagnosis

Diagnosis	Number of Patients
Depressive stupor	2
Schizo-affective depression	6
Recurrent unipolar depression	13
Bipolar (1 & 2)	9

Table 3.4. The time taken by lithium to resolve the depressive illness

	Number of patients
Response to lithium in less than one week	8
Response to lithium between 1 and 3 weeks	12
Response to lithium in 3-6 weeks	7
Slow lithium responders	3

It was found that the average duration of depressive episode prior to the addition of lithium was 6 months, and that the average time depressed following the addition of lithium was 2 weeks.

Table 3.5. The effect of lithium on ECT use

Number of patients	30
Number of patients given ECT prior to lithium	22
Total number of ECTs given before lithium	293
Number of patients treated with lithium and ECT	1
Number of ECTs given subsequent to lithium	0
Duration of follow-up on lithium	1-6 years
Average duration on lithium	2.8 years

DISCUSSION

This study shows that lithium has antidepressant activity, and that on thirty occasions depressive illness has responded to lithium. In seventeen instances the depression was of such severity as to necessitate the patients' admissions into hospital and in two of those patients the depression was such as to amount to a stuporous condition. Thirteen patients were treated on an out-patient basis. Lithium was found to resolve depression of marked and moderate severity in patients suffering from recurrent affective psychosis. Lithium-induced remissions usually occurred quickly, sometimes within 3 days of starting the therapy, and on average within 2 weeks of lithium being introduced. The use of lithium in the management of acute depression has been associated with a dramatic reduction in the amount of electroplexy required.

Two important investigations (8, 10) have been carried out by Mendels and were controlled trials. The first study demonstrated that lithium was as effective as desimipramine and the second trial compared lithium to placebo in 21 patients, 13 of whom showed definite improvements.

In contrast to these trials earlier investigations with lithium in depressive illness reported that lithium did not have any antidepressant activity. It is likely that the divergence in these findings is because lithium has antidepressant action only in a sub-group of patients, and that these patients are identified by the criteria listed below

1. Manic depressive illness
2. Family history of bipolar illness
3. "Endogenous" symptom pattern
4. "High" baseline plasma calcium/magnesium ratio
5. Initial increase in plasma magnesium and calcium concentrations with lithium treatment
6. "High" erythrocyte lithium to plasma ratio.

Depression in manic depressive illness, both unipolar and bipolar, where there have been at least two previous episodes with restoration of normal mental health between episodes is most likely to respond to lithium. The presence of a family history of affective illness in first degree relatives has been found to predict depression (11) responding to lithium, but it is of interest to note that in the present study only four of the thirty responders were found to have a positive family history. Endogenous symptom patterns, such as lack of apparent precipitating cause, inevitable course of the illness, self blame, poor concentration and suicidal thoughts or actions, are thought to characterise the mental state of depression likely to remit with lithium. Obsessional personality traits have also been found in depression responding to lithium (5).

A number of biochemical indicators have been put forward to help identify the depression likely to respond to lithium. Carmen *et al.* (12) stated that the pre-treatment calcium and magnesium ratio was related to subsequent antidepressant response to lithium carbonate, and a baseline ratio greater than 2.62 indicated a likely response to lithium. He also found that initial increase in magnesium and calcium during the first five days of lithium treatment accurately predicted response to the therapy.

Erythrocyte lithium to plasma lithium ratio has also been investigated (6) but as yet there is no general agreement on the usefulness of these findings. Some workers suggest that patients who respond to lithium treatment have a significantly higher erythrocyte lithium to plasma lithium ratio than patients who do not respond, and it has been pointed out that erythrocyte lithium concentrations correlate better with brain lithium concentrations than do plasma lithium levels. Recent observations (13) cast doubt on the validity of observations which would have us believe that the ratio of erythrocyte lithium to plasma lithium can predict the outcome of lithium treatment.

Effects of lithium, tricyclic and amphetamine drugs on the cholinesterases of dog blood and rat brain have been investigated (14). Both the tricyclic drugs and lithium appear to inhibit rat brain butyrylcholinesterase. Amphetamine drugs and antihistaminics moderately inhibit this enzyme but chlorpromazine does not. In the reversal of reserpine-induced hypothermia lithium can mimic both the tricyclic and amphetamine drugs. Although low doses of lithium tend to reverse tetrabenazine depression, increasing doses of lithium tend to reinforce the tetrabenazine depression. In general, lithium does not appear to share the pharmacological profile of the tricyclic antidepressant drugs and has not been found to protect against the convulsant effects of drugs such as eserine and nicotine.

The EEG profile has emerged as an important method of identifying drug action (15) and it has been shown that lithium-induced ECG changes resemble those seen after the administration of anticholinergic thymoleptic drugs and also the cholinergic hallucinogens, but there are differences. Lithium induces an increase in epileptic potential and an increase of synchronisation and rythmical activity, which are some of the characteristic changes seen after chlorpromazine.

In the evaluation of lithium's therapeutic activity close attention has to be paid to the serum lithium level and a short study of three cases has shown that this can be a critical factor in demonstrating the drug's effectiveness (16). This study indicated that raising the serum lithium by a margin of 0.1 mmol/l can be associated with the remission of depressive symptoms.

CASE REPORT

The patient, a 67 year old married woman, with a 20 year history of recurrent depressive disorder, and with a family history of affective illness in a first degree relative, was treated for an acute depressive illness of marked severity with lithium carbonate in September 1975. She had been on lithium carbonate from 1968 and had remained well until about

January 1975 when, in view of her 6 year remission, it had been agreed to discontinue lithium. Within a few months of stopping lithium the depression relapsed and by the time lithium was restarted she was semi-stuporous, anorexic, dehydrated and mildly uremic. She was markedly suspicious with a wild, psychotic look. She did not verbalize at any length and refused to co-operate in psychiatric examination.

Lithium treatment was begun on 6th September 1975 and by 10th September a dramatic improvement was noted, characterized by a return of normal speech and mood and a co-operative attitude. She was sufficiently recovered to be discharged from hospital on 16th September and when last seen on 22nd January 1977 she was found to be well and free of all depressive symptoms.

During the acute depressive illness the serum lithium level ranged from 1.82 to 0.91 mmol/1 on a daily dose of 800 mg lithium carbonate. At present she is maintained on 400 mg daily and her serum level was last noted to be 0.5 mmol/1.

References

1. Herrington R. N., Bruce, A., Johnstone, E. C. and Lader, M. H. (1974). *Lancet,* **ii**, 731
2. Herrington, R. N., Bruce, A., Johnstone, E. C. and Lader, M. H. (1976). *Psychol. Med.,* **6**, 673
3. Vojtechovsky, M. and Zkusenosti, S. (1957). *J. Psychiat. Res.,* **5**, 67
4. Bennie, E. H. (1975). *Lancet,* **i**, 216
5. Neubauer, H. and Bermingham, P. (1975). Paper deliver at the International Congress on Neurology and Psychiatry; Prague.
6. Mendels, J. (1975). Paper read at the Annual Meeting of the American Psychiatric Association.
7. Fieve, R. R., Platman, S. R. and Plutchick, R. R. (1968). *Am. J. Psychiat.,* **125**, 487
8. Mendels, J., Secunda, S. K. and Dyson, W. C. (1972). *Arch. Gen. Psychiat.,* **26**, 154
9. Coppen, A., Montgomery, R. K., Gupta, R. K. and Bailey, J. E. (1976). *Br. J. Psychiat.,* **128**, 479
10. Mendels, J. (1975). In F. N. Johnson (ed.). *Lithium Research and Therapy.* pp. 43-62 (London: Academic Press).
11. Mendlewicz, T., Fieve, R. R., Stallone, F. and Fleiss, J. L. (1972). *Lancet,* **i**, 599
12. Carmen, J. S., Post, R. M. and Teplitz, T. A. (1974). *Lancet,* **ii**, 1454
13. Marini, J. L. (1977). *Br. J. Psychiat.* **130**, 139
14. Perkinson, E., Ruchart, R. and Devanzo, J. P. (1969). *Proc. Soc. Exp. Biol. Med.,* **131**, 685
15. Itil, T. M. Personal communication.
16. Friedel, R. O. (1976). *Am. J. Psychiat.,* **133**, 976

4

The Use of Lithium in the Treatment of Schizo-affective Disorders

M. F. HUSSAIN and J. D. GOMERSALL

INTRODUCTION

The success with lithium in hypomanic states has led to therapeutic trials in a wide range of disorders characterized by strong affective components and periodic recurrence, where it has been noted that it could sometimes be of benefit (1). The cyclical course of manic depressive illness, also typical of some schizo-affective disorders, suggests that the latter may be amenable to modification with lithium. Three case histories are reported here, which throw light on the treatment of schizo-affective disorders with lithium carbonate in the form of a sustained release preparation (Priadel).

The term "schizo-affective" was introduced by Kasanin (2) in the 1930s to describe patients showing a mixture of affective and schizophrenic symptomatology. The condition has now been widely recognized and is included in the International Classification of Diseases (3) and standard texts (4). Several writers have reported the efficacy of lithium carbonate therapy in these states. Prien *et al.* (5) studied 83 patients with this condition and found that lithium carbonate and chlorpromazine were equally effective for both affective and schizophrenic symptomatology, in mildly active cases. Zall| *et al.* (6) showed improvement in nine out of ten schizo-affective patients, but in the manic symptomatology only, and a similar finding was shown in reports by Gottfries (7) and Tupin. (8). Egli (9) showed that there was a significant prophylactic action where the disorder was recurrent, but Angst *et al.* (10) found the prophylactic action less pronounced than in recurrent affective disorders. An earlier paper (11) had shown that lithium was prophylactically effective in a mixed group of affective and schizo-affective patients.

Other authors have not found that lithium is of value in this condition. Johnson *et al.* (12) in a comparative study of lithium carbonate and chlorpromazine in mania and schizo-affective disorders reported that, in mania, lithium was superior to chlorpromazine in its prophylactic effect but with schizo-affective disorders this finding was reversed. Johnson *et al.* (13) and Schou (14) showed that there was a well marked response in manic patients but that an admixture of cases with schizophrenic symptoms decreased the response to treatment.

The possibility of the co-existence of manic depressive and schizo-affective disorders as separate entities must be borne in mind, and it is interesting to note that Bratfos and Haug (15) noted that 3% of their group diagnosed as manic-depressive later developed schizophrenic symptoms.

CHOICE OF CASES

The three cases described were all given lithium carbonate after other treatments had failed to give satisfactory improvement. All had long-standing symptoms of a manic-depressive and schizophrenic nature which showed an irregular periodic recurrence. The dosage was adjusted to maintain a serum level within the therapeutic range; only one patient showed mild gastro-intestinal symptoms.

CASE REPORTS

Case No. 1:

This was a 47 year old male joiner whose illness was manifested by manic hypermotility, bizarre behaviour, thought disorder, lack of warmth and absorption in psychotic fantasy. An older brother of the patient had suffered a recurrent depressive illness and had committed suicide 12 years previously at the age of 43. The patient had had a happy childhood and was average in studies. On leaving school he began training as a joiner, marrying at the age of 25, his wife being a pleasant, competent woman, and the marriage relationship happy. They had three healthy grown up children. His pre-morbid personality, according to people who knew him, was described as hardworking, polite, frank and of average intelligence. Previous medical history revealed only a unilateral congenital ptosis and past history of gastric ulcer. He had had a road traffic accident at the age of 30 and was unconscious for 3 days.

At the ages of 17 and 21 he had suffered episodes of emotional disturbance resulting in short periods of out-patient treatment at a London Psychiatric Clinic. His first admission was at the age of 24 followed, up to the time he was started on lithium carbonate, by 15 admissions of increasing duration with shorter remissions between. His mental state was hypomanic or depressed with paranoid delusions, auditory hallucinations and frequent suicidal ideation and one suicidal attempt which mimicked his brother's successful attempt in jumping out of the first floor window.

Medication with various antidepressants and most major tranquillizers was given with minimal benefit, and for the last year he had been given regular weekly ECT which had prevented a relapse. Over the years he received well over one hundred ECT treatments.

In August 1975, in view of the ineffectiveness of other treatment, it was decided to start lithium carbonate (Priadel) for his schizo-affective disorder. An improvement within 2 weeks of starting this therapy was remarkable. His condition dramatically changed and the picture became one of harmonious behaviour, free from mood swings and other symptoms. Industrial rehabilitation was arranged and he was soon discharged and took up his old employment. The only problem was that a social worker was required to work with the family who had adjusted, as in cases of anticipated bereavement, to the patient being a chronic in-patient.

He was, however, re-admitted a year later with bizarre behaviour, restlessness, wanting to shop around excessively, being suspicious and deluded. It emerged that he had stopped his medication for the previous six weeks because his son was getting married and he thought that the drinking at the wedding reception might adversely interact with his lithium. He was re-admitted and re-started on lithium carbonate, showing rapid improvement. He has kept well since.

Case No. 2:

This was a 23 year old typist, who was first admitted in April 1974. She had left home to live with her boyfriend and was complaining that her thoughts were being wiped out of her mind and that she was being watched by hidden cameras and microphones. In June 1974 she took an overdose of Librium. She had insomnia and feelings of guilt, later on became talkative, showed mood swings and difficulty in concentration. In September 1974 she was re-admitted and a diagnosis of schizo-affective disorder was made.

Her family history showed that her father was 61 years old, retired and her mother prone to anxiety and domineering. Her elder sister was working in the USA and had a PhD in biochemistry. Her twin brother, whom she disliked, was described as having a labile mood. She had a past broken engagement, but a current boy friend.

During her previous admission she was treated with trifluoperazine, orphenadrine and ECT. In January 1977 on re-admission it was decided to give her haloperidol and lithium carbonate (Priadel). In two weeks it was possible to bring her excitement under sufficient control to render her condition manageable. She seemed well on her way to recovery and transition from hospital to normal life. Her mood disturbance was stabilized and she was no longer irritable. She is still keeping well on this treatment, though it is early to be sure of the prophylactic effect of lithium and to know if this will be still effective when haloperidol is withdrawn.

Case No. 3:
The third case was a pale, thin, 20 year old, unemployed girl who had become unmanageable with erratic behaviour, restlessness, mood swings, paranoid delusions and thought disorder. She had first been admitted 3 years previously when she had started to believe that men and girls were following her, and that her life was in danger, with references being made to her on television. She felt that a gang of men were spreading rumours about her being a nymphomaniac. She had flight of ideas and insomnia. Her family history showed that her father had had treatment for a schizophrenic illness and that her mother had been depressed though she had not had any treatment. Her mother felt that this girl had been showing some psychotic disturbance for the past 2 years prior to her admission.

Since the first admission a variety of tranquillizers and several courses of ECT had been given, all with very temporary benefit. She was frequently verbally aggressive and had attempted suicide.

In March 1977 she showed all the features of a schizo-affective disorder and was started on lithium carbonate. Improvement was evident after a few days, the incongruous expression disappeared and her aggressive, restless behaviour was replaced by an attitude of co-operation in a person with whom rapport could be established. Paranoid ideas rapidly diminished and she was soon discharged.

As in the second case, the follow up period has been short but treatment with lithium carbonate has been maintained with no sign of recurrence so far.

It is interesting to note that in this case it is possible that the schizophrenic and depressive aspects of the illness could have been inherited from father and mother respectively.

DISCUSSION

The decision to use lithium carbonate as a treatment in all these cases was based mainly on their resistance to other forms of therapy, though the fact that all three showed some degree of periodicity in their illness was an additional factor contributing to the decision.

It is not possible to say that natural remission did not play a part in these cases, though this would seem unlikely, at least in the first case reported, and the rapid improvement in all three leading to a return home was remarkable. The relapse of the first case on stopping lithium carbonate therapy is also noteworthy.

If lithium acts by counteracting a metabolic disorder of hereditary aetiology, then where other members of the family suffer a similar illness, this drug may be of value. It was unfortunate that the brother of the first patient (Case 1), died before this could be tested.

Further controlled study of lithium in schizo-affective states where it is not used as a last resort may help to give a more accurate picture.

References

1. Kerry, R. J. (1975). In: F. N. Johnson (ed.) *Lithium Research and Therapy* pp. 146. (London: Academic Press)
2. Kasanin, J. (1933). *Am. J. Psychiat.,* **90** 97
3. Stengel, E. (1959). *Bull. WHO,* **21**, 601
4. Mayer Gross, W., Slater, E. and Roth, M. (1967). *Clinical Psychiatry* (Baltimore: Williams and Wilkins)
5. Prien, R. F., Caffrey, E. M. and Klett, C. J. (1972). *Arch. Gen. Psychiat.,* **27**, 182
6. Zall, H., Therman, P. O. G. and Myers, J. M. (1968). *Am. J. Psychiat.,* **125**, 549
7. Gottfries, C. G. (1964). *Acta. Psychiat. Scand.* suppl. **203**, 157
8. Tupin, J. R. (1969). *Public Health Service Publication No. 1876,* U. S. Department of Health, Education and Welfare.
9. Egli, H. (1971). *Schweiz. Med. Wochenschr.,* **101**, 157
10. Angst. J., Weis, P., Grof, P., Baastrup, P. C. and Schou, M. (1970). *Br. J. Psychiat.,* **116**, 604
11. Angst, J., Dittrich, A. and Grof, P. (1969). *Int. Pharmacopsychiat.,* **2**, 1
12. Johnson, G., Gershon, S., Burdock, E. I., Floyd, F. and Hekimian, L. (1971). *Br. J. Psychiat.,* **119**, 267
13. Johnson, G., Gershon, S. and Hekimian, L. J. (1968). *Comprehens. Psychiat.,* **9**, 563
14. Schou, M., Juel-Nielson, N., Stromgren, E. and Voldby, H. (1954). *J. Neurol. Neurosurg.* Psychiat., **17**, 250
15. Bratfos, O. and Haug, J. O. (1968). *Acta. Psychiat. Scand.,* **44**, 89

5

A Double-blind Trial of Lithium Carbonate in Alcoholism

C. M. REYNOLDS, J. MERRY, J. BAILEY and A. COPPEN

INTRODUCTION

The incidence of alcoholism has increased steadily in recent years. This is borne out by statistics recently reported by the Advisory Committee on Alcoholism which was set up in March 1975. Between 1968 and 1973 the number of driving accidents involving drink rose by 27% per annum. Since 1969 wine consumption has almost doubled and spirit consumption has risen by 80%. Alcoholism will account for nearly 25% of all mental hospital patients by 1985 if admissions for alcoholic psychosis continue to rise at the present rate.

In the light of this rapidly escalating problem the difficulty of finding conclusive evidence that any of the many treatment measures used to combat alcoholism has been therapeutically effective (1) emphasizes the need for further investigations.

There is a high incidence of depressive symptomatology in alcoholics and their relatives, and it is well known that suicide is a common outcome in these patients (2). This association between affective disorders and alcoholism has been fully documented (3-7) and it was with this in mind that the present investigation was initiated. If the hypothesis is correct that affective morbidity contributes to the drinking behaviour of some problem drinkers, then it is logical to treat the depressive symptoms with the most effective therapeutic agent available. Although the efficacy of chronic administration of tricyclic antidepressants is open to question, that of lithium salts is not. There is much well controlled evidence that lithium salts reduce very considerably the morbidity of unipolar and bipolar affective illness (8-10). Lithium has also proved superior, in the prevention of recurrent depression, to a tetracyclic antidepressant (Maprotiline) which is of the same efficacy as amitriptyline and other established tricyclics (11).

The chronic and recurrent nature of alcoholism would suggest that lithium is the most rational therapeutic agent currently available to investigate in this context. A previous study (12) was inconclusive and a double-blind study by Kline *et al.* (13) reported a significant beneficial effect from lithium which, however, did not appear to be related to affective disturbance. The present double-blind prospective investigation was prompted by these considerations. A preliminary report on this work has been published (14).

METHOD

The patients were selected from those admitted to a regional alcoholism unit. These patients are in themselves a selected group in that they have been referred for this form of treatment, and have been considered to have some degree of motivation. The unit in this study admits more than 100 patients per year, of whom approximately 25% are readmissions. After an initial period of "drying out", the patient spends 6 weeks or more in the unit where treatment consists of group psychotherapy and social rehabilitation. As part of treatment all patients are advised to abstain completely from alcohol.

All those entering the study were diagnosed as alcoholic using the WHO definition (1952) (15) and the Glossary of Mental Disorders Classification (16), after consideration of the history and clinical findings. Care was taken to exclude those suffering from a primary affective disorder with secondary alcoholism. Those suffering from physical disorders contraindicating the use of lithium were also excluded.

On admission to the unit the purpose of the trial was discussed, and those wishing to participate, and who showed interest and motivation, were familiarised with the procedure to be followed.

CLASSIFICATION

When the staff were satisfied that a patient was fully detoxified and had ceased taking all medication, he was asked to complete the Beck self-rating inventory for depression (17). This was done in the morning before commencing ward activities and was subsequently repeated 1 week later. The mean of these results was used to classify the patients into two groups — depressive and non-depressive; the cut-off point on the depression inventory score being 15 or more for depressives.

All the patients were then randomly assigned to receive either lithium or placebo tablets on a double-blind basis. Patients attended an outpatient clinic held in the MRC neuropsychiatric unit at West Park Hospital. The clinic was conducted on well tried principles, having been involved in double-blind trials of lithium on numerous previous occasions (10). At each 6-weekly attendance, after initially more frequent visits while the serum lithium level was being stabilized, patients were asked to complete the Beck depressive inventory, and were assessed separately by an independent rater who noted the number of days on which they had been drinking, together with those days on which they were incapacitated by alcohol. This incapacity was taken to be an inability to carry out everyday tasks which would be done under normal circumstances, for example attending work for a full day, shopping, housework and usual social activities. At the same time the rater noted the affective morbidity on a three-point scale without reference to the Beck score. These results were recorded on a data sheet modified from previous lithium studies (10).

An independent coordinator not concerned with rating the patient was assigned to adjust the dosage of lithium to maintain the serum level between 0.8 and 1.2 mmol/l. On each occasion that it was necessary to adjust the dosage, a placebo patient's dose was also changed. The coordinator also supervized the weighing of each patient, kept the Beck inventory scores and noted side effects. At each assessment the coordinator kept a blood sample which was analysed for blood alcohol without the patient's knowledge.

Patients who failed to attend were followed up whenever possible by direct contact and a further appointment was given. At each visit seven weeks supply of medication was given to facilitate continuity of therapy. Those who attended regularly were asked to complete the Marke-Nyman temperament scale (18).

RESULTS

Table 5.1 shows the general details of those patients entering the trial. Of the 71 patients originally started on the trial, only 40 completed it to the satisfaction of the investigators. The mean age for the lithium group was 44.9 years and that for the placebo group 45.3, the mean time on the trial being 41.0 and 42.8 weeks respectively. Serum lithium levels were consistently maintained within the therapeutic range. The first month on the trial was discounted when assessing the results of treatment.

High dropout rates have been noted in previous investigations of this type involving alcoholics (19) and a double-blind technique. In this study 33 of the original patients dropped out, 16 of whom were in the depressive

Table 5.1. General details of patients and drop-outs

	Started on trial	Completed trial					Time on trial (weeks)		Lithium level (mmol/l)	
			Age (yrs)		Sex					
	N	N	Mean	SE	M	F	Mean	SE	Mean	SE
Lithium Group										
Non-depressed	18	11	48.8	2.4	10	1	40.9	6.0	0.91	0.05
Depressed	18	9	40.0	3.5	6	3	41.0	7.2	0.80	0.03
All patients	36	20	44.9	2.2	16	4	41.0	4.5	0.86	0.03
Placebo Group										
Non-depressed	19	11	44.6	3.5	8	3	41.3	5.2	—	—
Depressed	16	7	46.6	6.3	3	4	45.1	6.6	—	—
All patients	35	18	45.3	3.1	11	7	42.8	4.0	—	—

Table 5.2. Days spent drinking

	N	Number of days with drinking		Per cent time on trial drinking	
		Mean	SE	Mean	SE
Lithium Group					
All patients	20	9.5	5.1	4.9	3.0
Depressed patients only	9	1.3*	1.0	0.9*	0.8
Placebo Group	18	20.7	14.5	5.8	3.7
All patients	7	48.1*	36.6	13.2**	9.2
Depressed patients only					

*Lithium vs. Placebo $p < 0{\cdot}01$ (after log transformation)

**Lithium vs. Placebo $p < 0{\cdot}05$ (after angular transformation)

There was no significant difference in the drinking habits between non-depressed patients on lithium and non-depressed patients on placebo group. Of the 33 patients, 18 completed less than 4 weeks on the trial, and only seven completed 3 months. The vast majority of these were drinking at the time of, or soon after, dropout, but several showed evidence of poor motivation. A few moved out of the area completely, including one man who emigrated but had remained abstinent a year later. Two patients went to prison for offences involving drink (one committed before treatment), and another two eventually died as a result of overdoses of drugs and alcohol. The poor motivation of this group is further indicated by the fact that only four of the 33 subsequently sought readmission to the alcoholic unit; this apart, the dropout group did not differ in any fundamental way to that of the patients reported in this study.

Table 5.2 shows the number of days on which the patients took an alcoholic drink. The depressed patients on placebo drank on significantly more days than those on lithium, but there was no significant difference in the drinking habits of the non-depressed groups whether they were on lithium or not. Table 5.3 shows that of the nine depressed patients in the lithium group, six did not drink at all during the trial, whereas of the seven depressed patients on placebo, not one remained totally abstinent.

Table 5.3. Alcoholic morbidity

	Days drinking	
	Some	None
Depressed patients in Lithium Group	3	6
Depressed patients in Placebo Group	7	0

Fisher's Exact Probability Test: $p < 0.025$

	Days drinking	
	Some	None
Non-depressed patients in Placebo Group	4	7
Depressed patients in Placebo Group	7	0

Fisher's Exact Probability Test: $p < 0.025$

Table 5.4 indicates that the depressed group was incapacitated by alcohol on significantly fewer days when treated with lithium as opposed to placebo.

Table 5.5 indicates the depression ratings on patients. The mean baseline Beck inventory score for the depressed patients on lithium was 20.5 and on placebo 18.7. During the course of the trial the clinical ratings for affective morbidity made by the independent assessor were found to correlate closely with the Beck inventory scores. There was an overall but not statistically significant improvement in Beck inventory scores at the end of the trial, the percentage improvement for lithium-treated depressives was 60% as opposed to 40% for placebo.

Table 5·4. Days incapacitated by alcohol

	N	Number of days incapacitated Mean	SE	Per cent time on trial incapacitated Mean	SE
Lithium Group					
All patients	20	4.9	2.3	2.7	1.6
Depressed patients only	9	0.7	0.4	0.4*	0.3
Placebo Group					
All patients	20	3.7	1.3	1.2	0.4
Depressed patients only	7	5.1**	2.2	1.5*	0.6

*Lithium vs. Placebo $p < 0.05$ (after angular transformation)
**Lithium vs. Placebo $p < 0.05$ (after log transformation)

Table 5·5. Depression ratings on patients

		Beck Depression Inventory					
		Baseline		End of trial		Per-cent improvement	
	N	Mean	SE	Mean	SE	Mean	SE
Lithium Group							
All patients	20	13.8	1.7	6.4	1.1	33.7	17.9
Depressed patients only	9	20.5	1.9	6.7	1.7	60.2	13.1
Placebo Group							
All patients	18	12.2	1.6	7.8	1.3	25.5	12.6
Depressed patients only	7	18.7	1.9	10.6	1.8	40.4	12.3

DISCUSSION

One of the most striking findings at the outset of this investigation was that using the Beck depressive inventory; almost half the patients fell into the depressive group, and this was in accordance with the independent clinical ratings.

We know that only a proportion, probably about 35%, of alcoholics are referred at some stage of their illness to a Regional Alcoholic Unit. It is likely that those who actively seek treatment in this way are fairly well motivated and have a reasonable degree of insight. They may, therefore, not be entirely representative of alcoholics as a whole, but the fairly liberal admission policy of this particular unit and the high dropout recorded would suggest that this group has many of the characteristics of the majority of alcoholics who have contact with the psychiatric and medical services.

It is probable that all the patients considerably underestimated their alcohol intake, but there was no reason to suppose that this was any different in the lithium treated as opposed to placebo treated groups. This view is further substantiated by the complete failure to detect alcohol in any of the 6-weekly blood samples which were taken from every patient. It seems probable that patients particularly avoided drinking just prior to this interview surmising (correctly) that a test for blood alcohol was likely to be performed.

Note has already been taken of the high dropout rate, which was to be expected, but out of the original group of 71, 34 fell into the depressive group, and 16 of these (22%) were willing to carry on with lithium for a period of approximately 1 year. The Marke-Nyman Temperament Scale did not indicate any features which related to dropout or treatment outcome. Following recent reports, untoward side-effects from lithium therapy were monitored (20-22) but none was found except in one case where a male patient in the non-depressive group developed mild hyperthyroidism.

We recognize that a careful follow-up clinic such as that used in this study, wth regular appointmnets, blood tests, weighing, clinical interviews, questionnaires and group-cohesive influences and structuring must have in itself a powerful therapeutic effect, but nevertheless a clear advantage could be demonstrated for those depressed alcoholics who were treated with lithium compared with those who had placebo. Not only was there a significantly higher morbidity in those depressive alcoholics who were on placebo, but these findings indicate that lithium reduced the drinking and resulting incapacity of those patients classified as depressive alcoholics when taken over a period of several months. These findings would therefore suggest that there is a considerable number of alcoholic patients who would show a substantial advantage from long-term lithium therapy.

References

1. Wallgren H. and Barry M. (1970). In: *Actions of Alcohol* Vol. 11. (Amsterdam: Elsevier Publishing Co.)
2. Kessel, N. and Grossman, G. (1961). *Br. Med. J.,* **ii**, 1671
3. Winokur G. and Pitts, F.N. (1965). *J. Psychiat. Res.* **3**, 113
4. Wilkins, R.M. (1974). *The Hidden Alcoholic in General Practice.* (London)
5. Freed, E.X. (1970). *Q.J. Stud. Alcohol,* **31**, 62
6. Rathod, N.H. (1964). *Public Health,* **78**, 181
7. Barraclough, B., Bunch, J., Nelson, B. and Sainsbury, P. (1974). *Br. J. Psychiat.,* **125**, 355
8. Baastrup, P.C., Poulsen, J.C., Schou, M., Thomsen, K. and Amdisen, A. (1970). *Lancet,* **ii**, 326
9. Coppen, A., Noguera, R., Bailey, J., Burns, B., Swani, M., Hare, E. and Gardner, R. (1971). *Lancet,* **ii**, 275
10. Coppen, A., Peet, M., Bailey, J., Noguera, R. Burns, B., Swani, M.S., Maggs, R. and Gardner, R. (1973). *Psychiat. Neurol. Neurochir.* (Amst.), **76**, 501
11. Coppen, A., Montgomery, S. A., Gupta, R. K. and Bailey, J.E. (1976). *Br. J. Psychiat.,* **128**, 479
12. Fries, H. (1969). *Acta Psychiat. Scand. Suppl.,* 207
13. Kline, N.S., Wren, J.C. Cooper, T.B., Varga, E. and Canal, O. (1974). *Am. J. Med. Sci.,* **268**, 15
14. Merry, J., Reynolds, C.M., Bailey, J. and Coppen, A. (1976). *Lancet,* **ii**, 481
15. WHO Expert Committee on Mental Health (1952). Alcohol sub-committee second report. WHO technical report series 48
16. Studies on medical and population subjects, No. 22. *A Glossary of Mental Disorders.* HMSO (1968)
17. Beck, A. T., Ward, C.H., Mendelson, U., Mock, J. and Erbough, J. (1961). *Arch. Gen. Psychiat.,* **4**, 561
18. Coppen, A. (1966). *Br. J. Med. Psychol.,* **39**, 55
19. Edwards, G. (1970). In: E. Popham (ed.) *Alcohol and Alcoholism, p.* 173 (Toronto: University of Toronto Press)
20. Crowe, M.J., Lloyd, G.G., Block, S. and Rosser, R.M. (1973). *Psychol. Med.,* 3, 337
21. Hullin, R.P., McDonald, R. and Allsopp, M.N.E. (1975). *Br. J. Psychiat.,* **126**, 281
22. Rosser, R.M. (1967). *Br. J. Psychiat.,* **128, 61**

6

Lithium and Reduced Consumption of Drugs of Abuse

H. STEINBERG and T. M. McMILLAN

INTRODUCTION

During this decade the clinical use of lithium has greatly increased, and so has cognate research (1-3); as is illustrated by the contents of this volume, the range of approaches is broad.

We have been concerned with analysing the effects of lithium on forms of animal behaviour, and have chosen aspects which may be relevant to clinical problems.

In earlier work approximations to affective disorders were mainly studied — drug-induced 'mania' in rats and mice was reduced or abolished by lithium treatment (4) — and more recently we have found that lithium can markedly reduce the voluntary consumption of solutions of morphine (5) and of alcohol in rats (6).

Reduced consumption of drugs of abuse in man as a result of lithium treatment has been reported, particularly in opiate addicts (7,8) and in alcholics (9-11), but the published literature is as yet small, often inconclusive and apt to be scattered. Since the effectiveness of lithium in affective disorders is clearly established (12) it has been suggested that its beneficial effects in drug dependence occur especially where latent or manifest depression is also involved (13). Lithium has in fact been reported to be particularly helpful in depressed alcoholics in whom it can reduce incapacitating alcohol consumption (9), but how far effects of this kind are mediated by reduction of depression either during periods of drinking or after withdrawal is difficult to assess. It has, for example, been reported that some alcoholics who reduce or stop drinking after lithium treatment continue to appear depressed (10). 'Euphoria' has also been considered in relation to the effects of lithium in drug abuse, in the sense that its anti-manic effects in affective disorders might be paralleled by anti-euphoric effects in drug addiction and so lead to less rewarding and hence reduced consumption (14). This has not been borne out in one study where lithium appeared to have no effect on morphine-induced euphoria in opiate addicts (8). Clinical investigations with addicts are beset by methodological and practical problems, including difficulties over appropriate controls and environmental factors. High drop-out rates are common, despite strong initial motivation; these drop-out rates may be aggravated by the absence of immediately obvious therapeutic effects of lithium (7,13). At the present time the use of lithium in the treatment of drug abuse including alcoholism, though increasing, does not appear to be widespread.

Recent interest in the similarities between effects of alcohol and of opiates, especially in relation to dependence, has led to speculation about common mechanisms of action (15). Naloxone, which is generally regarded as an almost pure opiate antagonist, has also been shown to inhibit convulsions following ethanol withdrawal in ethanol dependent mice (16); however, also in ethanol-dependent mice, it failed to induce withdrawal jumping, which typically occurs after the withdrawal of opiates (17). Further, it has been reported that morphine injections can suppress alcohol drinking in laboratory rats, regardless of whether access to alcohol solutions had lasted 1 or 32 days (18). The effects of morphine on the 'alcohol deprivation effect' have also been studied (19): if rats which have had prolonged access to alcohol are deprived of it for several days they will, when alcohol again becomes available, drink much more of it than before, at least initially; but if morphine is given during the deprivation interval either 'passively' or by self-administration, the alcohol deprivation effect is suppressed. That opiates and alcohol are often used as substitutes for each other by man has of course long been known (15).

In recent years we have examined the effects of lithium administration on the drinking of morphine and of alcohol solutions by laboratory rats.

Adult male hooded rats, singly housed, fed ad libitum and experimentally naive were used. In order to encourage the consumption of drug solutions and induce preferences as rapidly as possible, animals were deprived of fluid for a number of hours each day before being given access to fluids. Fluids were available through two 300 ml plastic drinking bottles with metal spouts; the positions of the bottles were varied to allow for side preferences. Solutions of both LiCl and NaCl were isotonic with plasma (0.154M) and were injected i.p. in a volume of 13 ml/kg/rat, giving a dose of 2 mmol/kg. This dose of LiCl was chosen because in previous experiments it had been found to be behaviourally effective and without manifest toxic effects (29).

Experiments with morphine (5)

Rats were first accustomed to satisfying their thirst during a daily 3-hour drinking period (12.00-15.00), and were then made dependent on morphine in the form of a morphine-sucrose solution (0.5 mg/ml morphine hydrochloride + 10% w/v sucrose) which was presented as their only source of fluid for 6 weeks. Within a few days they had learned to consume more of this solution than they had previously drunk of water, and after 6 weeks of this 'forced' drinking the strength of their preference was tested by giving them daily choices between morphine-sucrose solution and sucrose solution or tap water. On average, the preference for morphine-sucrose solution when given in competition with plain water was markedly greater (approximately 90% of total fluid intake) than with sucrose solution (approximately 57%). Daily injections of 2 mmol/kg LiCl substantially decreased the amounts of morphine solution consumed relative to saline injected controls, and the amounts drunk of sucrose solution or tap water increased. Morphine-sucrose drinking was reduced already after the first lithium injection in the morphine-sucrose vs. sucrose solution group, but consistent reduction was delayed by about 12 days in the morphine-sucrose vs. tap water group, possibly because the degree of dependence was based on a much greater intake of morphine (Figures 6.1 and 6.2). Further experiments with a quinine-sucrose solution adjusted as far as possible to match the bitterness of the morphine-sucrose solution suggested that the lithium effect was independent of taste.

Experiments with alcohol (6)

For 14 days before the first experiment was to begin, the rats were only allowed access to drinking water for 6 hours (10.00-16.00) daily. A daily choice procedure between alcohol solution and water was used from the first day of the experiment onwards. The concentration of alcohol was increased by 1% steps on every third day up to 6%, and then remained at this level.

One group of the animals was, in addition, injected i.p. with 2 mmol/kg LiCl during two separate periods: days 18 and days 28-36 of the experiment; these were designated the 'alcohol naive' group. The second group received injections of 2 mmol/kg NaCl on days 1-18 and 2 mmol/kg LiCl

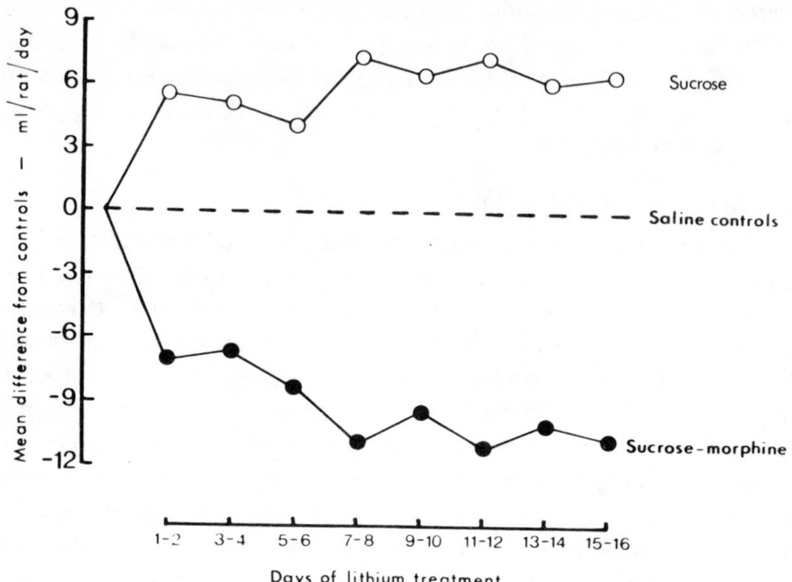

Figure 6.1. Addicted rats which were given daily choices between solutions of 10% sucrose + 0.5 mg/ml morphine hydrochloride (sucrose-morphine, ● and 10% sucrose alone (sucrose, O), were injected daily with either 13 ml/kg of isotonic saline or with 2 mmol/kg of LiCl (n = 7 per group). Lithium-treated rats reduced their consumption of sucrose-morphine from an average of 23 ml/day to 15 ml/day (saline controls increased theirs slightly and increased their consumption of sucrose solution). The results are represented as mean differences from the controls (————)

on days 28-36, and as clear and consistent preferences for alcohol had emerged, they could be regarded as 'alcohol experienced' by day 28. Neither group was injected during days 19-27. In this way the saline-injected 'alcohol experienced' group acted as controls for the lithium-injected 'alcohol naive' group between days 1-27, but became a second, experimental, i.e. lithium-injected, group in its own right between days 28 and 36.

Polydipsia, as expected, was found to occur in lithium-treated animals and led to an average increase in total fluid intake of the order of 65% as compared with pre-experimental consumption.

On day 36, 3 hours after the last injection, serum lithium levels were found to be 0.61 ± 0.17 mmol/l (mean and standard deviation) for the 'naive' group, and 0.83 ± 0.15 mmol/l for the 'experienced' group. These values are within the lower limits of the usually quoted therapeutic range in man (12). Figure 6.3 shows that alcohol drinking was reduced both in 'alcohol naive' and 'alcohol experienced' rats during lithium treatment.

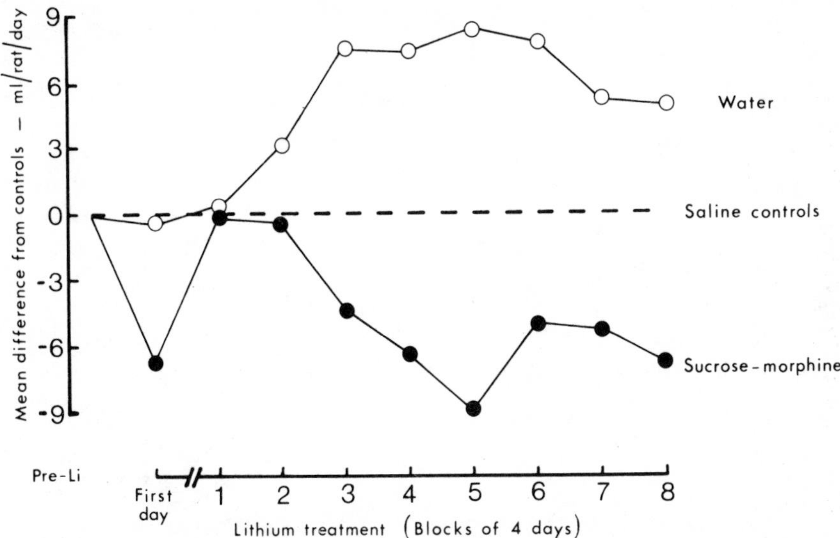

Figure 6.2. Addicted rats which were given daily choices between sucrose-morphine (●) and tap water (O) instead of sucrose solution as in Figure 6.1, were injected with 2 mmol/kg of isotonic LiCl (n = 9) or 13 ml/kg of saline (n = 8). Lithium-treated rats reduced their sucrose-morphine consumption consistently only after some 12 days. The results are presented as differences between LiCl and saline controls (————————)

Reduced alcohol consumption was maintained in the 'naive' group during days 19-27 when lithium was no longer given; this is consistent with one finding in the literature (22) but not with others where alcohol intake rapidly increased when lithium administration stopped (23-25). In the 'experienced' group which had not had lithium before, alcohol drinking had, by the fourth day of injections (i.e. day 31 of the experiment), dropped from approximately 70% to 35%; alcohol drinking in the 'naive' group continued at its already lowered level and, if anything, declined further during the same period. It had, however, taken 9 days of lithium injections before a significant reduction in alcohol drinking occurred in the 'naive' group, (from approximately 50 to 28%); this was a much longer delay than in the 'experienced' group. A further experiment was devised to examine whether the delay in the 'naive' animals might have been due to the lower concentration of alcohol available to them at this time. The procedure was essentially similar to that of days 1 to 18 in the first experiment, except that the concentration of alcohol remained at 3% instead of being increased to 6%. A small but statistically non-significant preference for alcohol solution developed in saline injected animals; there was a reduction in alcohol solution drinking in the lithium treated rats, but

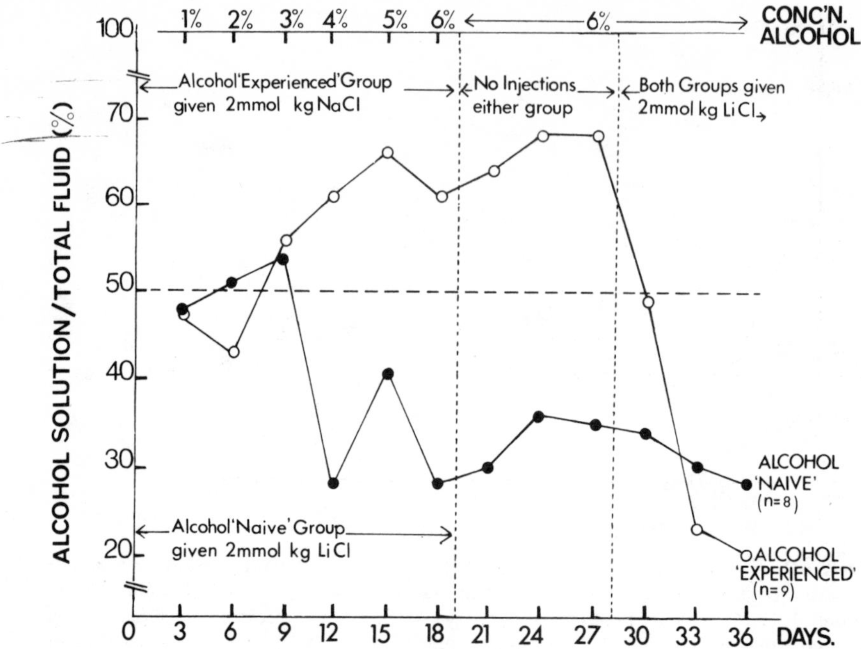

Figure 6.3. Lithium reduces alcohol consumption in rats. Rats were given daily choices between alcohol solutions and water. Lithium injections led to a substantial reduction in alcohol drinking both in alcohol naive rats on day 10, after 9 days of lithium ingestion, and in rats which had a previously established preference for alcohol, i.e. which were alcohol 'experienced' on day 31 after 3 days of lithium injection. The reduction persisted between days 19 and 27 after lithium had been stopped in the 'naive' group. Each point on the graphs represents mean values for 8 or 9 rats averaged over three days

this was again not significant. These findings suggest that, in short term alcohol drinking experiments at least, whether or not a preference for or a reduction in alcohol drinking occurs is partly dependent on the concentration of alcohol available.

Loss of body weight during lithium administration was found in both these experiments (maximum 8% in the first, and 15% in the second experiment) However, relations between weight loss and alcohol drinking are unclear since alcohol drinking decreased most in the first experiment while weight loss was greater in the second experiment where reduction of alcohol drinking was insignificant.

CONCLUSIONS

The two sets of experiments from our laboratory which we have described show that lithium is effective in reducing voluntary consumption of morphine and alcohol solutions in laboratory rats; the reductions are marked, consistent and, in the case of alcohol, occur not only in animals with established preferences for alcohol solutions but also in animals which are being exposed to alcohol for the first time: this seems to represent a new finding. In the context of our results and of the literature to which we have referred, the possible role of lithium in the prevention and treatment of drug dependence would appear to merit serious attention.

ACKNOWLEDGEMENTS

We thank Professor J. W. Black and Drs P. E. Harrison-Read and D. H. Jenkinson and Mr Michael Tomkiewicz for discussion, Miss Jane Allsop for experimental and Mr A. Davis for statistical help, and the Medical Council on Alcoholism, the Foundations Fund for Research in Psychiatry and the Medical Research Council for financial support.

References

1. Mendels, J. and Secunda, S.K. (eds.) (1972). *Lithium in Medicine* (London: Gordon and Breach)
2. Gershon, S. and Shopsin, B. (eds.) (1973). *Lithium : Its Role in Psychiatric Research and Treatment* (New York : Plenum Press)
3. Johnson, F.N. (ed.) (1975). *Lithium Research and Therapy* (London: Academic Press)
4. Davies, C., Sanger, D.J., Steinberg, H., Tomkiewicz, M. and U'Prichard, D.C. (1974). *Psychopharmacologia,* **36**, 263
5. Tomkiewicz, M. and Steinberg, H. (1974). *Nature,* **252**, 227
6. McMillan, T. and Steinberg, H. (Submitted for publication)
7. Altamura, A.C. (1975). *Acta Psychiat Scand.,* **52**, 312
8. Jasinski, D.R., Nutt, J.G., Haertzen, C.A., Griffith, J.D. and Bunney, W.E. (1977). *Science,* **195**, 582
9. Merry, J., Reynolds, C.M., Bailey, J. and Coppen, A. (1976). *Lancet,* **ii**, 481
10. Kline, N.S., Wren, J.C., Cooper, T.B., Varga, E. and Canal, O. (1974). *Am. J. Med. Sci.,* **268**, 15
11. Sellers, E.M., Cooper, S.D., Zilm, D.H. and Shanks, C. (1976). *Clin Pharmacol. Ther.,* **20**, 199
12. Schou, M. (1968). *J. Psychiat. Res.,* **6**, 67
13. Flemenbaum, A. (1974). *Dis.Nerv. Syst.* **35**, 281
14. Bunney Jr, W.E., Goodwin, D.K. and Murphy, D.L. (1972). *Arch.Gen. Psychiat.,* **27**, 312
15. Blum, K., Hamilton, M.G. and Wallace, J.E. (1976). In: K. Blum (ed.) *Alcohol and Opiates: Neurochemical and Behavioral Mechanisms,* pp 203-236 (New York: Academic Press)
16. Blum, K., Futterman, S., Wallace, J.E. and Schwertner, H.A. (1977). *Nature* **265**, 49
17. Goldstein, A. and Judson, B.A. (1971). *Science,* **172**, 290
18. Sinclair, J.D. (1974). *Pharmacol. Biochem. Behav.,* **2**, 409
19. Sinclair, J.S., Adkins, J. and Walker, S. (1973). *Nature* **246**, 254
20. Lester, D. and Freed, E.X. (1973). *Parmacol. Biochem. Behav.,* **1**, 103
21. Meisch, R.A. (1977). In: T. Thompson and P.B. Dews (eds.) *Advances in Behavioral Pharmacology* Vol 1 pp. 35-84 (New York: Academic Press)
22. Sinclair, J.D. (1974). *Med. Biol.,* **52**, 133

23. Sinclair, J.D. (1975). In: J.D. Sinclair and K. Kiianma (eds). Satellite Symposium, 6th Int. Congr. Pharm. Vol. 1 pp. 119-142
24. Ho, A.K.S. and Tsai, C.S. (1975). *J. Pharm. Pharmacol.,* **27,** 58
25. McCaughran, J.A. and Corcoran, M.E. (1977). *J. Pharm. Pharmacol.,* **29,** 120
26. Wise, R.A. (1973). *Psychopharmacologia,* **29,** 203
27. Amitz, Z., Stern, M.H. and Wise, R.A. (1970). *Psychopharmacologia,* **17,** 367
28. Kumar, R., Steinberg, H. and Stolerman, I.P. (1968). *Nature* **218,** 564
29. Harrison-Read, P.E. and Steinberg, H. (1971). *Nature New Biol.,* **232,** 120

7

The Antiaggressive Effects of Lithium

E. P. WORRALL

INTRODUCTION

In animals lithium has been shown to affect a variety of aggressive behaviours, reducing isolation-induced aggression in mice (1), foot shock elicited aggression in rats (1) and territorial aggressive behaviour in Siamese fighting fish (2) and rats (3). These are specific effects and are not associated with a general depression of motor behaviour.

A large number of reports have claimed that lithium has an antiaggressive effect in man in patients not suffering from manic-depressive psychosis. These claims have covered a wide variety of patients in a variety of clinical settings but include a single blind (4) and a double-blind (5) study on non-psychotic imprisoned violent offenders; an open study on a group of aggressive prisoners half of whom were diagnosed as suffering from schizophrenia and the other half described as sociopathic (6); a single case study in a female aggressive psychopath (7); a single-blind study on a mixed group of hospital inpatients all of whom were described as hyperaggressive and some of whom were epileptic (the formal diagnosis in this group included schizophrenia and a personality disorder but none were diagnosed as manic-depressive) (8); another single case report of a female aggressive psychopath described as having 'severe sadistic and masochistic traits and violently self-destructive' (9); a double-blind study of the effects on aggression in patients suffering from Huntington's chorea (10); an open study on aggressive adolescent mental defectives (11); a single case study of self-directed aggression in a self-mutilating mental defective (12); and finally a double-blind study on aggressive non-manic-depressive severely subnormal females (13).

There are a number of problems in proving that lithium has a general antiaggressive effect in man. Firstly, the aggressive behaviour in question has to be adequately defined and measured Secondly, there must be reasonable proof that the patients studied are not manic-depressive. Thirdly, it must be shown that any antiaggressive effect is not just part of a toxic effect. Lastly, and ideally, subjects should not receive other psychotropic drugs when the antiaggressive effects are being studied.

DEFINING AND MEASURING AGGRESSION

In animal work there are clear and specific models for measuring behaviour which is regarded as aggressive. In man the term is used much more widely to embrace a variety of behaviour including deliberate physical assault on others (and possibly on self) and verbal or motor behaviour which carries the threat of such assault. As pointed out by Marini and Sheard (14) in psychiatric practice the term is sometimes used in a wider and looser sense to include also behaviour which is simply assertive and striving. The studies quoted earlier however have only included patients showing aggressive behaviour in the more restricted sense of physical violence or the implied threat of such violence. Such aggressive behaviour in man, when it is neither the result of underlying psychotic illness or a direct component of a psychomotor seizure, may or may not be regarded as abnormal and is related to both fixed characteristics in an individual and to chance external events. The animal models of aggression have not so far been particularly useful in providing a vocabulary and a frame of reference for further defining the factors which determine aggressive behaviour in man. The internal fixed individual characteristics certainly exist but are poorly understood. They include such things as long-term effects of early learning and rather loose syndromes such as the American concept of episodic discontrol (15). The chance external factors are legion but include the behaviour of the victim, pharmacological effects on both the aggressive individual and his victim — particularly effects of alcohol (16) and even the weather (for example, American Negro mob violence being particularly prevalent in hot summer weather). Since the internal factors can often only be inferred from past behaviour and since the external factors are often chance events there is a quite different strategy required in looking at the effects of lithium on this behaviour and inherent difficulties which are not found in looking at the effects of lithium on psychotic illness. Assumptions can be made when assessing the effects of lithium in manic-depression which cannot be made when looking at the antiaggressive effects. In particular, in psychotic patients, the clinician at an interview can reliably judge the presence or absence of illness and using appropriate rating scales can assess its severity, whereas in assessing aggressive behaviour there may be no abnormalities at interview and the investigator may have to rely entirely on reports by others. The subject himself is likely to be an unreliable witness to actual events and rating scales of subjective feelings of anger, hostility and aggression may bear little relation to actual behaviour. Consequently, nearly all studies have been conducted on either imprisoned offenders or hospital inpatients with ratings of behaviour made by prison officers or nursing staff. Furthermore, the difficulties in obtaining subjects who are sufficiently frequently aggressive to allow for any significant effects of lithium to be demonstrated account for the relatively small numbers of patients in many of the studies. Consequently because of the eccentric nature of most of the patients, and the setting in which their aggression was measured, the aggressive behaviour shown by these subjects may not have a great deal of clinical significance for the mass of aggressive behaviour shown in the community at large. An adequate outpatient study demonstrating the clinical efficacy of lithium as an antiaggressive agent has yet to be done.

As well as measuring the occurrence of aggressive episodes, the degree of aggression also requires to be estimated. Clearly there is a difference between a threatening posture, or even a barrage of verbal abuse, and an actual physical assault.

THE PROBLEM OF DIAGNOSIS

There must be reasonable proof that the patients studied are not manic-depressives in whom the diagnosis has been missed. In practice this is not difficult. However the notion that lithium is a specific treatment for manic-depression has led some critics to suspect the antiaggressive work. It is true that, since the advent of lithium, diagnostic practice in some centres has changed and psychotic patients who would once have been diagnosed for example as excited schizophrenics are now diagnosed as suffering from mania and given lithium (17). However, this practice is likely to be more prevalent in the United States than it is in Britain, and in Scotland in particular, where the label of manic-depression has always been given very readily to any psychotic patient where there was a suspicion of a persistent mood disturbance or even to patients who would be regarded as neurotic elsewhere. Lithium, however, is not a panacea even in classical manic-depression and it would seem unwise to include response to lithium as a defining characteristic of manic-depressive illness.

SPECIFIC EFFECT OR TOXICITY

It must be shown that any antiaggressive effect of lithium is not just part of a generalised toxic reaction. Toxicity could occur either if the serum lithium levels were well above the "normal" range or if non-manic-depressives tolerated lithium particularly badly. In the absence of brain damage there is no good clinical evidence to support the latter possibility. Brain-damaged patients, however, do seem to be unusually likely to develop neurotoxicity at lithium levels within the therapeutic range and lithium has been shown to increase intellectual impairment in Huntington's chorea (18). Work done on brain-damaged patients, therefore, even in the absence of overt signs of toxicity may be under suspicion. Such patients, apart from Huntington's chorea patients themselves, would include many of the mental defectives (11,12,13), the epileptics of Morrison *et al.* (8) and some of the aggressive prisoners studied by Tupin *et al.* In this last study one of the features of their lithium responsive group was "a strong suggestion of brain damage" (6). Indeed, the well-known association between abnormal EEGs and aggressive psychopathy must put under suspicion many of the frequently aggressive prison inmates who have been studied.

INTERACTION WITH OTHER DRUGS

Ideally, an unequivocal antiaggressive effect of lithium should be demonstrated when patients are not receiving other psychotropic drugs. This is an impossible requirement if epileptics are used as the subjects and in the sort of inpatients who are studied it is also a difficult requirement. Nevertheless, the importance of this has been highlighted by at least one trial which claimed that the antiaggressive effects of lithium only occurred when the drug was used in combination with haloperidol (10). Although the figure provided in this report charting aggressive behaviour of one of these patients did suggest that one patient at least had less "angry outbursts" when on lithium alone compared to placebo.

THE WORK OF SHEARD

The work done by Sheard and colleagues comes nearest to meeting and overcoming these four problems. They have investigated the effect of lithium on non-psychotic violent prisoners (4,5,14,19). In their latest work (5), a double-blind study, they demonstrated a clear advantage of lithium over placebo in reducing aggressive behaviour. Aggression was assessed from the routine reports of the prison staff who recorded aggressive behaviour sufficient to warrant official action such as loss of privileges and isolation. The study design therefore allowed for measurement of presence or absence of aggressive acts regarded as serious by the prison staff but otherwise not of any gradation or degree of aggression. Their patients were not regarded by them as suffering from other than personality disorder and did not receive any other psychotropic medication during the time of the study. The mean serum lithium levels which they recorded were well within the therapeutic range even allowing for the fact that they were 24-hour lithium levels in young, physically healthy subjects. There was no clinical evidence of toxicity during the study and in a variety of psychometric tests measuring speed and power in motor skills and cognitive tasks they claimed that lithium produced no impairment. Furthermore, as in the study by Tupin *et al.* (6) there was no significant improvement in other antisocial behaviour in these prisoners to parallel the improvement in aggression. All these findings suggested that the antiaggressive effect was specific and not a sign of generalised sub-clinical neurotoxicity.

ANTIAGGRESSIVE EFFECT IN MENTAL DEFECTIVES

I will now discuss a study conducted by Worrall, Moody and Naylor in Strathmartin Hospital, Dundee, in the context of the four problems mentioned above. Our subjects were eight severely mentally retarded inpatients in one ward in a mental deficiency hospital. The study was designed to be double blind, seven patients were studied over 16 weeks and one patient was studied over 8 weeks. The subjects received lithium or placebo alternately for intervals of 4 weeks during the investigation period. The patients were chosen for the trial as all had shown frequent aggressive behaviour over many years despite receiving a variety of other psychotropic drugs and all presented a nursing problem. Seven of these patients were known regularly to assault other patients or nursing staff, the eighth patient severely scratched her own face or damaged ward furnishings when frustrated. Some of the external stimuli determining the aggression in some of these patients was known and included; for example, retaliatory aggression on receiving threats from other patients and being in close proximity to other patients or nursing staff in a confined space: aggressive behaviour in subjects of normal intelligence has a relationship with body buffer zones and it is known that aggressive offenders have larger body buffer zones than normal (20). In one of the patients, however, the aggression was completely unpredictable and she would attack other patients without any obvious provocation and the nursing staff regarded her as being sadistic. Because the aggressive behaviour in these patients consisted of brief, discrete episodes without any regular periodicity an attempt was made to record as accurately as possible nearly every aggressive event. All nursing staff in contact with the patients recorded their aggressive behaviour on a simple 7 point scale over three periods of time during waking hours, namely 8.00 to 12.00, 12.00 to 17.00 and 17.00 to 21.00. Prior to the start of the trial this rating scale had been shown to have high inter-rater reliability. As well as measuring the occurrence of an aggressive episode the rating scale also allowed for a simple measure of the degree of aggression shown to be made. Each patient therefore ended up with three aggression scores per day for the length of the trial. The design of this study was such that it was in effect 8 single case studies in patients sharing the same environment.

In regard to the problem of missing a diagnosis of manic-depression there were a number of factors which seemed to make this unlikely. Both of the clinicians involved in the trial had as their main interest manic-depressive illness; the diagnostic practice in the hospital was to diagnose functional psychosis in behaviourally disturbed mental defectives whenever this seemed likely. In particular the investigators were acquainted with the work of Reid (21) who had, from work done by him in the hospital, described criteria for diagnosing manic-depression in defectives and indeed a trial of the effects of lithium on mental defectives with manic-depression as defined by these criteria had been separately carried out in the hospital (22). Only one of the patients in the antiaggressive study was known to have a family history of manic-depressive illness and she was not only non-responsive to the lithium but became more aggressive whilst on the active drug. For these reasons I do not think the patients in this study could be reasonably regarded as suffering from a typical manic-depressive illness.

There was a problem about ruling out the effects of generalised toxicity in our patients. Although the mean plasma lithium levels for six of the patients were well within the therapeutic range the two other patients whose mean plasma lithium levels were at the upper end of the therapeutic range did develop unequivocal evidence of serious neurotoxicity and had to be withdrawn from the trial. Although none of the other patients showed any clinical evidence of neurotoxicity this was a brain-damaged group and the problem of sub-clinical toxicity shown only as an antiaggressive effect remains a possibility.

In assessing the effect of lithium in our patients we ignored the aggression scores for the first week of each lithium and placebo period — regarding these as build-up and wash-out phases respectively. Looking at the remaining scores, three of our patients were less aggressive whilst on lithium, one was more aggressive and the other three were unchanged. In each individual patient comparing the aggression score on placebo to the equivalent period on lithium by means of a Wilcoxon Matched-pairs-ranks test two of the responders were significantly less aggressive $p < 0.001$, the scores for the third apparent responder did not reach significance. The patient who was more aggressive had scores which were significant at $p < 0.001$ (Table 7.1).

Table 7.1. Lithium effects on aggression

Age	Mental deficiency diagnosis	Mean plasma lithium-level mmol/l	Effect on aggression	Significance
42	Phenylketonuria	0.76	Greatly deceased	$p < 0.001$
33	Idiopathic MD	0.77	Greatly decreased	$p < 0.001$
39	Post-encephalitic brain damage	0.87	Decreased	N.S.
35	Phenylketonuria	0.93	Increased	$p < 0.001$
44	Idiopathic MD	0.74	Unchanged	
54	Idiopathic MD	0.87	Unchanged	
57	Epiloia	1.38	Neurotoxicity. Withdrawn from trial	
51	Down's syndrome	1.16	Neurotoxicity. Withdrawn from trial	

The problem of potentiation of lithium by other drugs was not resolved by our trial as psychotropic medication being prescribed for our patients before the trial was continued unchanged throughout the trial.

Figure 7.1 illustrates the response of one patient who improved on lithium and shows the mean weekly aggression scores over the 16 weeks of the trial. Our two patients who unequivocally responded to lithium, in common with some of the other reports, did so by the end of the first or beginning of the second week of medication (6,8,7,12).

Again in common with our trial two of the other reports (although they did not make any comments in detail) did state that some of their patients became more aggressive whilst on lithium (6,7). The variability in response to the antiaggressive effects of lithium does suggest that there are underlying patient characteristics which determine the antiaggressive

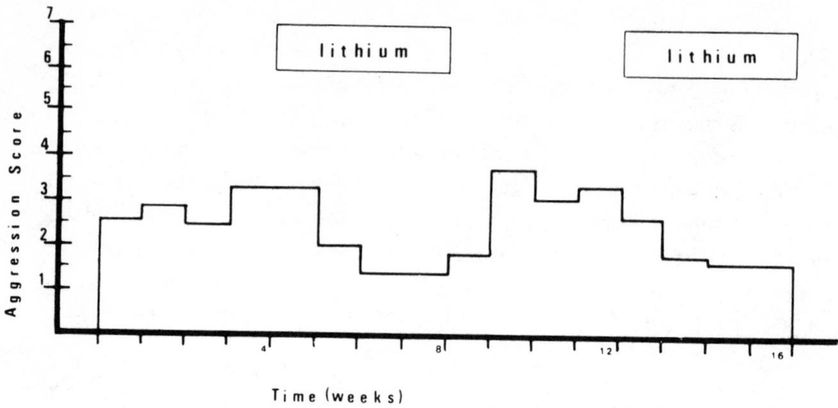

Figure 7.1 Effect of lithium treatment on aggression scores in a single patient over a 16-week period

response. What these characteristics are is not clear.

Some investigators have suggested that it is primarily the affect of anger which is reduced by the lithium and they have commented on the fact that their patients became more "reflective" and did not immediately respond with aggression in situations which previously provoked them (6,7). Our patients were too retarded to allow us to make any comparable inferences. I have myself however been impressed by this feature in one patient. This was a woman of normal intelligence who presented the problem of frequent self-mutilation; she had the typical features of this syndrome as described by Simpson (23). Before embarking on possibly useless long-term treatment with lithium I tried to assess the effects of lithium against placebo on her self-directed aggression over a 10 week period on a double blind basis. During the second week of lithium administration, when talking about her feelings of cutting herself she said quite spontaneously "Before, it was all impulse; now I feel like it but you seem to be able to think about it and control it. Before I would just have done it".

References

1. Sheard, M.H. (1970). *Nature (London),* **228**, 284
2. Weischer, M-L. (1969). *Psychopharmacologia,* **15**, 245
3. Sheard, M.H. (1973). *Agressologie,* **14**, 323
4. Sheard, M.H. (1971). *Nature (London),***230,** 113
5. Sheard, M.H. Marini, J.L., Bridges, C.I. and Wagner, E. (1976). Am. *J. Psychiat.,* **133,** 1409
6. Tupin, J.P., Smith, D.B., Clanon, T.L., Kim, L.I., Nugent, A. and Groupe, A. (1973). *Comprehens. Psychiat.* **14,** 311
7. Shader, R.I., Jackson, A.H. and Dodes, L.M. (1974). *Psychopharmacologia,* **40,** 17

8. Morrison, D.D., Erwin, C.W., Gianturco, D.T. and Gerber, C.J. (1973). *Dis. Nen. Sys.,* **34,** 186
9. Baastrup, P.C. (1969). *Acta Psychiat. Scand.,* Suppl. **207,** 12
10. Leonard, B.E. (1974). *Lancet,* **ii,** 1208
11. Dostal, T. (1971). In: *Proceedings of the 4th U.E.P. Congress,* Stockholm, pp491-498. (Stockholm: Almqvist and Wiksell)
12. Cooper, A.F. and Fowlie, H.C. (1973). *Br. J. Psychiat.,* **122,** 370
13. Worrall, E.P., Moody, J.P. and Naylor, G.J. (1975). *Br. J. Psychiat.,* **126,** 464
14. Marini, J.L. and Sheard, M.H. (1977). Acta Psychiat, Scand., **55,** 269
15. Monroe, R.R. (1970). *Episodic Behaviour Diorders.* (Cambridge Massachusetts: Havard University Press)
16. Gillies, H. (1976). *Br. J. Psychiat.,* **128,** 105
17. Taylor, M.A. and Abrams, R. (1973). *Arch. Gen. Psychiat.,* **29,** 520
18. Aminoff, M.J. (1975). *Lancet,* **i,**107
19. Sheard, M.H. (1975). *J. Nerv. Ment. Dis.,* **160,** 108
20. Kinzel, F.A. (1970). *Am. J. Psychiat.,* **127,** 59
21. Reid, A.H. (1972). *Br. J. Psychiat.,* **120,** 205
22. Naylor, G.J., Donald, J.M., Le Poidevin, D. and Reid, A.H. (1974). *Br. J. Psychiat.,* **124,** 52
23. Simpson, M.A. (1976) *Br. J. Hosp. Med.,* **16,** 430

8

The Efficacy of Lithium in the Treatment of Emotional Disturbance in Children and Adolescents

B. LENA, S. J. SURTEES and R. MAGGS

INTRODUCTION

Lithium is well established in the treatment of manic depressive illness in adults. However, its usefulness in the treatment of psychiatric disturbance in children and adolescents is not clear.

Van Krevelen and Van Voorst (1) reported favourable results with lithium in treating a 14-year-old boy who suffered from a 'periodic psychosis with longer manic and shorter depressive phases'. In 1969 Annell published her results after using lithium in the treatment of 'periodic psychosis'. In one report (2) of a total sample of 12, aged from 10 to 18, only two showed typical mania. The others had periods of mental disorders of other kinds which, according to her, came on suddenly and disappeared suddenly. Eleven out of twelve responded favourably to the drug, and she made an attempt to maintain serum lithium levels in the recommended therapeutic range for adults. Eight of the sample were 15 and over. She also (3) reported on eight cases, all first admitted for psychiatric treatment, under the age of 10 years and who all showed a favourable response to lithium. There was no typical manic depressive illness occurring in this sample. Although Annell gives case histories of the children treated, her investigations were uncontrolled.

Frommer (4) reported good results with 'hypomanic' children. The doses used were relatively small ranging from 100 mg to 250 mg. No mention is made of any attempt to regulate the dose to attain the recommended serum levels. Forsmann and Walinder (5) reporting on their results of using lithium on 'atypical indications' refer to a 15-year-old girl who had previously been treated for anorexia nervosa, who showed a favourable response to lithium. Dyson and Barcai (6) in a non-blind cross-over study, treated two children of parents who were lithium responders. These children aged 8 and 11, showed the following symptoms: over-activity, explosive anger, followed by guilt; distractability and short-attention span which improved while the children were treated with lithium Whitehead and Clark (7) treated seven hyperactive children whose ages ranged from 5 to 9, with either lithium, placebo or thioridazine at any one period, and comparisons were made. Lithium was found to be no better than placebo. Thioridazine reduced the activity in all cases; the difference, however, was not 'marked'. They do not refer to any attempts to correlate the dose of lithium to its recommended therapeutic range in the serum. Dostal and Zvolsky (8) treated 14 severely retarded, aggressive male adolescents whose ages ranged from 11 years to 17 years who had been previously resistant to phenothiazines. Serum lithium levels ranged from 0.30 to 0.95 mmol/l. A significant 'affect damping' and 'antiaggressive effect' was observed but treatment was complicated by excessive polydipsia and polyuria. Campbell *et al.* (9) in a controlled cross-over investigation used lithium and chlorpromazine in 10 'hyperactive severely disturbed' children of 3-6 years of age. No significant changes were noted except in the case of a 6-year-old boy who indulged in self-mutilating behaviour. Serum lithium levels ranged from 0.25 to 1.19 mmol/l. Gram and Rafaelsen (10) in a double-blind cross-over trial using a total sample of 18 children found significant improvement, particularly at school, with lithium treatment. These children were psychotic with mixed diagnoses. Greenhill *et al.* (11) in a double-blind cross-over investigation used lithium, dextroamphetamine and placebo on nine severely hyperactive children, who previously had not responded to drug psychotherapy. The ages ranged from 9 to 14 and serum lithium levels were maintained in the range of 0.8-1.2 mmol/l. Only two chidren improved and these differed from the seven who did not, in that they showed affective symptoms.

Berg (12) described a 14-year-old girl suffering from bipolar manic depressive psychosis who was treated with a relatively large dose of lithium 2.4 g daily (serum lithium level: 1 mmol/l). Her hypomania however did not respond to lithium treatment. Lena and O'Brien (13) reported the case of a 9-year-old-boy who responded well on lithium after other forms of treatment were found to be ineffective.

It is probable that manic depressive illness as it occurs in adults is rare in children (14). It has, however, been suggested that manic depressive illness could occur in children in atypical forms and may not often be diagnosed (2).

The following investigation was designed to investigate whether lithium is better than placebo in producing a significant improvement in children and adolescents suffering from episodic mood and behaviour disturbance.

METHOD

A double-blind cross-over trial has been set up, each patient being on lithium or placebo for a period of 8 weeks; the total duration therefore being 16 weeks. Children and adolescents between the ages of 8 and 16 are included. Those with any renal or thyroid dysfunction or any other organic disease are not included in the trial. Some subjects are randomly allocated to commence on lithium then crossing over to placebo, whilst the others are initially on placebo, subsequently crossing over to lithium. Lithium is administered in tablets of 400 mg strength in a sustained release preparation, the dose being adjusted to achieve a serum lithium level of 0.7 to 1.2 mmol/l. This is always carried out by the same member of the team (SJS). The side effects of lithium are explained to the parents and they are given specific instructions to contact one member of the team (RM) if the child shows any of the serious side effects or toxic symptoms. The parents have access to this member of the team both at his hospital and at his home.

Thyroid function is monitored monthly and renal function at fortnightly to monthly intervals. Any of the children or adolescents showing impairment of either thyroid or renal function or any significant toxic symptoms are taken out of the trial.

The child and parents are assessed by the member of the team who remains blind (BL), at weekly intervals during the four months' period. Information is being collected fortnightly to monthly during this period from the teachers with the help of questionnaires.

Biochemical investigations are carried out as shown in Table 8.1.

RESULTS

The total number of children and adolescents participating is eleven. Their ages range from 9 years to 15 years. We have now completed our findings on five of these. Although a severe degree of emotional disturbance exists in all the children and most of their families, none of the children has dropped out so far for any reason in spite of the heavy

Table 8.1. Biochemical investigations

Week:	*0	1	2	4	6	8	9	10	12	14	16
Serum lithium	✓	✓	✓	✓	✓	✓	✓	✓	✓	✓	✓
Urea/electrolytes	✓			✓		✓			✓		✓
Serum creatinine	✓			✓		✓			✓		✓
T4/T3 uptake	✓			✓		✓			✓		✓
Latex LE	✓										✓
MSU	✓		✓	✓	✓	✓		✓	✓	✓	✓
Hb. WBC. DC	✓										✓

(*Week 0 = initial 2-4 week period for gathering baseline data).

commitment involved in hospital attendance. The children appear to be tolerating lithium reasonably well.

Two of the five, a boy aged 12 and a girl aged 14, have shown marked improvement while on lithium. Two other boys, aged 10 and 14, showed moderate improvement during the period on lithium. The other boy aged 9, although showing moderate improvement throughout the survey, was, according to the parents, better behaved while on placebo. In the case of the 14-year-old girl who showed marked improvement and the 10-year-old boy who showed moderate improvement while on lithium, progress at home was also associated with progress at school. Within a few days to weeks after the completion of the survey there has been a relapse in the case of the 14-year-old girl and of the 12-year-old boy who had shown marked improvement while on lithium.

Throughout the survey, thyroid function of these five patients remained unimpaired. Renal function too was not affected excepting in the case of the 14-year-old girl who on occasions had proteinuria.

The investigation is still proceeding and the significance of these early results requires further analysis.

ACKNOWLEDGEMENT

BL is grateful to Dr P. Barker for his encouragement, and the West Midland Regional Health Authority for their support in the preliminary work which preceeded this survey. We are grateful to Dr K.R.D. Porter for his encouragement, the South-East Thames Regional Health Authority for their sponsorship, the Delandale Laboratories for their assistance and to Mr M. Bastable and the Staff of the Pathology Department for their cooperation.

References

1. Krevelen, D.A. Van and Voorst, J.A. Van. (1959). *Acta Paedo-psychiat.,* **26**, 148
2. Annell, A-L. (1969). *Acta Psychiat. Scand.* Suppl. **207**, 19
3. Annell, A-L. (1969). *Acta Paedo-psychiat.,* **36**, 292
4. Frommer, E.A. (1968). In: A. Coppen and A. Walk (eds.) *Recent Developments in Affective Disorders.*
5. Forrsman, M. and Walinder, J. (1969). *Acta Psychiat. Scand.* Supple. **207**, 34
6. Dyson, W.L. and Barcai, A. (1970). *Curr. Ther. Res.* **12**, 286
7. Whitehead, P.L. and Clark, L.D. (1970). *Am. J. Psychiat.,* **127**, 824
8. Dostal, T. and Zvolsky, P. (1970). *Int. Pharmacopsychiatry,* **5**, 203
9. Campbell, M., Fish, B., Korein, J., Shapiro, T., Collins, P. and Kohn, C. (1972). *J. Autism Child. Schiz* **2**, 234
10. Gram, L.F. and Rafaelsen, O.J. (1972). *Acta Psychiat. Scand.,* **48**, 253
11. Greenhill, L.L., Rieder, R.O., Wender, P.H., Buchsbaum, M. and Zahn, T.P. (1973). *Arch. Gen. Psychiat.,* **28**, 636
12. Berg, A. (1974). *Br. J. Psychiat.,* **125**, 416
13. Lena, B. and O'Brien, E.M.D. (19/5). *Lancet,* ii, 1307
14. Scott, P. and Anthony, E.J. (1960). *J. Child. Psychol. Psychiat.,* **1**, 53

Part III:
Metabolic Effects

Introduction

The most infuriating question which can be (and frequently is) asked of those who employ lithium in treatment or who carry out research into its effects, is 'How does lithium really work?' When this question meets with a blank look followed, after a quick intake of breath, with a vague and evasive reply, a second question rapidly follows: 'Well, what exactly does lithium *do* in the body?' The answer to this second question is easy: one simply takes — quite at random — any biochemical system and claims that lithium has an effect on that. And the chances are that one will be right.

In Chapter 9 Dr Birch presents an impressive review of the metabolic effects which lithium is known to have, a review which, as he says, will provide a ready entrée into the literature for anyone new to the area. Dr Shaw, in Chapter 10 takes us through some recent thoughts on the relationship between tryptophan metabolism and the aetiology of mood disorders. There is no doubt that work of this kind has the strongest implications for our understanding of those biochemical effects of lithium which lie behind its therapeutic actions, and in the following chapter Dr Collard explores the relationship between 5-hydroxytryptamine metabolism and lithium: the relationship between tryptophan and 5-hydroxytryptamine metabolism is, of course, very close.

Dr Lazarus (Chapter 12) reports on human and animal studies which examine the effects of lithium on carbohydrate metabolism, a theme continued in Chapter 13 by Dr Plenge and in Chapter 14 by Dr Vendsborg.

The importance of cAMP and its associated biochemicals in the control of a wide variety of metabolic systems is only now being fully recognized; the report by Dr Geisler and his associates on the interaction between lithium and adenylate cyclase is therefore particularly interesting (Chapter 15).

It might be expected that amongst its many metabolic effects, lithium would influence membrane transport processes, particularly since the related alkali metals, sodium and potassium, are known to be involved at this level. Dr Martin, in Chapter 16, deals with the question of choline uptake by erythocytes and platelets. In Chapter 17 Professor Dick and his colleagues examine sodium transport across membranes, and Dr Glen, in the following chapter, presents an account of the exciting work being done in his unit in relation to lithium effects on membrane ATPases.

Whilst lithium has clear affinities with the other alkali metals, it has additional similarities to the alkaline earth metals, calcium and magnesium. Dr Christiansen and his associates deal with this issue in Chapter 19 and the topic is also the subject of Chapter 20 written by Dr Srinivasan and associates. Dr Hariharasubramanian returns, in Chapter 21, to the alkali metal actions of lithium.

Whatever the final picture may be of the biochemical effects of lithium, the information recorded in these chapters will surely figure largely in it. We may be sure that there are surprises in store for us in this area of lithium research, but at the moment the studies which are recorded here provide sound guidelines for the directions which future investigations may profitably take.

9

Metabolic Effects of Lithium

N. J. BIRCH

INTRODUCTION

Scope and limitations

Since 1957, when Schou published a review of the whole field of lithium research (1), the rate of progress has accelerated to such an extent that this comprehensive approach is no longer possible and the attempt to define the boundaries of current knowledge has led to the publication of compilations of reviews of specific areas (2-4). One of the features of the biology and pharmacology of lithium is the breadth of the range of its effects. In this review, I have therefore concentrated on examples of very recent work in particular areas of metabolism at different levels of organization. My objectives have been to illustrate the range of processes and degrees of organization affected by lithium, to give an up to date survey of work within the purview of metabolism and to provide a ready entrée into the literature. I have been selective rather than comprehensive but have attempted to give points of entry into the major areas of current research activity.

A number of *caveats* must be borne in mind when considering the lithium literature. Much of the earlier work was done for toxicological purposes and the concentrations of lithium used (up to 150 mmol/l) do not bear any useful relationship to those observed in humans or animals during lithium treatment, nor even to terminal toxicity. The range of lithium concentration considered to be pharmacologically relevant (5) is less than 5 mmol/l in body fluids (usually around 1 mmol/l), and not more than 10 mmol/kg in tissues, though, with the exception of the renal tubule where higher local concentrations may occur, this level is reached only in impending toxicity and the usual range is 0.5-5.0 mmol/kg wet weight of tissue. Frequently, lithium has been used to replace sodium in physiological solutions in studies of membrane phenomena. As recently as 1976, reports (6,7) have appeared in highly respected journals of studies in which sodium was replaced by 148 mmol/l Li and 118.5 mmol/l Li and the results were discussed in terms of decreased extracellular sodium. The authors gave no evidence that they were aware that lithium has pharmacological effects at one hundredth of these concentrations or that other workers might have used the metal for purposes other than as 'ersatz sodium'. Conversely, since the efficacy of lithium has been recognized, experiments from many disciplines have been reported to have relevance to its mode of action with scant regard for the conditions under which it is used in patients.

One must distinguish between studies carried out in animals and those in man since it may not necessarily be legitimate to extrapolate from one to the other. Furthermore it is important to consider as two distinct entities the acute affects and those which occur only after long-term administration of lithium. Since different dosage schedules produce different circadian fluctuations in tissue concentrations it may not be possible to describe a true equilibrium state. However, in man, 'equilibrium' is often used to denote the steady state at which the 24 hour excretion of lithium is equal to its intake.

The reviews already cited (1-5) together with those on pharmacological (8) and biochemical (9) aspects and two colloquia (10,11) cover the majority of the literature until late 1975. Schou has published a comprehensive bibliography of lithium which is periodically updated (12-15).

METABOLISM IN THE WHOLE ANIMAL

Mode of administration of lithium and pharmacokinetic factors

It is often difficult to compare directly reports of lithium effects in animals because of differences in mode of administration. Much of the acute experimentation on animals has used classical pharmacological techniques of intraperitoneal or subcutaneous injection. However with a simple ion such as lithium this produces a very rapid peak in the plasma concentration which is quite unlike that occurring in the human patient using exclusively oral administration. It might be argued that some of the effects obtained are a result of brief periods of exposure to extremely high lithium concentrations in those tissues which have an extensive blood supply. After 28 days two groups of rats treated with lithium either by intraperitoneal injection or by administration of a similar dose in the drinking fluid had markedly different tissue concentrations of lithium (16).

Olesen (17) has investigated the plasma concentration curve in rats following different routes of lithium dosage and concludes that administration in the diet produced the most constant diurnal plasma lithium pattern. However, this study did not test the administration of lithium by drinking fluid. Schou (5) has said that this route is not practical since polyuria-polydipsia develops leading to increased fluid intake and ultimately toxicity. My own experience is at variance with this since both in metabolic cage studies (16,18) and recently, in extensive long-term studies, there has been no evidence of progressive toxicity and very little increase in water intake in rats receiving lithium chloride in the drinking fluid compared with their tap water treated controls (Table 9.1).

The fundamental difference is in definition of objectives. My experiments have attempted over periods of up to one year to reproduce the dose received and pattern of intake of human subjects during prophylaxis. I have therefore tried to give a dose of approximately 1 mmol/kg/day. The objective of many other groups is to maintain a plasma lithium concentration which is comparable to that found in humans during prophylaxis. However, the rat has a rather more efficient kidney than man and requires a higher dose to maintain that level; that dose now being toxic to the animal without additional sodium. Thomsen has shown in a series of elegant studies, firstly that it is possible to maintain rats at quite high plasma lithium concentrations provided sufficient supplementary sodium is given (19,20), that if given access to supplementary sodium chloride rats regulate their sodium intake according to the lithium dose administered (21), and recently that addition of supplementary potassium prevents lithium induced sodium loss (22). These studies are directed towards the understanding of lithium toxicity (23,24) and not the mode of action in the prophylaxis of recurrent affective disorders. The dilemma in animal experimentation is whether to try to mimic human dosage on a body weight basis or to mimic human plasma concentrations of the drug. Ultimately, one can never reproduce exactly the human situation since the tissue pharmacockinetics varies between species because relationships between the various 'metabolic compartments' are peculiar to each species.

The question of mode of administration of lithium is crucial. We are able to treat rats in the long term without producing polyuria. Polyuria is also not considered to be a problem amongst the 150 patients at our out-patient clinic. It is therefore always surprising to meet colleagues who consider polyuria to be expected as a side effect in much the same way that we expect hypothyroidism. We have recently carried out a profile study of our out-patients (25,26) and were impressed by the number of patients who were maintained without relapse on relatively low levels of lithium (plasma lithium of about 0.5 mmol/l). Perhaps we should consider polyuria to be a warning of potential toxicity and reconsider the question of optimal lithium levels for prophylaxis.

Table 9.1 Approximate fluid intake of groups of rats receiving either 10 mmol/l lithium chloride or tap water

Fluid intake (ml/animal/week)	Time at which the group of rats was killed (weeks after Li started) 5	13	26	52
Control	244(13)	262(12)	240(10)	243(13)
Lithium	241(17)	229(16)	215(13)	235(10)

Fluid intake was monitored by recording, on a chart for each cage of three or four animals, the dates on which the drinking fluid bottle (550 ml) was refilled. 100 female Wistar weanling rats commenced the study simultaneously. Ten animals were removed from each treatment group for tissue analysis at 5, 13 and 26 weeks. The numbers of animals for which the mean was calculated is given in brackets and varies because some rearrangement of cages occurred after each sampling

Weight changes following lithium

One of the areas of considerable interest to clinicians is the tendency for a number of patients receiving lithium prophylactically to gain weight, sometimes dramatically (27). Dempsey *et al.* (28) have reported recently the successful treatment of weight gain by individually designed, low calorie diets with particular emphasis on adequate sodium and potassium intake. The salt supplementation is essential to avoid intoxications such as that reported by Furlong (29).

The origin of the weight gain is obscure (28) though lithium is known to have effects on electrolyte and water metabolism (30), thyroid function (31), and lipid and carbohydrate metabolism (30), all of which may contribute. The weight gain has also been attributed to the improvement in affect and general health following stabilization (27).

Mellerup and Rafaelsen (32) describe the conditions under which weight gain is seen in lithium treated rats and humans and discuss in detail the various aspects of carbohydrate metabolism which contribute to this gain. They also stress that not all lithium treated patients show this gain. It may be that there is a sub-group of manic depressive subjects who are predisposed to weight gain under certain circumstances.

Various reports indicate that continued weight gain in growing rats is a sensitive indicator of lithium treatment since toxicity leads to a failure to grow (24,33,34). Opitz (34) has shown that an additional increase in body weight in some lithium treated rats is due to increased food intake which is reversed, and the gained weight lost, on discontinuation of lithium. Using intraperitoneal injection, he has shown that toxic doses of lithium immediately result in decreased food and water intake and hence loss of body weight. He notes that this effect is more pronounced in male than female rats. It may be that we should distinguish between failure of growth in immature rats and loss or gain of weight in mature animals.

What, therefore, is the relevance of rat studies to human weight gain? Plenge (33) has emphasised that in order to show weight gain during lithium administration to rats, it is necessary to keep them quiet and isolated from external disturbances. Environmental factors therefore play a part and in the human we should consider the relationships between food intake, activity and metabolic rate. Caloric intake is influenced by physiological hunger, psychological factors such as drive and motivation and by the type of food which is preferred, can be afforded and is physically accessible. Activity and metabolic expenditure are exceptionally difficult to measure in humans since most accurate measures of energy usage restrict the activity of the individual in some way. Since we are considering psychogenically induced changes, this would negate the purpose of the experiment. Johnson has recently reviewed the relevance of animal experimentation in investigating the behavioral effects of lithium (35) and perhaps some light may be thrown on the weight gain problem when we are able to recognize whether lithium at low concentration specifically stimulates hunger centres, inhibits satiety centres or merely resets the 'glucostat'.

Changes in water and electrolyte balance may also contribute to the weight gain in the redistribution of the major ions and changes in total electrolyte balance which have been described following lithium (16).

Carbohydrate metabolism

Mellerup, Plenge and Rafaelsen (36) have described an insulin-like action of lithium and drawn attention to earlier views of the relationship between manic-depressive psychoses and diabetes mellitus. In a series of studies in rats they have shown that lithium causes increases in glucose uptake and glycogen synthesis in muscle, brain and adipose tissue and causes weight gain. Changes in phosphate metabolism have also been observed and these and the changes in calcium and magnesium (37) are considered to be secondary to the carbohydrate changes. The *in vitro* studies of Haugaard *et al.* (38) confirm that lithium increases glucose utilization and glycogen synthesis in rat hemidiaphragms. Lithium has also been shown to affect, *in vitro*, a number of enzymes involved in carbohydrate metabolism (32).

Lazarus *et al.* (39) have recently reported acute studies of lithium on carbohydrate metabolism 3 h after moderately high doses of lithium were given to rats by intraperitoneal injection, (2-10 mmol/kg body weight: the units printed in the original paper are incorrect). Though they agree with the increase in muscle glycogen found by other workers (36,38) they found a decrease in liver glycogen which agrees with early acute studies of Plenge (40) but contrasts with an increase in liver glycogen found by Krulik and Zvolsky (41) in a 10 day treatment experiment. Lazarus *et al.* (39) were unable to establish a relationship between liver glycogen and plasma glucagon in actuely treated animals.

The glucose tolerance curve of patients receiving lithium has been studied by several groups and a pattern seems to emerge that it is abnormal in the initial stages of prophylaxis (42,43,44). Shopsin *et al.* (44) found a decreased tolerance while the others found an increase. Vendsborg and Prytz (45) have shown that after 6 months of lithium treatment the situation has reverted to a normal response. This is substantially in agreement with Gordon and van der Velde (46) who found no difference in glucose tolerance between lithium-treated and non-treated manic depressives though both had reduced tolerance, compared with normals, after being subjected to a 3 day fast. An earlier study by Mellerup *et al.* (47) showed lower serum insulin in drug-free manic depressives compared with both normal controls and lithium treated patients. There was no difference in serum insulin during lithium therapy between patients who had gained weight and those who had not.

Control of metabolism

Control of whole body metabolism occurs at the highest levels by the integrative action of the nervous and endocrine systems which regulate the metabolic relationships between the various tissues either quickly but briefly, in the case of nervous control, or with a slower but sustained response by the endocrines. This is largely a matter of cell economics since the energy requirements of the nervous control put a high price on speedy response. Individual cells, however, exert a large degree of autonomous control and this occurs in a hierarchy of subcellular organisation which uses maximum economy in energy expenditure. Hence enzymes which are used infrequently or with varying demand are synthesized as a response to substrate, the inducible enzymes. These enzymes are regulated by the genetic material since the genes responsible for their synthesis are usually under repression which is reversed when substrate becomes available. Thus there is characteristically a lag between presence of substrate and the arrival of enzyme. The regulatory enzyme whose concentration is more or less constant, is the next most autonomous level of control and this may be regulated by product or substrate inhibition and be activated by its own substrates. This enzyme is often to be found at branch points in metabolic pathways where it may be sensitive to two or more activators or inhibitors which act as switches. The most autonomous control in all enzymes is provided by the optimal conditions of the enzymes itself. Hence pH, concentrations of substrate, product and any required cofactor are the critical factors in the close chemical milieu of the enzyme.

I have surveyed this hierarchy because I think that it is essential to keep in mind continually the multiplicity of potential sites at which lithium might have its effects on metabolism. Research tends to have concentrated in a few well defined areas, on intelligent guesses of where the particularly vulnerable parts of processes might be and at points at which several control systems meet. This latter is responsible for the particularly large amount of work on adenyl cyclase and cyclic 3-5-adenosine monophosphate (48-50) whose ubiquity of action may be soon rivalled by the prostaglandins (51-54).

Much of the recent literature of lithium and metabolism is systems oriented. I intend, therefore, to move immediately to the subcellular aspects so that the systems may be later considered in the light of what has been said about their constituents.

METABOLISM AT SUBCELLULAR LEVELS

Introduction

The literature of effects of lithium on enzymes is vast. This has come about, not because of any desire of the experimentalists to elucidate the mode of action of lithium but because, to the biochemist, metal ions have been merely tools, differing sizes of socket spanner to be fitted to the various rachet devices and extension pieces to adjust the 'real' mechanism, the ^{12}C containing part of the process.

This failure of biochemists to realise the significance of metals is slowly being eroded with the recognition of the role of calcium in neurosecretory processes and in cell regulation (55). Most of the *in vitro* studies of lithium and enzymes have had as their main objective the elucidation of some part of the enzyme mechanism. Lithium was included, at high concentration, as part of a series of cations, usually Group I alkali metals, to test the effect of different sizes of cofactor or inhibitor. *In vivo* studies by contrast have often been directed at the understanding of lithium and by their nature have been forced to use lithium concentrations which are tolerated by the organism if only in the short term.

The most significant and comprehensive review of this area was written as recently as 1975 by Dr Susan Johnson (56). In this section I will concentrate on work published during the last two years and on enzymes which are at the critical points of metabolic pathways which might be expected to have controlling functions.

A valuable additional viewpoint has become apparent recently with the interest of inorganic chemists in biological processes (57,58). This interest was harnessed in a symposium organized by the Neurosciences Research Program in USA when physical and inorganic chemists met with neuroscientists and clinicians to discuss the neurobiology of lithium (4). R.J.P. Williams, in this country, has recently made contributions towards the theory of the mode of action (59,60). Though there is often a conceptual barrier to be overcome, it is important that these dialogues should be continued and that biochemists should also be persuaded to regard lithium as not just another piece of mobile charge, but as a drug which has marked effects at the same molar concentrations as those at which ATP appears *in vivo* in the cell, Perhaps it is rather an obvious point, but one which is not often emphasized, that the concentration of lithium in cells during prophylaxis (1-5 mmol/l) is of similar order to the concentrations of magnesium (5-10 mmol/l), sodium (5-10 mmol/l) and 10 000 times more than calcium (less than 10-4 mmol/l) (61).

Relationship of lithium to other ions

The review of Johnson (56) was written primarily from the point of view that lithium should be compared to the alkali metals (Group I in the periodic table). I have suggested that the chemistry, and hence biochemistry, of lithium might be better described in terms of the 'diagonal relationship' between elements in the first row of the periodic table and the second and subsequent row elements in the following group (18,62,63). In this way lithium might be considered to have actions resembling, or competing with, the Group II elements magnesium and calcium. Early studies confirmed that lithium did indeed have effects on magnesium and calcium distribution (16,18) and these were supported by other studies published almost simultaneously (64,65). Since then much effort has been directed towards the Li-Mg-Ca relationship and support for the concept has grown (59,66) though there is still much which is controversial.

From a theoretical chemical standpoint, Williams has demonstrated that lithium could readily displace calcium from sites on membranes (61). Since the concentration of lithium is so much more than calcium within the cell, lithium might displace some calcium even though its association constant is lower. Indeed since its bond lengths are potentially more variable than magnesium, it has fewer orbitals and is thus less restricted, it might displace bound magnesium. Eisenman (67) has suggested that the really unique property of lithium is its potential ability to interact with both monovalent and divalent dependent processes at the concentrations at which it is clinically effective. Eigen (68) has suggested that both calcium and magnesium are good candidates for interaction with lithium.

Magnesium dependent enzymes

A large number of biological processes are magnesium dependent (69,70), among them a very significant number of enzymes (71). If lithium were to have some effect on the function of key enzymes the overall metabolic significance might be enormous. Schou (9) has listed a number of reported effects of lithium.

One of the major pathways controlling energy availability in the organism is, of course, glycolysis. It is interesting to note that on this pathway of some 13 steps, no less than 8 are dependent on magnesium in some way. One can readily see that even a small increment or decrement in activity along the whole pathway might lead to drastic changes in total energy flow, particularly in an organ as uniquely sensitive as the brain. Similarly, a relatively small change in an enzyme at a critical point in the path could lead to imbalance of the switching between alternative pathways. With this in mind we set out to do some preliminary studies on readily available magnesium dependent enzymes.

The preliminary results were encouraging since of five enzymes investigated, three were found to be inhibited by moderate concentrations of lithium (72). Of those which were inhibited, pyruvate kinase and hexokinase had previously been reported to be affected by lithium (73,74) though at higher concentrations. Alkaline phosphates, also inhibited, had not been previously studied. Neither glucose-6-phosphate dehydrogenase nor 3-phospho-glycerate kinase was affected by lithium.

It appeared that perhaps we were seeing a competition between lithium and magnesium, not actually at the enzyme, but in the form of a complex with the substrate nucleotides adenosine diphosphate (ADP) and adenosine triphosphate (ATP). We carried out studies to determine the association constants for the complexes ATP-Mg, ATP-Li, ADP-Mg, ADP-Li using an elegant technique of Sephadex chromatography derived from the work of Colman (75). We concluded that though there was no direct competition between lithium and magnesium for the same sites on the nucleotide, there was evidence of a possible ternary complex of the type Li-Mg-ADP (76). We are currently attempting to confirm this by physical techniques.

It became clear that our finding of *in vitro* effects of lithium on pyruvate kinase was not necessarily applicable to the *in vivo* situation. Pscheidt and Meltzer (77) were unable to replicate our findings in the serum of lithium treated patients though it is likely that the variety of the enzyme present in human plasma is different from that in rabbit muscle, as in our experiments, since both L and M forms are known. However, support for the concept of a lithium effect on magnesium dependent enzymes has come from the work of Kadis (78.79) on L-alanine aminotransferase and from Essman (80) who has shown changes in 5-hydroxytryptamine content and turnover in the brains of lithium treated, magnesium deficient mice.

In vivo studies have also shown lithium effects on inducible enzymes of the liver (81) (glucokinase, tyrosine aminotransferase, tryptophan oxygenase), on induction of drug metabolising enzymes of the liver (82,83), on neural enzymes (84), (acid phosphatase, alkaline phosphatase, aryl sulphatase and cholinesterase) and on RNA synthesis in brain (85,86). Acetyl choline synthesis has been shown to be inhibited by lithium *in vitro* and *in vivo* (87) and the action of lithium on acetylcholinesterase has been studied *in vivo* (88). Vizi (87) has said that the impairment by lithium of acetyl choline synthesis might be attributed to effects on (1) the uptake of choline, (2) acetyl-coenzyme-A synthetase, (3) glucose-pyruvate transformations and that (2) and (3) are likely to be the most important. (One should, perhaps, note that all three processes are magnesium dependent). Abreu and Abreu have shown effects of lithium on aconitase (89) and succinate dehydrogenase (90) in brains of lithium treated mice.

In vitro studies of RNA synthesis in mammary gland explants (91) and in rat brain homogenates (86,92) have been reported. DNA polymerase is inhibited by high concentrations of lithium (93-95). Allosteric effects of lithium, amongst other ions, have been shown on rabbit liver fructose-1.6 -diphosphate (96). Agar *et al.* have shown an inhibition of red cell enolase by lithium (97).

Studies on ATPases have been inconclusive. Gupta and Crollini (98) were unable to show lithium effects on Na^+K^+ATPase, which is Mg^{++} dependent. However, lithium has been shown to stimulate (99,100) or inhibit (101) different ATPases and to alter the sub-cellular distribution of others (102). Choi and Taylor (103) were unable to show an effect on Ca^{++} ATPase in red cell fragments. The wide range of ATPase preparations used, their mode of preparation and species variation probably account for many of the differences and one must not draw mechanistic conclusions by interspecific extrapolation.

This very brief survey shows, therefore, that magnesium requiring enzymes are affected by lithium and that a very wide variety of such enzymes exists. Furthermore, the metabolic control aspects of these enzymes should be emphasised. The control varies from those enzymes which are purely autonomous, through those which are induced and extends to those which actually control the expression and replication of the genetic material. Lithium has been reported to cause surface changes in human lymphocyte chromosomes (104) and it is used in experimental embryology at high concentrations to cause developmental abnormalities in primitive chordates. An irreversible effect of lithium in human erythrocytes has recently been reported (105) in which the choline transport mechanism is inhibited by about 90%. This effect is species specific. It is conceivable that the lack of chromosomal material in the red cell might result in an effect which is 'normally' overcome by induction of synthetic enzymes for an alternative pathway.

We have recently extended our original studies to confirm the previous findings and to try to define the mode of inhibition of pyruvate kinase and hexokinase. We have not been able to confirm the inhibition of hexokinase which we found earlier (72) and which has also been reported by other workers (74,106) and furthermore we are unable to account for the discrepancy. Further studies are required. However, we have confirmed the findings with pyruvate kinase and have extended them to consider other aspects (107).

The interaction of lithium with all of the substrates of rabbit muscle pyruvate kinase, phospho enol pyruvate (PEP), adenosine diphosphate (ADP), Mg^{++} and K^+ was examined. The results indicate that lithium is competitive with respect to ADP binding to the enzyme and non-competitive with respect to all other substrates. Under the normal assay conditions (85 mmol/l Tris hydrochloride buffer pH 7.5, 0.5 mmol/l PEP, 10 mmol/l $MgCl_2$, 5 mmol/l ADP, 20 mmol/l KCl, 0.25 mmol/l NADH and excess lactate dehydrogenase) the inhibition due to 10 mmol/l lithium chloride was between 16 and 24%. This was less than previously reported

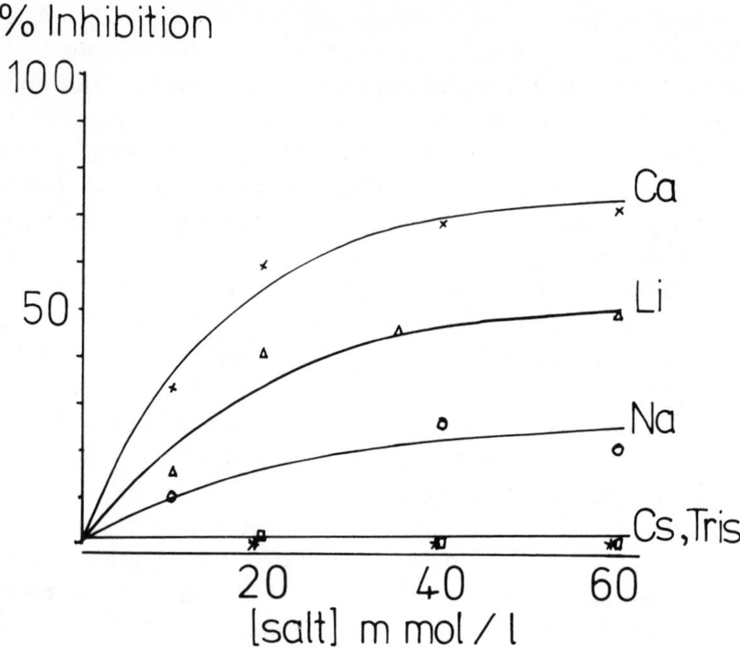

Figure 9.1 The effect of differing concentrations of ions on the inhibition of pyruvate kinase

(72). However, at concentrations of ADP of 1.0-1.5 mmol/l, i.e. at levels usually obtaining in the cell, the inhibition is markedly increased, up to an inhibition of twice that at 5 mmol/l ADP. We have specifically excluded the possibility that an ionic strength or general ion effect has occurred. In fact inhibition is limited to the ions calcium, lithium and sodium (Figure 9.1). Caesium and Tris were tested at concentrations up to 200 mmol/l.

Kinetic investigations showed that the calcium inhibition was of a similar type of lithium (Table 9.2) and that the inhibition for both was similar at both high (100 mmol/l) and low (20 mmol/l) concentrations of potassium.

We have shown inhibition due to lithium concentrations of from 5 mmol/l and above. The clinical significance of this is open to question though undoubtedly a small inhibition occurs below this concentration. However, this is one enzyme, chosen almost at random, in which inhibition does occur at concentrations not entirely beyond the pharmacological range. It is almost certain that other enzymes will be more sensitive than this. In a series such as glycolysis, an inhibition of 5% occurring in successive enzymes would produce a very large change in energy balance.

Table 9.2. Inhibition of pyruvate kinase. Effects of lithium and calcium on various substrates

	Inhibitor	
Substrate	Li^+	Ca^+
K^+	n.c.	n.c.
Mg^{++}	n.c.	
Phospho enol pyruvate	n.c.	n.c.
ADP (20 mmol/IK^+)	comp	comp
ADP (100 mmol/IK^+)	comp	comp

n.c. = non-competitive with respect to the substrate
comp = competitive with respect to the substrate

Adenyl cyclase and cyclic 3′5′ adenosine monophosphate (cyclic AMP)

The pivotal position of cyclic AMP and adenyl cyclase (adenylate cyclase) in current thinking of endocrinological and neurotransmitter action ensures that the effects of lithium on this system have been extensively studied. A recent comprehensive review is that of Forn (108). Both Eccleston and Somerville survey the early literature in a symposium previously cited (10).

Perhaps the two most seminal papers in the literature of lithium and cyclic AMP were those of Dousa and Hechter (109) and of Abdulla and Hamadah (110), the one on tissue actions of lithium on adenyl cyclase, the other on the excretion of cyclic AMP by periodic psychotic patients. These papers, both published in 1970, were marginally ahead of other investigators.

The role of adenyl cyclase and cyclic AMP as second messenger in the mechanism of action of hormones (111) has led to a variety of studies of lithium effects associated with various endocrinological effects. I will only provide signposts to some of the various groups who are particularly involved in this area. Geisler and his colleagues have investigated both clinical studies on CSF cyclic AMP (50) and studies on glucagon stimulated (112) and vasopressin stimulated (113) adenyl cyclase and plasma concentrations of cyclic AMP in lithium treated rats (114). Frazer *et al.* have reported an adrenaline stimulated cyclic AMP accumulation (115). Wang *et al.* (116) and Murphy *et al.* (52) reported effects of lithium on prostaglandin stimulated adenyl cyclase. Others have reported (117,118) on aspects of PTH stimulated adenyl cyclase. Ebstein and his colleagues have reported an inhibition by lithium of adrenaline stimulated cyclic AMP release in human subjects (119).

The results reported to date can be divided into two main categories. It appears that lithium does have an effect on the cellular function of adenyl cyclase under a variety of stimuli, there being some doubt whether there is a specific adenyl cyclase for each stimulating species or different receptor specificities at different sites. The clinical results are much less clear cut and it may be that to attempt to follow cellular function of cyclic AMP by following its excretion or concentration in body fluids is too optimistic an approach. I should like to record in passing that both adenyl cyclase, the synthetic enzyme and specific phosphodiesterase, the degradive enzyme for cyclic AMP are magnesium dependent.

Subcellular particles and lithium

In contrast to the study of adenyl cyclase and cyclic AMP the study of subcellular particles and their response to lithium has been neglected. Most of the studies published are comparable to much of the *in vitro* enzyme work, they are the side product of studies carried out at high concentrations of lithium for purposes other than the study of lithium. A study of the interaction of alkali metal ions, including lithium, with eukaryotic ribosomes used a concentration of 1M LiCl (120). Similarly a study of lithium on mitochondrial citrate uptake was not relevant to the clinical problem (121).

A study of heart mitochondria, however, showed a stimulation of calcium efflux by 5-10 mmol/l Li though it was only about one third as effective as sodium (122). Effects of lithium on ribosomes have been shown by Rillema and Smith (91) and also by Reboud (123). The uptake and effects of lithium in mitochondria has been reviewed by Johnson (56) though her literature survey over a period from 1959 to 1974 found only twelve references.

One might predict, particularly with the current interest in calcium transport at mitochondria and in the sarcoplasmic reticulum, that the whole area of subcellular particles could be a very rich research area for lithium pharmacologists.

LITHIUM AND THE METABOLISM OF TISSUES

Introduction

'Metabolism' can be interpreted in many ways. At one end of the spectrum the patient, gaining weight at the menopause, asks, "Is it my metabolism, Doctor?" meaning the sum total of all physiological change resulting from the endocrinological readjustment. At the other extreme there is a myopic sub-species of molecular biologist, previously undescribed, to whom metabolism is the transcription, forward or reverse, normal or aberrant and replication of a small section of a single gene controlling rhubarbolysis in a bacteriophage called Hic74962ØF2, of which he has the only known culture.

With regard to metabolism at levels above the 'Intermediary Metabolism' of the biochemistry texts I shall be selective. Other authors in this congress will be dealing with the nervous system and endocrinology, thyroid function, membrane phenomena and the erythrocyte, pharmacokinetics, lithium absorbtion and excretion. Since I have already mentioned overall energy balance I will deal very briefly with the brain and then concentrate on factors influencing mineral metabolism and the metabolism of kidney and bone.

Metabolism in the nervous system

Some mention must be made of the amine hypotheses of affective illness and the role of lithium since they dominate the research activities of so many research groups. The literature on this aspect of 'Metabolism' is probably larger than the total of the rest. The evidence for the catecholamine and indoleamine hypotheses and lithium action has been reviewed by many workers (124-127). Much of the evidence is conflicting, perhaps not surprisingly when one considers the complexities of the relationships and their inextricable dependence upon each other. The variety of techniques, *in vitro* model systems, pharmacological insults, dosage ranges and different species of animal all make comparisons extremely difficult and it is only to the eye of an *aficionado* that the clear line of progress is visible.

Shaw (127), in his review of lithium and amine metabolism, has said, "Although patterns may be discerned in the various experiments it is most difficult to say which are the most significant, or even which are the most valid, observations. As stated above, many of the effects may be secondary to toxic processes or to the stress of being in a toxic state". He concludes, "It is manifestly not possible, at this time, to make any definite statement about the mechanisms whereby lithium brings about its effects on amine metabolism." I will not, therefore, enter this particular arena.

However, there are a few neurochemical findings to which I would like to draw attention since they may have a bearing on the biochemistry of the brain during lithium treatment. Organisciak and Klingman have shown that chronic lithium reduced the total quantity of ATP and phosphocreatine in rat superior cervical ganglia after stimulation (128). In a later study, these workers showed that ganglia from lithium treated rats had reduced uptake of labelled pyruvic acid into the lipid fractions, particularly the sphingolipids (129).

A recent study by Edelfors (130) has shown decreases in the hexosamine and total protein of brains from lithium treated rats while the content of hyaluronic acid was increased. This is the first report of changes in brain macromolecules after lithium. This is interesting when considered with our early finding of decreased sodium and magnesium content after 28 days of lithium treatment in rats (16).

We have carried out some studies using column chromatography on Sephadex G-10 to determine whether or not lithium might form a complex with the postulated Mg-ATP-noradrenaline transmitter complex at the synapse (131,132). A sample of 14 micromol ATP and 14 micromol noradrenaline was eluted from a column (40 × 1.5 cm) of Sephadex G-10 previously buffered with the eluant, a solution of 114 mmol/l LiCl, 114 mmol/l $MgCl_2$ in 108 mmol/l triethanolamine hydrochloride buffer at pH 7.4 (133). Since this method had been successfully used to determine the binding of lithium and magnesium to ADP and ATP (76) we expected to be able to test easily whether this might be a site of lithium interaction at the synaptic level. However, not only were we unable to demonstrate a lithium complex with ATP-noradrenaline but we were unable to show the ternary Mg-ATP-noradrenaline complex reported by Rajan *et al.* (132). We repeated the study using a similar buffered eluant but containing only the magnesium chloride. The result is seen in Figure 9.2. It is clear that two species appear to be present, the ATP-Mg complex which we have previously shown (76) and noradrenaline with, in some runs, a suspicion of an ATP peak at the same point. However, on reconsideration of the work of Rajan *et al.* we found that the complex which they describe was determined by potentiometric titration and occurred at a pH of 9.0-9.5. The physiological significance of this to the synapse must be doubtful but it does draw attention to the ease with which *in vitro* studies may be extrapolated to *in vivo* situations and then become accepted by others as valid.

Effects of lithium on calcium and magnesium metabolism

Calcium and magnesium are present in the body in large quantities, the largest concentration being in bone. Magnesium is also present intracellularly throughout the body where it is second to potassium in concentration. Heaton (134,71), has proposed that the intracellular magnesium concentration may act as a regulator of a number of enzymes whose K_m (concentration at which half maximal reaction velocity occurs) is in the region of the normal intracellular concentration of 5 mmol/l Mg. Intracellular calcium concentration is rather low, 10^{-4} mmol/l, and is closely

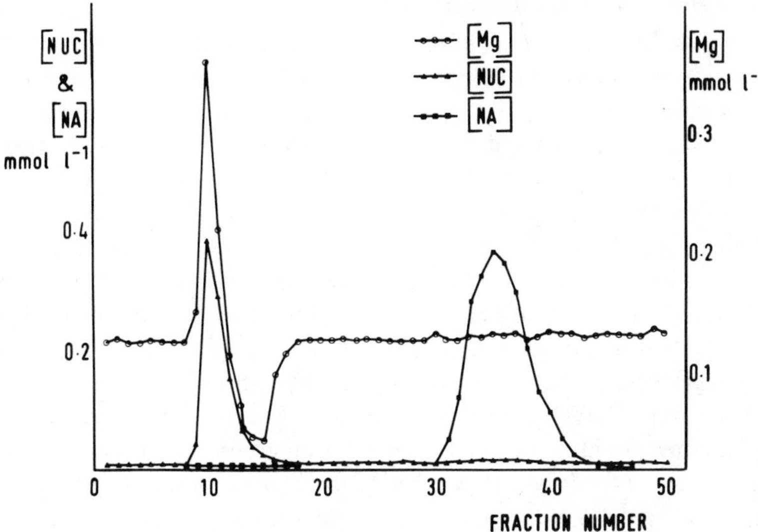

Figure 9.2. Elution profile of ATP (NUC) + noradrenaline (NA) by triethanolamine hydrochloride buffer, pH 7.4, containing $MgCl_2$, from a column (1.5 × 40 cm) of Sephadex G-100. For conditions see text

regulated by homeostatic mechanisms (135).

Discussion of the role of alkaline earth metals in lithium pharmacology falls naturally into three parts. Firstly there are reports of calcium and magnesium metabolism in the affective disorders and the effects of ECT. Secondly lithium has been shown in animal and human experiments to affect calcium and magnesium distribution and excretion. Finally lithium has effects on mineralized tissues.

Calcium, magnesium and the affective disorders

Calcium metabolism has been studied after the use of electroconvulsive therapy (136) when it was shown that ECT, or imiprimine, caused decreased plasma calcium and increased retention of calcium due to increased gut absorbtion and decreased urinary excretion. This early report has been confirmed very recently (137) when CSF calcium was also found to be decreased though only after the first three or four treatments. Carman *et al.* (137) have reviewed the early literature of calcium and the affective disorders and point out that extensive studies have never been carried out. There have been sporadic reports of differences between calcium and magnesium plasma levels in different mood states (138-140).

Lithium and alkaline earth metals

Lithium has been shown to have quite marked effects on calcium and magnesium metabolism. Mellerup *et al.* (141) have recently reported a study of effects of lithium on diurnal rhythms of the alkaline earths and phosphate and have reviewed the literature. They found decreased urinary calcium overnight and increased excretion of magnesium during the day. The most common finding after lithium in rat and man is raised plasma magnesium (16,18,37,62,142,143-146). Calcium in plasma has been reported to be increased (37,143,145) or decreased (147) or not to change (18,37,146). The variety of results with calcium may be a measure of the diurnal fluctuation rather than an effect of lithium.

In a metabolic profile study of 90 long-term lithium treated subjects (25,26) we were unable to establish that there was any difference between the mean for plasma calcium in the lithium group and normal values. Dunner *et al.* (148) found that after long term treatment there was no evidence of raised plasma magnesium and they suggest that regulatory mechanisms have reversed the acute effects observed by other workers. Our findings in the profile group were that there was no correlation between plasma lithium and plasma magnesium but that in the post menopausal female group the mean magnesium was higher than that of controls though not outside the normal range (26). Gerner *et al.*(149) have extensively reviewed the literature and investigated the role of parathormone on the lithium effect in patients and conclude that slight alteration of the PTH response is seen during lithium therapy.

Various studies have reported increased and decreased excretion of calcium and magnesium (150-153) after lithium in man and Carman *et al.* (150) have proposed that calcium excretion could be used as a test for predicting the antidepresent response to lithium.

In animals increased excretion of calcium has been almost universally observed (16,18,64,143). It is possible that dietary factors may be important in the differential response.

Arruda *et al.* (154) have carefully studied the endocrinology and effects of lithium on phosphate excretion in dogs. The conclude that, *in vivo*, lithium blocks the PTH sensitive adenylcyclase in renal cortex but also may interfere at a step distal to 3′5′ AMP since phosphaturia was reduced in both PTH and 3′5′AMP treated animals. Steele (118) has independently confirmed the PTH result in rats and additionally showed that vasopressin induced phosphaturia was blocked by lithium. Earlier work had showed that neither PTH magnesium nor calcium was able to alter lithium reabsorbtion in rat kidney (155,156).

These results therefore suggest that the effects of lithium on alkaline earth metals at the kidney are mediated by the cyclic 3′5′AMP system and that this is blocked by lithium. However, many of these studies were carried out acutely and it may be that the relevance to the long term effects in patients is that adaptation does indeed occur and that a new set point is fixed in the relationship between the systems controlling alkaline earth metabolism.

Lithium and bone

Lithium accumulates in bone (16,18,157,158) to a higher concentration that in any other tissue with the possible exception of thyroid (5), and is also retained after discontinuation of administration both in rat and man (157,158). About 60% of bone lithium must be sequestered in the bone mineral and indeed the concentration of lithium in the bone of growing rats bears a striking relationship with the rate of bone growth, suggesting that lithium is laid down during mineralization. The metabolic significance of this lithium, held in the bone for long periods, is difficult to assess.

It has been shown that after lithium treatment for 28 days, 28 lithium treated rats had decreased bone sodium and calcium when compared with 56 control animals by correlation coefficients and also by analysis of variance. Two reports have challenged this finding. Henneman and Zimmerberg (159) gave at first low, then highly toxic and finally well tolerated concentrations of lithium in drinking fluids of rats for 7, 3 and 30 days respectively. On the evidence of separated metaphyses from *six* (6) treated and *three* (3) control animals they state that, 'The data *clearly demonstrated* (my *italics*) that the chronic administration of LiCl . . . fails to modify serum calcium and inorganic phosphorus, metaphyseal bone mineral salts and organic matrix content, total hydroxyproline, calcium content or cellularity'.

In contrast, a careful study by Bellwinkel *et al.* (160) used two different doses, 0.5 mmol/kg/day and 2.5 mmol/kg/day and a control group, all of eight animals. However, all administrations were by once daily subcutaneous injection and it has already been stressed that this mode of dosage leads to a very sharp peak in plasma lithium (17) followed by a low plasma lithium for the rest of the 24 hour period. Our findings (16) were not visible by t test. Only by using the much more powerful statistical techniques of correlation coefficients and analysis of variance in a large number of rats were we able to demonstrate the bone sodium and calcium effects. It is not justifiable to compare our findings with these other reports. Mellerup and Plenge (161) have reported in their latest long-term study (8 weeks) that they confirm their earlier short-term findings (37,65) in bone. Lithium caused reduced uptake of radioactive phosphate, magnesium and calcium when determined simultaneously in rats. This is not incompatible with our findings.

We have been concerned that lithium might cause loss of mineral or lack of mineralization in bone in patients, particularly since we confirmed in post-mortem samples the presence of lithium some nine months after discontinuation of therapy (158). We have therefore carried out in rats and humans a number of studies to confirm or deny this effect. Initial studies of patients' hand radiographs, subjected to morphometric measurement (162), suggested that some of them might be considered to have lowered bone density. However, when the data from 74 lithium treated patients was analysed only four out of thirty seven postmenopausal subjects were found to have a metacarpal index (cortical area/total area) of more than two standard deviations below age and sex matched control means. The mean of treated subjects was almost identical to control values obtained in over 1000 subjects (163). Measurements of phalanges, radius and ulna gave similar results. The distribution of all other results was normal.

We repeated the hand radiographs two years later in 37 of the original group. In 14 of the 26 postmenopausal females there was a significant decrease in cortical width ($p < 0.05$). Bone loss is, however, a normal feature of ageing after the menopause and the mean rate of loss was closely comparable to that in psychiatrically normal control populations (163).

These results suggest that lithium does not cause accelerated bone loss in mature humans. However, Christiansen, Baastrup and Transbol (144,145) have reported decreased bone mineral content of the forearm in lithium treated patients. They have also shown a rise in serum parathormone, Mg and Ca after the initiation of lithium therapy (164) and also an elevated plasma parathormone, Mg and Ca in patients stabilized on lithium (165).

We have also attempted to replicate our earlier findings (16) in rats using long-term treated immature animals. One hundred weanling Wistar rats were divided into two groups and received either tap water or 10 mmol/l LiCl. The results of water intake are in Table 9.1. Animals were killed in groups of ten control and ten lithium treated at 3 weeks, 3 months, 6 months and 1 year. Brain, muscle, both femora, both forelegs, skull and plasma were taken from each animal. Morphometric measures were made of both femora after antero-posterior contact radiographs had been taken. The results of the group of 24 treated and 24 control animals taken at 1 year are presently available (Table 9.3). Tissue analyses await completion of the morphometry.

There is a significant decrease in femoral total width in the lithium treated group. This may be interpreted as an effect on total bone growth. Further studies may reveal whether or not it is a progressive change. Meanwhile, we are concerned at the intermittent reports of lithium use in children and would advise caution in its use in persons of immature bone structure.

Table 9.3 Radiology morphometry: mid shaft rat femur

Combined data	Total	Medulla	Cortex
Control (n = 48)	0.771 ±0.043	0.395 ±0.034	0.376 ±0.031
Lithium treated			
(n = 48) (1 year)	0.734 ±0.045	0.375 ±0.037	0.359 ±0.032
t test	$p < 0.0025$	0.05	0.05

Data from 24 control and 24 lithium treated rats. Left and right femora combined to provide a sample of 48 of each ('*F*' test between left and right femora not significant). Total width and medullary width (cm) was determined and cortical width estimated by difference

Measurement of fluxes of lithium; a new technique

It would be a great advance if we were able to measure the rate of turnover of lithium in bone and cells, which, of course, is relatively easy for sodium, potassium, calcium and magnesium, all of which have suitable radioisotopes. Lithium has three radioactive isotopes; ^{5}Li, half life 10^{-21} s, ^{8}Li, half life 0.8 s, ^{9}Li half life 0.2 s. It is difficult to do studies on lithium in which two-way fluxes are involved (166).

The stable isotope ^{6}Li occurs with a natural abundance of about 7% in normal lithium salts. It is also available relatively cheaply at about 95% enrichment since it is used in the nuclear power industry. It is not radioactive and would not be expected to be more toxic than ^{7}Li, and is already present in the lithium carbonate which we give to patients. The determination is possible by mass spectrometry but this is very costly.

We have developed a method, based on that for determination of lithium enrichment in reactor materials (167) using atomic absorbtion spectroscopy. The resolution of the atomic absorbtion spectrometer is not sufficient to resolve the isotopic shift of 0.015 nm. However, by the use of two hollow cathode lamps, one for ^{6}Li and the other ^{7}Li it is possible to determine the 6/7 absorbance ratio at a given concentration. The calibration is logarithmic and a family of concentration curves is generated against isotopic ratio. Presently we are unable to determine ^{6}LI at sufficiently low concentration for *in vivo* studies but we are investigating means by which we can increase our sensitivity.

We have maintained rats on ^{6}Li in drinking fluid for one year with no evidence of toxic affects.

Lithium and the kidney

We are concerned about recent reports of long term renal effects of lithium (168-170), in which tubular damage, reduced concentrating ability, focal necrosis and fibrosis have been reported. I wish only to report that in our series of lithium treated patients there is no evidence of a developing renal failure. In our recent profile study of this group (25,26,171), 90 subjects at that time, we have no evidence of a correlation, positive or negative, between duration of lithium treatment and any of the following· (a) clearance of lithium, creatinine, sodium, potassium, calcium, magnesium, phosphate, chloride, urea; (b) urine excretion rate of any of these; (c) urine volume/time, urine volume/urine creatinine. Chages in some of these measures would be expected in progressive damage. We have not noticed in rats the granular scarring and cysts reported in human post mortem samples.

CONCLUSIONS

Much remains to be learned of the metabolic effects of lithium and perhaps one should continuously suggest to colleagues who have specific biochemical or physiological techniques that they try a little lithium, just to see what happens. However, it is essential to do this at pharmacological concentrations. Lithium research in this area is still at the stamp-collecting stage.

ACKNOWLEDGEMENTS

I wish to thank especially Mrs Joyce Eastwood who has wrought this manuscript from very base metal. I am very grateful to Dr R.P. Hullin for comments on parts of the script. N.J.B. is supported by the Medical Research Council.

References

1. Schou, M. (1957). *Pharmacol Rev.*, **9**, 17
2. Gershon, S. and Shopsin, B., (eds.) (1973). *Lithium: Its role in Psychiatric Research and Treatment.* (New York: Plenum Press)
3. Johnson, F.N. (ed.) (1975). *Lithium Research and Therapy.* (London: Academic Press)
4. Bunney, W.E. and Murphy, D.L. (eds.) (1976). *The Neurobiology of Lithium.* Boston, Neurosciences Research Program Bulletin, **14**, 111
5. Schou, M. (1976). *Ann. Rev. Pharmacol. Toxicol.*, **16**, 231
6. Ullrich, K.J., Rumrich, G., Klöss, S. (1976). *Pflügers Archiv.*, **364**, 223

7. Crawford, A. (1975). *J. Physiol. (Lond),* **246,** 109
8. Davis, J.M. and Fann, W.E. (1971). *Ann. Rev. Pharmacol.,* **11,** 285
9. Schou, M. (1973). *Biochem, Soc. Trans.,* **1,** 81
10. Iverson, L.L. and Rose, S.P.R. (eds.) (1973). Biochemistry and Mental Illness. London, the Biochemical Society. *Biochem. Soc. Spec. Publ.* 251 pp
11. Cremer, J.E. (1973). *Biochem. Soc. Trans.,* **1,** 73
12. Schou, M. (1969). *Psychopharmacol. Bull.,* **5,** 33
13. Schou, M (1972). *Psychopharmacol. Bull.,* **8,** 36-62
14. Schou, M (1976). *Psychopharmacol. Bull.,* **12,** 49, 69 and 86
15. Schou, M. (1976). *Neuropsychobiol.,* **2,** 161
16. Birch, N.J., Jenner, F.A. (1973). Br. J. Pharmacol., **47,** 586
17. Olesen, O.V., Schou, M., Thomsen, K. (1976). *Neuropsychobiologie,* **2,** 134
18. Birch, N.J. (1971). *A Study of the Effects of Lithium Salts on the Distribution and Excretion of Other Ions.* Ph.D. Thesis, University of Sheffield.
19. Thomsen, K. (1973). *Acta Pharmacol. Toxicol.,* **33,** 92
20. Thomsen, K. and Olesen, O.V. (1974). *Int. Pharmacopsychiat.,* **9,** 118
21. Thomsen, k., Jensen, J. and Olesen, O.V. (1974). *Acta Pharmacol. Toxicol.,* **35,** 337
22. Olesen, O.V. and Thomsen, K. (1976). *Neuropsychobiologie,* **2,** 112
23. Thomsen, K. (1976). *J. Pharmacol. Exp. Ther.,* **199,** 483
24. Thomsen, K., Olesen, O.V., Jensen, J. and Schou, M. (1976). *Current Developments* in *Psychopharmacology* Vol. 3 (New York; Spectrum Pub. Inc.)
25. Birch, N.J., Greenfield, A.A. and Hullin, R.P. (1974). *Br. J. Pharmacol.,* **52,** 443P
26. Birch, N.J., Greenfield, A.A. and Hullin, R.P. (1977). *Psychol. Med.* (in press)
27. Kerry, R.J., Liebling, L.I. and Owen, G. (1970). *Acta psychiat. scand.,* **46,** 238-243
28. Dempsey, G.M., Dunner, D.L., Fieve, R.R., Farkas, T. and Wong, J. (1976). *Am. J. Psychiat.,* **133,** 1082
29. Furlong, F.W. (1973). *Can. Psychiat. Assoc. J.,* **18,** 75
30. Jenner, F.A. (1973). see ref. **10,** 101
31. Wolff, J. (1976). See ref. **4,** 178
32. Mellerup, E.T. and Rafaelsen, O.J. (1975). see ref. **3,** 381
33. Plenge, P.K., Mellerup, E.T. and Rafaelsen, O.J. (1973). *Int. Pharmacopsychiat.,* **8,** 234
34. Opitz, K. and Schafter, G. (1976). *Int. Pharmacopsychiat.,* **11,** 197
35. Johnson, F.N. (1976). *Comp. Psychiat.,* **17,** 591
36. Mellerup, E.T., Plenge, P. and Rafaelsen, O.J. (1974). *Dan. Med. Bull.* **21,** 88
37. Mellerup, E.T., Plenge, P. and Rafaelsen, O.J. (1973). *Biochem. Soc. Trans.,* **1,** 109
38. Haugaard, E.S., Frazer, A., Mendels, J. and Haugaard, N. (1975). *Biochem. Pharmacol.,* **24,** 1187
39. Lazarus, J.H., Riley, M. and Hayes, T.M. (1975). *Biochem. Pharmacol.,* **24,** 1820
40. Plenge, P., Mellerup, E.T. and Rafealsen, O.J. (1970). *J. Psychiat. Res.,* **8,** 29
41. Krulik, R., Zwolsky, p. (1970). *Activ. Nerv. Suppl.,* **12,** 279
41. Vendsborg, P.B. and Rafaelsen, O.J. (1973). *Acta Psychiat, Scand.,* **49,** 601
43. Van der Velde, C.D. and Gordon, M.W. (1969). *Arch. Gen. Psychiat.,* **21,** 478
44. Shopsin, B., Stern, S. and Gershon, S, (1972). *Arch. Gen. Psychiat.,* **26,** 566
45. Vendsborg, P.B. and Prytz, S. (1976). *Acta Psychiat. Scand.,* **53,** 64
46. Gordon, M.W. and van der Velde, C.D. (1974). *Nature, (London),* **247,** 160
47. Mellerup, E.T., Gronland Thomsen, H., Bjorum, N. and Rafaelsen, O.J. (1972). *Acta Psychiat. Scand.,* **48,** 332
48. Somerville, A.R. (1973). see Ref. **10,** 127
49. Forn, J. and Valdecasas, F.G. (1971). *Biochem. Pharmacol.,* **20,** 2773
50. Geisler, A., Bech, P., Johannesen, M. and Rafaelsen, O.J. (1976). *Neuropsychobiologie,* **2,** 211
51. Samuelsson, B., Granström, E., Green, K., Hamberg, M. and Hammarström, S. (1975). *Ann. Rev. Biochem.,* **44,** 669

52. Murphy, D.L., Donnelly, C. and Moskowitz, J. (1973). *Clin. Pharmacol. Ther.,* **14**, 810
53. Horrobin, D.F., Mtabaji, J.P. and Manku, M.S. (1976). *Med. Hypotheses,* **2**, 219
54. Horrobin, D.F., Mtabaji, J.P. and Robinson, C.J. (1976). *J. Physiol.* (*Lond*), **260**, 60P
55. Smellie, R.M.S. (ed.) (1974). *Calcium and Cell Regulation.* London, Biochemical Society Biochem. Soc. Symp., **39**, 151
56. Johnson, S. (1975). see Ref. **3**, 533
57. Hughes, M.N. (1972). *The Inorganic Chemistry of Biological Processes,* (London: Academic Press)
58. Eichhorn, G.L. (ed.) (1975). *Inorganic Biochemistry* Vols 1 & 2, (Amsterdam: Elsevier Scientific Pub.)
59. Williams, R.J.P. (1973). see Ref. **2**, 15
60. Frausto da Silva, J.J.R. and Williams, R.J.P. (1976). *Nature,* (*London*), **263**, 237
61. Williams, R.J.P. (1976). see Ref. **4**, 145
62. Birch, N.J. (1970). *Br. J. Psychiat.,* **116**, 461
63. Birch, N.J. (1973). *Biol. Psychiat.,* **7**, 269
64. Gotfredsen, F.F. and Rafaelsen, O.J. (1970). *Int. Pharmacopsychiat.,* **5**, 242
65. Mellerup, R.T., Plenge, P., Ziegler, R. and Rafaelsen, O.J. (1970). *Int. Pharmacopsychiat,* **5**, 258
66. Rafaelsen, O.J., Mellerup, E.T. and Shapiro, R.W. (1975). *Psychopharmacol. Comm.,* **1**, 611
67. Eisenman, G. (1976). see Ref. **4**, 154
68. Eigen, M. (1976). see Ref. **4**, 142
69. Wacker, W.E.C. and Parisi, A.F. (1968). *N. Engl. J. Med.,* **278**, 658, 712 and 722
70. Aikawa, J.K. (1976). In A.S. Prasad (ed.) *Trace Elements in Human Health and Disease.* vol II pp. 47-78 (New York: Academic Press)
71. Heaton, F.W. (1973). *Biochem. Soc. Trans.,* **1**, 67
72. Birch, N.J., Hullin, R.P., Inie, R.A. and Leaf, F.C. (1974). *Br. J. Pharmacol.,* **52**, 139P
73. Kachmar, J.F. and Boyer, P.D. (1953). *J. Biol. Chem.,* **200**, 669
74. Balan, G., Cernatescu, D., Trandafirescu, M. and Ababei, L. (1970). *Proc. C.I.N.P. VII,* Prague, p. 19
75. Colman, R.F. (1972). *Analyt. Biochem.,* **46**, 358
76. Birch, N.J. and Goulding, I. (1975). *Analyt. Biochem.,* **66**, 293
77. Pscheidt, G.R. and Meltzer, H.Y. (1975). *Lancet,* **i**, 932
78. Kadis, B. (1974). *Lancet,* **ii**, 1209
79. Kadis, B. (1977). *Bioinorganic Chem.,* (In press)
80. Essman, W. B. (1975). *Lancet,* **ii**, 547
81. Grier, G.W., Davis, L.C. and Pfeifer, W.D. (1976). *Horm. Metab. Res.,* **8**, 379
82. Parmar, S.S., Ali, B., Spencer, H. and Auyong, T.K. (1974). *J. Pharm. Pharmacol.,* **27**, 131
83. Ali, B., Spencer, H., Auyoung, T.K. and Parmar, S.S. (1975). *J. Pharm. Pharmacol.,* **27**, 131
84. Bera, H. and Chatterjee, G.C. (1976). *Biochem. Pharmacol.,* **25**, 1554
85. Dewar, A.J. and Reading, H.W. (1971). *Psychol. Med.,* **1**, 254
86. Dewar, A.J. and Reading, H.W. (1974). *Biochem. Pharmacol.,* **23**, 369
87. Vizi, E.S. (1975). see Ref. **3**, 391
88. Simpson, L.L. (1974). *Psycnopharmacologie,* **38**, 145
89. Abreu, L.A. and Abreu, R.R. (1973). *Experientia,* **29**, 446
90. Abreu, L.A. and Abreu, R.R. (1972). *Nature New Biol.,* **236**, 254
91. Rillema, J.A. and Smith, R.D. (1975). *Proc. Soc. Exp. Biol. Med.* **149**, 573
92. Dewar, A.J. and Reading, H.W. (1973). *I.R.C.S.* (**73-3**), 3-8-1
93. Howk, R. and Wang, T.Y. (1969). *Arch. Biochem. Biophys.,* **133**, 238
94. Bishop, C.C. and Gill, J.E. (1971). *Biochem. Biophys. Acta,* **227**, 97

95. Lazarus, L.H. and Kitron, N. (1974). *Lancet*, **ii**, 226
96. Nakashima, K. and Tuboi, S. (1976). *J. Biol. Chem.*, **251**, 4315
97. Agar, N.S., Gruca, M.A., Gupta, J.D. and Harley, J.D. (1975). *Lancet*, **i**, 1040
98. Gupta, J.D. and Crollini, C. (1975). *Lancet*, **i**, 216
99. Gutman, Y., Hockman, S. and Wald, H. (1973). *Biochem. Biophys. Acta.*, **298**, 284
100. Tobin, t., Akera, T., Han, S.S. and Brody, T.M. (1974). *Molec. Pharmacol.*, **10**, 501
101. Ploeger, E.J. (1974). *Arch. Int. Pharmacodyn.*, **210**, 374
102. Reading, H.W., Dewar. A.J. and Kinloch, N. (1974). *Biochem. Soc. Trans.*, **2**, 507
103. Choi, S.J. and Taylor, M.A. (1976). *Lancet*, **ii**, 1080
104. Marfey, S.P. and Li, M.G. (1975). *Z. Naturforsch.* **30**, 304
105. Lingsch, C. and Martin, K. (1976). *Br. J. Pharmacol.* **57**, 323
106. Balan, G., Cernatescu, D., Trandafirescu, M. and Ababei, L. (1974). *Revta Med-chir. Soc. Med. Iasi*, **78**, 901
107. O'Brien, M.J., Allin, C.J., Birch, N.J. and Hullin, R.P. (1977). *Br. J. Pharmacol.* (In press)
108. Forn, J. (1975). see Ref. **3**, 485
109. Dousa, T., Hechter, O. (1970). *Lancet*, **i**, 834
110. Abdulla, Y.H. and Hamadah, K. (1970). *Lancet*, **i**, 378
111. Singer, I. (1976). see Ref. **4**, 175
112. Geisler, A., Vendsborg, P.B., Johaneesen, M., Klysner, R. and Thomsen, J. (1976). *Acta Pharmacol. Toxicol*, **38**, 433
113. Christensen, S. and Geisler, A. (1977). *Acta Pharmacol. Toxical.*, **40**, 447
114. Christensen, S., Geisler, A., Badawi, I. and Madsen, S.N. (1977). *Acta Pharmacol. Toxicol*, **40**, 447
115. Frazer, A., Haugaard, E.S., Mendels, J. and Haugaard, N. (1975). *Biochem. Pharmacol.*, **24**, 2273
116. Wang, Y.C., Pandey, G.N., Mendels, J. and Frazer, A. (1974). *Biochem. Pharmacol.*, **22**, 845
117. Spiegel, A.M., Gerner, R.H., Murphy, D.L. and Aurbach, G.D. (1976). *J. Clin. Endocrinol. Metabol.*, **43**, 1390
118. Steele, T.H. (1976). *J. Pharmacol. Exp. Ther.* **197**, 206
119. Ebstein, R., Belmaker, R., Grunhaus, L. and Rimon, R. (1976). *Nature, (London)*, **259**, 411
120. Welfle, H., Henkel, B. and Bielka, H. (1976). *Acta Biol. Med. Ger.*, **35**, 401
121. Gyorgi, S. and Harris, E.J. (1975). *Acad. Sci. Hung.* **10**, 57
122. Crompton, M., Capano, M. and Carafoli, E. (1976). *Eur. J. Biochem.*, **69**, 453
123. Reboud, A.M., Buisson, M., Madjar, J.J. and Reboud, J.P. (1975). *Biochimie*, **57**, 295
124. Goodwin, F.K. and Sack, R.L. (1973). In E. Usdin and S.H. Snyder (eds.) *Frontiers of Catecholamine Research* pp. 1157-1164 (Oxford: Pergamon Press)
125. Schildkraut, J.J. (1974). *J. Nerv. Ment. Dis.*, **158**, 348
126. Murphy, D.L., Mandell, A.J. and Bloom, F.E. (1976). see Ref. **4**, 165
127. Shaw, D.M. (1975). see Ref. **3**, 411
128. Organischiak, D.T. and Klingman, J.D. (1974). *J. Neurochem.*, **22**, 341
129. Organisciak, D.T. and Klingman, J.D. (1976). *Brain Res.*, **115**, 467
130. Edelfors, S. (1977). *Acta Pharmacol. Toxicol.*, **40**, 126
131. Rajan, K.S., Davis, J.M., Colburn, R.W. and Jarke, F.H. (1972). *J. Neurochem.*, **19**, 1099
132. Rajan, K.S., Davis, J.M. and Colburn, R.W. (1976). *Abstracts. 2nd Internat. Symp. Magnesium*, Montreal, p 70
133. Birch, N.J., Janik, A.C., Inie, R.A. and Hullin, R.P. (1976). *Biochem. Soc. Trans.* **4**, 757
134. Heaton, F.W. (1976). *Abstracts 2nd Internat Symp. Magnesium*, Montreal. P. 5
135. Wacker, W.E.C. and Williams, R.J.P. (1968). *J. Theor. Biol.*, **20**, 65
136. Faragalla, F.F. and Flach, F.F. (1970). *J. Nerv. Ment. Dis.*, **151**, 120

137. Carman, J.S., Post, R.M., Goodwin, F.K. and Bunney, W.E. (1977). *Biol. Psychiat.,* **12,** 5
138. Cade, J.F.J. (1964). *Med. J. Aust.,* **1,** 195
139. Naylor, G.J., Fleming, L.W., Stewart, W.K., McNamee, H.B., le Poidevin, D. (1972). *Br. J. Psychiat.,* **120,** 683
140. Herzberg, L. and Bold, A.M. (1972). *Lancet,* **i,** 128
141. Mellerup, E.T., Lauritsen, B., Dan, H. and Rafaelsen, O.J. (1976). *Acta Psychiat. Scand.,* **53,** 360
142. Nielsen, J. (1964). *Acta Psychiat. Scand.,* **40,** 190
143. Andreoli, V.M., Villani, F. and Brambilla, G. (1972). *Psychopharmacologia,* **25,** 77
144. Christiansen, C., Baastrup, P.C. and Transbøl, I. (1976). *Lancet,* **ii,** 969
145. Christiansen, C., Baastrup, P.C. and Transbøl, I. (1976). *Neuropsychobiol.* **1,** 344
146. Aronoff, M.S., Evens, R.G. and Durell, J. (1971). *J. Psychiat. Res.* **8,** 139
147. Tupin, J.P., Schlagenhauf, G.K. and Creson, D.L. (1968). *Am. J. Psychiat.,* **125,** 536
148. Dunner, D.L., Meltzer, H.L., Schreiner, H.C. and Feigelson, J.L. (1975). *Acta Psychiat. Scand.,* **51,** 104
149. Gerner, R.H., Post, R.M., Spiegel, A.M. and Murphy, D.L. (1977). *Biol. Psychiat.,* **12,** 145
150. Carman, J.S., Post, R.M., Teplitz, T.A. and Goodwin, F.K. (1974). *Lancet,* **ii,** 1454
151. Crammer, J. (1975). *Lancet,* **i,** 215
152. Bjorum, N., Hornum, I., Mellerup, E.T., Plenge, P.K. and Rafaelsen, O.J. (1975). *Lancet,* **i,** 1243
153. Miller, P.D., Dubovsky, S.L., McDonald, K.M. and Schrier, R.W. (1976). *Clin. Res.,* **24,** 156A
154. Arruda, J.A.L., Richardson, J.M., Wolfson, J.A., Nascimento, L., Rademacher, D.R. and Kurtzman, N. A. (1975). Administration and phosphate excretion. *Am. J. Physiol.,* **231,** 1140
155. Steele, T.H. and Dudgeon, K.L. (1974). *Kidney Int.* **5,** 196
156. Steele, T.H., Manuel, M.A., Newton, M. and Boner, G.(1975). *Am. J. Med., Sci.,* **269,** 349
157. Birch, N.J. and Hullin, R.P. (1972). *Life Sci.,* **11,** 1095
158. Birch, N.J. (1974). *Clin. Sci. Mol. Med.,* **46,** 409
159. Henneman, D., Zimmerberg, J.J. (1974). *Endocrinology,* **94,** 915
160. Bellwinkel, S., Schäfer, A., Minne, H. and Ziegler, R. (1975).*Int. Pharmacopsychiat.,* **10, 9**
161. Mellerup, E.T. and Plenge, P. (1976). *Int. Pharmacopysychiat.,* **11,** 190
162. Nordin, B.E.C. (ed.) (1976). *Calcium, Phosphate and Magnesium Metabolism.* (Edinburgh: Churchill-Livingstone.)
163. Horsman, A. (1976). see Ref. **162,** 357
164. Christiansen, C., Baastrup, P.C. and Transbol, I. (1977). (Submitted for publication)
165. Christiansen, C., Baastrup, P.C., Lindgren, P. and Transbol, I. (1977). (Submitted for publication)
166. Dolman, D.E.M. and Edmonds, C.J. (1976). *J. Physiol.,* **259,** 759
167. Wheat, J.A. (1971). *Appl. Spectrosc.,* **25,** 328
168. Hestbech, J., Hansen, H.E., Amdisen, A. and Olsen, S. (1977). *Kidney Int.* (In Press)
169. Hansen, H.E., Hestbech, J., Amdisen, A. and Olsen, S. (1977). *Proc. Eur. Dialysis Transpl. Assoc.* **14,** (In Press)
170. Amdisen, A (1977). Personal communication.
171. Birch, N.J., Greenfield, A.A. and Hullin, R.P. (1977). (Submitted for publication)

10

Tryptophan Metabolism and the Aetiology of Affective Disorder

D. M. SHAW

Currently many groups are reassessing the hypotheses advanced to explain the basis of depressive illness. We also have been taking part in this exercise and one of the hypotheses we have been pursuing is that there is an abnormality in peripheral tryptophan metabolism in affective disorders.

The method chosen to pursue this hypothesis was multiple compartmental analysis which gives data on a 'freely available' pool of tryptophan in the body. Up to now, we have studied mostly patients suffering from unipolar affective disorder, either during an episode or after clinical recovery. Some of the patients had had no antidepressant drug therapy for a minimum of one week and none had had neuroleptics in the preceding month. Some patients were studied during treatment with lithium, with tricyclic drugs or with monoamineoxidase inhibitors. Data were collected from volunteers who were without personal or family history of psychiatric illness or alcoholism. The volunteers and patients were fasted overnight and throughout the test which lasted until early afternoon. Briefly, blood was taken from an indwelling venous cannula at about 0930 and ^{3}H-l-tryptophan was injected via another vein. Venous blood samples were taken at intervals over several hours. Plasma from these samples was assayed for tryptophan concentration and specific activity of the amino acid.

The data were subjected to multicompartmental analysis, the best fit for

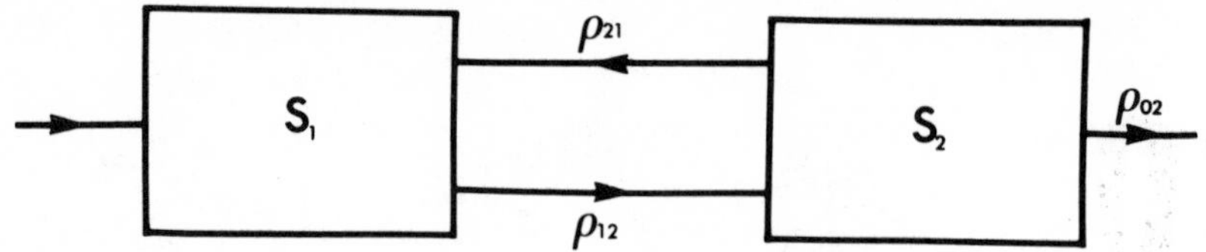

S = concentration of tryptophan (nMol.ml^{-1})

ρ = flux of tryptophan (nMol. ml^{-1}min^{-1})

Figure 10.1 Two compartmental model

the observed values being a two compartment model with through fluxes and a return flux from the second to the first compartment.

The results from drug-treated versus 'drug free' patients showed no significant drug effects. The absence of a drug effect allowed comparisons between values from control individuals, unipolar patients (ill) and unipolar patients (after recovery) irrespective of drug treatments. The two compartments delineated by the study were considered tentatively to be extra- and intra-cellular pools of available tryptophan. The amounts of tryptophan in these compartments, the fluxes between them and the exit fluxes tended to be reduced in depressed patients whether they were ill or whether they had recovered. The results suggested therefore that in unipolar affective disorder there was an illness-independent abnormality with regard to the amino acid tryptophan in the two main compartments of the body (1).

The magnitude of the changes observed was not sufficient to make it likely that metabolic processes in the body would be affected severely and, indeed, although there were statistically significant changes, there was some overlap with the values seen in the normal controls.

It was possible, however, that the low values for concentrations and fluxes of tryptophan in the patients could be the indicants of a degree of biochemical vulnerability — a difficulty in maintaining the tryptophan pool at normal levels in the body (2).

This could be exacerbated, for instance, by stress, which would result in the production of cortisol, the induction of tryptophan pyrrolase (3) and increased losses of tryptophan via degradation of the amino acid in the liver. This occurrence in the presence of an already partially depleted pool, could give rise to a 'tryptophan famine' in the body.

When considering the possible effects of such a 'tryptophan famine' on the brain, it should be remembered that the blood supplies only about two thirds of the amino acids needed by the brain, the remainder coming from recycling (4). Of the essential amino acids, tryptophan is present in the smallest amounts in the body, and its concentration in non-bound form in plasma and interstitial fluid is very low indeed. In addition, entry to the brain by amino acids is competitive so that increases or relative increases in the amounts of other amino acids, especially the aromatic ones, can decrease the entry of tryptophan to the brain (5). Clearly, therefore, a tryptophan deficit in the body could easily put the entry of this compound to the brain in jeopardy.

The great majority of the cells in the brain might tolerate some degree of deficiency of this amino acid but the serotoninergic neurones could be uniquely vulnerable in this situation. They are the only neurones having a dual need for tryptophan, for protein synthesis and for production of 5-HT.

We became interested, therefore, in the possibility that unipolar depressive illness could be due to a temporary failure in the supply of tryptophan to the brain, giving rise to reduction in protein synthesis in 5-HT neurones and ultimately leading to a disruption of serotoninergic function (2). Such a hypothesis would imply that the 'exacerbated defect' (i.e. the failure in supply of tryptophan) might antecede the appearance of the clinical symptoms and indeed might have been corrected or partially rectified when the episode has begun.

In examining the feasibility of such a hypothesis, it is important to remember that only cell bodies of 5-HT cells and possibly their synaptic bulbs will be involved. Data on metabolic processes in the brain are derived from collections of glia, nerve endings, axons and cell bodies from a variety of cells. Some glial cells, neurones or fragments of neurones will have their idiosyncratic biochemical characteristics, while only a variable fraction of the total will be representative of the particular cells of interest —in the present case, serotoninergic neurones.

With these provisos in mind, therefore, we can look at some of the published data of relevance to 5-HT neurones:-

1. 5-HT is synthesized by both cell bodies and nerve terminals and it used to be thought that most was produced distally, in the synaptic bulbs. It is likely that the contrary is true — there is ahigher turnover of 5-HT in the cell bodies than in the terminals (6). Most of the protein produced by the cells also is in the cell body, so that there could be competition for tryptophan at this site. Additional competition for tryptophan could occur where serotoninergic bulb and cell bodies were located together to the

detriment probably of the supply of amino acid to the former (7).

2. The rate of entry of tryptophan into rat brain is in the region of 1.76 nmol/min/g brain (3). One assay for tryptophan concentration of brain gave a value of 11.3 micromol/100 g protein (8), so that assuming an average protein turnover of 0.7%/h (4) and a protein content of the brain of 80 mg/g brain (9), the calculated figure for tryptophan turnover is in the region of 1 nmol/min/g brain. This figure is based on average protein turnover rates and gives rather high estimates.

3. A more realistic estimate should be obtained from the rate of entry of tryptophan into brain protein in rats during infusion of labelled tryptophan, and estimates using this technique gave a range of 4-8 micro g-tryptophan/h/g brain (10). A mean of 6 micro g tryptophan/h/g brain gives a rate of incorporation of tryptophan into brain protein of 0.5 nmol/min/g.

4. The figures for protein turnover are the sum total of that occurring in neurones and glia, whereas the data for neuronal tissue synthesizing 5-HT gives an overall value for what is in fact the activity of only a proportion of the cells present, as discussed above. Thus any such figure underestimates the *local* requirements for tryptophan of processes synthesizing 5-HT in the neurones.

Reported data for 5-HT turnover in dorsal and median raphe have been given as 16-45 ng 5-HT/mg protein/h (6). Assuming a content of protein of 8 g/100 g brain (9), values for turnover lie between 0.1 and 0.4 nmol/min/g brain. If a half or a third of the tissue studied were actively engaged in synthesizing 5-HT, this could make competition for tryptophan between the processes producing 5-HT and protein a likely event, since the needs for tryptophan of the two pathways are of comparable magnitudes.

Of course, calculation based on data from several sources is subject to considerable distortion, but the exercise has been performed only to show that the variables concerned are of the right order to allow competition for tryptophan to take place in 5-HT neurones.

Thus, there is evidence for an observed peripheral abnormality in the peripheral disposition of tryptophan which, if exacerbated, could lead to a fall in the rate of synthesis of protein in 5-HT neurones. The hypothesis therefore is feasible; one possible outcome would be a gradual reduction in the release of 5-HT, and this in turn would lead to the development of supersensitivity at the post-synaptic receptors (2).

This is an interesting possibility because we now have a number of observations either of affective illness or of areas of knowledge relevant to these disorders which have to be reconciled (11).

These observations include the following:-

1. Acute depletion of 5-HT or catecholamines did not replicate the depressive syndrome, and attempts to treat depressive illness by potentiation of catecholamines have failed (12-14). Tricyclic antidepressants produce rapid changes in aminergic function in animals yet have a progressive but slow antidepressant activity. It is unlikely therefore that depression is due to just a simple 'lack of amines'.

2. Two secondary amine tricyclic antidepressants had an inverted 'U' shaped plasma level-response curve indicating that only in a middle range of plasma levels was there an optimal therapeutic effect (15-18). With two tertiary amine tricyclics there were no indications of an upper limit to increasing response to rising plasma levels (19-21). Secondary amine tricyclics block the reuptake of amine at the presynaptic membrane of mostly noradrenergic neurones (22), while tertiary amine tricyclics act mostly at 5-HT neurones (23) (and to some extent on noradrenergic neurones via their secondary amine metabolites).

3. Monoamineoxidase inhibitors increase the availability of 5-HT, NA and dopamine in the brain but favour the serotoninergic pathway by supplying an excess of the precursor of 5-HT, tryptophan accelerated recovery (24). Overflow conditions at serotoninergic synapses, therefore, are therapeutically optimal.

4. Recovery from depression during treatment with imipramine was continuous when the synthesis of NA was inhibited but ceased when the production of 5-HT was blocked (25). From this study, it seems that the integrity of the 5-HT pathway is essential for recovery during treatment with this drug.

5. Mianserin is an antidepressant which blocks 5-HT receptors (26). Nine patients treated with pizotifen (which also blocks 5-HT receptors) and maprotiline had a good rate of recovery (11).

6. Withdrawal of pizotifen, given for the treatment of migraine, was followed by depressive symptoms in some patients (27).

7. A decrease in sex drive (28,29) and food intake (30) occur during increased 5-HT activity in animals, whilst loss of appetitie for sex and food are prominent symptoms of depressive illness.

The most likely common denominator for these observations is that depression may be associated with 5-HT overactivity. If so, some anti-depressants might function by potentiating noradrenergic function to produce 'balance' in aminergic activity. Others might function by inducing tachyphylaxis in already overactive serotoninergic pathways or by allowing 5-HT supersensitivity to subside.

References

1. Shaw, D.M., Tidmarsh, S.F., Johnson, A.L., Michalakeas, A., Macsweeney, D.A., Hewland, R., Francis, A., Riley, E. and Blazek, R. (1977). (In preparation)
2. Shaw, D.M., Riley, G., Tidmarsh, S., Blazek, R. (1976). *Lancet,* **i**, 363.
3. Kenney, F.T. (1970). In: *Mammalian Protein Metabolism,* pp. 131-176. (New York: Academic Press)
4. Pratt, O.E. (1975). In: *Transport Phenomena in the Nervous System,* pp.55-76. (New York: Plenum Press)
5. Lajtha, A. (1974). In: *Aromatic Amino Acids in the Brain,* pp. 25-49. (Amsterdam: Associated Scientific Publishers)
6. Neckers, L.M. and Meek, J.L. (1976). *Life Sci.* **19**, 1579
7. Mosko, S.S., Haubrich, D. and Jacobs, B.L. (1977). *Brain Res.,* **119**, 269
8. Gaitonde, M.K. and Tovey, T. (1970). *Biochem. J.,* **117**, 907
9. Richter, D. (1970). In: *Protein Metabolism of the Nervous System,* pp. 241-257. (New York: Plenum Press)
10. Blazek, R. (1977). (Personal Communication)
11. Shaw, D.M., Riley, G.J., Michalakeas, A.C. Timdarsh, S.F., Blazek, R. and Johnson, A.L. (1977). *Lancet,* (In press)
12. Mendels, J. and Fraser, A. (1974). *Arch. Gen. Psychiat.,* **30**, 447
13. Mendels, J., Stinnett, J.L., Burns, D. and Frazer, A. (1975). *Arch. Gen. Psychiat.,* **32**, 22
14. Goodwin, F.K., Post, R.M. and Kotin, J. (1972). *Psychopharmacologia,* **26**, Suppl. 82
15. Asberg, M., Cronholm, B., Sjoquist, F. and Tuck, D. (1971). *Br. Med. J., 3,* 331
16. Kragh-Sørensen, P., Asberg, M. and Hansens, C.E. (1973). *Lancet,* **i**, 113
17. Kragh-Sørensen, P., Hansen, C.E., Baastrup, P.C. and Hvidberg, E.F. (1976). *Pharmacopsych.,* **9**, 27
18. Whyte, S.F., Macdonald, A.J., Naylor, G.J. and Moody, J.P. (1976). *Br. J. Psychiat.,* **128**, 384
19. Braithwaite, R.A., Goulding, R., Theano, G., Bailey, J. and Coppen, A. (1972). *Lancet,* **i**, 1297
20. Gram, L.F., Reisby, N., Ibsen, I., Nagy, A., Dencker, S.J., Beck, P., Petersen, G.O. and Christiansen, J. (1976). *Clin. Pharmacol. Therapeut.* **19**, 318
21. Glassman, A.H., Perel, J.M., Shostak, M., Kantor, S.J. and Fleiss, J.L. (1977). *Arch. Gen. Psychiat.,* **34**, 197
22. Carlsson, A., Corrodi, H, Fuxe, K. and Hokfelt, T. (1969). *Eur. J. Pharmacol.,* **5**, 367
23. Carlsson, A., Corrodi, H., Fuxe, K. and Hokfelt, T. (1969). *Eur. J. Pharmacol.* **5**, 357
24. Coppen, A., Shaw, D.M. and Farrell, J.P. (1963). *Lancet,* **i**, 79
25. Friedman, E., Shopsin, B., Goldstein, M. and Gershon, S. (1974). *J. Pharm. Pharmacol.,* **26**, 995

26. Kopera, H. (1975). In: *Depressive Illness and Experiences with a New Antidepressant Drug GB94,* pp. 26-43. (Amsterdam: Excerpta Medica)
27. Hughes, R.C. and Foster, J.B. (1971). *Curr. Therap. Res.* **13,** 63
28. Gessa, G.L. and Tagliamonte, A. (1974). In: *Advances in Biochemical Psychopharmacology,* Vol. 11, pp. 217-228. (New York: Raven Press)
29. Everitt, B.J. (1976). Communication to British Association for Psychopharmacology, November 6th, 1976
30. Blundell, J. (1977). Communication to joint meeting of British Association for Psychopharmacology and The Society for Studying Obesity. April 1st, 1977

11

Lithium Effects on Brain 5-Hydroxytryptamine Metabolism

K. J. COLLARD

GENERAL INTRODUCTION

The metabolism of 5-hydroxytryptamine (5-HT) in the rat forebrain may be accelerated by two experimental procedures, the administration of a large dose of the precursor amino acid L-tryptophan (1), and by the electrical stimulation of the nucleus raphe medianus (2,3). The increase in the production of the major 5-HT metabolite 5-hydroxyindole acetic acid (5-HIAA) following raphe stimulation is believed to result from the metabolism of 5-HT which has been released extraneuronally and returned to cells for metabolism, whilst that produced following tryptophan loading is derived predominantly from the metabolism of 5-HT which remains within the intracellular compartment (4).

Since mania may be associated with an increase in the biochemical or bioelectric activity of 5-HT neurones (5), the effect of lithium on the accelerated metabolism of 5-HT under these two experimental situations has been investigated.

TRYPTOPHAN STUDY

Introduction

Earlier studies in this laboratory had shown that the acceleration of 5-HT production following tryptophan administration (100 mg/kg i.p.) was reduced by both 5 and 10 day lithium treatment (0.75 mmol/kg i.p. per day). The 5-HIAA concentration following tryptophan was unaffected by 5-day Li treatment. In the 10-day group however, the reduction in 5-HT was accompanied by an increase in 5-HIAA (6,7). This change in the pattern of 5-hydroxyindole production from a tryptophan load caused by 10-day lithium treatment has been interpreted as being due to an increase in the deamination of 5-HT (6,7). This finding extends previous reports of an increased production of deaminated metabolites of noradrenaline following both acute and chronic treatment with lithium (8,9), and supports the previous suggestion that the catabolism of 5-HT in mouse brain may be increased by lithium treatment (10).

An increase in the deamination of 5-HT may be brought about by a direct effect on the deaminating enzyme monoamine oxidase (MAO), or indirectly due to an effect of the storage process which protects 5-HT from deamination. MAO is believed to be present in the brain in great excess (11). It is considered therefore that the activity of the enzyme would have to be markedly increased in order to have any significant effect on the deamination of 5-HT. It is more likely that lithium is making 5-HT more accessible to the enzyme possibly by increasing the amount of free cytoplasmic 5-HT as a result of an impairment of the storage mechanism.

To examine these interpretations further, the effect of lithium on the sub-synaptosomal distribution of 5-HT and on MAO activity was investigated.

Methods

The effect of lithium on the subsynaptosomal distribution of accumulated ^{14}C-5-HT.

Rats were treated with lithium (0.75 mmol/kg i.p. per day, administered as isotonic 0.15 M LiCl) or saline for 5 or 10 days. 24 hours after the last dose of lithium or saline, synaptosomes were isolated from the forebrain essentially by the method of Kurokawa *et al.* (12). In this study however, a greater yield of synaptosomes was obtained by using 2.5% Ficoll rather than 3.0% in the middle band of the density gradient. Synaptosomal suspensions in Krebs solution were incubated for 10 minutes at 37°C in 1×10^{-7}M ^{14}C-5HT (specific activity 28 mCi/mmol). Following incubation, the synaptosomes were washed in Krebs solution and osmotically disrupted by suspension in distilled deionised water (13). The suspension was then centrfuged at 10 000 × g for 20 min to remove synaptosomal ghosts, myelin and mitochondria. The resulting supernatant was centrifuged at 100 000 × g for 60 min to yield a pellet rich in vesicles and a supernatant containing the soluble component of the synaptosomes (14).

The pellet of vesicles was resuspended in 0.4 N perchloric acid (PCA), and the 5-HT extracted essentially by the ion exchange method used previously in whole brain studies (4) but scaled down by using 5 × 50 mm columns of amberlite CG 50 H resin. A sample of supernatant was removed for estimation of total radioactivity, and 5-HT was extracted in 0.4 N PCA from a second sample and separated from its acid and neutral metabolites by ion exchange chromatography (4). Subtraction of the amount of 5-HT from total radioactivity gave a measure of the amount of 5-HT metabolites present in the supernatant. The radioactivity of all samples was measured by liquid scintillation counting. Protein concentration was measured by the method of Lowry *et al.* (15).

The effect of lithium on monoamine oxidase activity.

Monoamine oxidase activity in mitochondrial fractions from rat forebrain was measured by the method of Harada and Nagatsu (16) using 5-HT as substrate. Two studies were conducted. In one study, animals were pre-treated for 5 or 10 days with lithium or saline and mitochondrial fractions were removed for estimation of MAO activity. In the second study, lithium was added *in vitro* to mitochondrial fractions obtained from untreated rats. The amount of lithium added to the mitochondrial suspension was calculated from the known concentration of lithium in the forebrain of treated rats (70 ± 0.5 micromol/kg brain tissue), and the proportion of whole brain lithium found in the primary mitochondrial fraction by DeFeudis (17). The final concentration of lithium in the mitochondrial suspensions was 6×10^{-7}M and 8×10^{-7}M.

Results

The effect of lithium on the sybsynaptosomal distribution of accumulated ^{14}C-5-HT.

The results of this study are shown in Table 11.1.

The amount of 5-HT in the vesicle fraction, considered to be a major functional store of 5-HT was unaffected by treatment with lithium for either 5 or 10 days. Similarly, treatment with lithium for 5 days had no effect on the concentration of 5-HT and 5-HT metabolites in the supernatant (cytosol) phase. Treatment with lithium for 10 days, however, significantly reduced the concentration of 5-HT in the cytosol and proportionately but not significantly increased the concentration of 5-HT metabolites.

Table 11.1. The concentration of ^{14}C-5-HT and ^{14}C-5-HT metabolites in the vesicle fraction and supernatant (cytosol) of synaptosomes from lithium treated and saline treated animals.

	Treatment period	5-hydroxyindole concentration (pmol/mg protein) Lithium	Saline
Vesicular 5-HT (18)	5 days	26.80 ± 5.08	25.11 ± 5.60
	10 days	21.28 ± 4.95	17.98 ± 3.50
Supernatant 5-HT (16)	5 days	46.38 ± 3.66	40.14 ± 5.21
	10 days	35.35 ± 2.32	47.71 ± 4.64*
Supernatant metabolites (17)	5 days	29.21 ± 6.68	37.62 ± 6.92
	10 days	42.52 ± 6.89	30.36 ± 5.83

Results are expressed as the mean ± SEM and analysed by the Student's t test. Numbers in parentheses indicate the number of animals in each group (*$p < 0.05$).

The effect of lithium on monoamine oxidase activity.

The results of this study are shown in Tables 11.2 and 11.3. Treatment with lithium for either 5 or 10 days had no significant effect on forebrain MAO activity (Table 11.2). Similarly, the addition of lithium to mitochondrial suspensions *in vitro* had no effect on MAO (Table 11.3).

Table 11.2. The effect of lithium treatment for 5 or 10 days on forebrain mitochondrial monoamine oxidase activity

Duration of Li+ treatment	NH_4^+ production (nmol/mg protein/min) Control	Lithium
5 days	1.148 ± 0.135	1.060 ± 0.132
10 days	1.188 ± 0.118	1.052 ± 0.152

Enzyme activity is expressed as the mean NH_4^+ production (nmol/mg protein/min) ±SEM of 10 animals and analysed by the Student's t test

Table 11.3. The effect of lithium in vitro on the activity of forebrain MAO

NH_4^+ production (nmol/mg protein/min)			
Control (Na^+ 6 × 10^{-7}M)	Lithium (6 × 10^{-7}M)	Control (Na^+ 8 × 10^{-7}M)	Lithium 8 × 10^{-7}M
0.945 ± 0.103	0.914 ± 0.127	0.896 ± 0.094	0.856 ± 0.078

MAO activity is expressed as the mean NH_4^+ production (nmol/mg protein/min) ± SEM of 10 animals and analysed by the Student's t test

Discussion

The decrease in the concentration of 5-HT in the cytosol phase of the synaptosome was accompanied by an increase in the concentration of 5-HT metabolites which again provides evidence of and increase in the deamination of 5-HT following 10 day lithium treatment. However, this increase in deamination occurred without any observed effect on that fraction of the synaptosome considered to be a major site of 5-HT storage, namely the vesicles. In addition, the increased deamination of 5-HT also occurred without any measureable effect on the deaminating enzyme MAO. It is possible therefore that lithium may affect a 5-HT store outside the vesicle fraction. In addition to the vesicles, the 5-HT terminal contains a protein which is present in the cytosol and which can bind 5-HT by a high affinity process (18). This protein has a number of characteristics suggesting that it may be a storage site of 5-HT in the nerve terminal (19). The importance of this protein in synaptic function is as yet unknown. However, it is possible that the increase in 5-HT deamination following lithium treatment may be related to an effect on this binding protein.

RAPHE STIMULATION STUDY

Introduction

As mentioned previously, activation of ascending 5-HT pathways in rat brain by electrical stimulation of the nucleus raphe medianus increases the metabolism of 5-HT in the forebrain. The increased production of 5-HIAA by raphe stimulation is believed to result from the metabolism of 5-HT which has been released extraneuronally and returned to cells for metabolism (4). In the present study this technique has been used to examine the effect of lithium on 5-HT release in the rat forebrain. In order to clarify the interpretation of the data obtained in this study, the interaction of lithium and chlorimipramine on 5-HT uptake by synaptosomes was also studied.

Methods

The effect of lithium on the change in forebrain 5-hydroxyindole concentrations induced by raphe stimulation.

Two groups of 36 animals received treatment with lithium or saline for 10 days as described for previous studies. 24 h after the final injection of lithium or saline, half of the animals in each group received chlorimipramine (5 mg/kg/i.p.), while the others received an equivalent volume of saline. 3 hours after the injection of chlorimipramine or saline, pairs of animals from each of the four subgroups (saline alone, saline plus chlorimipramine, lithium alone and lithium plus chlorimipramine) received raphe stimulation or sham treatment as described previously (4,20). Following raphe stimulation or sham treatment each forebrain was removed for estimation of 5-HT and 5-HIAA(4).

The paired design was employed in order to minimise the effects of the within day and between day variation in 5-hydroxyindoles (21-23) and the effect of drug treatments was analysed by the paired t test.

The effect of lithium and chlorimipramine on 5-HT uptake into synaptosomes.

Synaptosomes were prepared from whole forebrain by the method previously described (16). Two uptake studies were conducted. In the first study, animals were pretreated with lithium and chlorimipramine as described in the stimulation study, and synaptosomes were prepared three and a half hours after the injection of chlorimipramine (a time corresponding to the time at which raphe stimulation was applied). In the second study lithium and chlorimipramine were added *in vitro* to synaptosomal suspensions prepared from untreated animals. The amount of lithium added to the synaptosomal suspension in the *in vitro* study was calculated on the basis of the work of DeFeudis (17) as described previously. The final concentration of lithium in the incubation medium was 2.5×10^{-8}M and 3.3×10^{-8}M. The final concentration of chlorimipramine in the incubation medium was 4×10^{-7}M, a concentration known to inhibit 5-HT uptake by about 50% (24).

In both studies, synaptosomal suspensions were incubated for 10 minutes at 37 °C with 1×10^{-7}M ^{14}C-5-HT (specific activity 27 mCi/mmol) in Krebs solution containing iproniazid phosphate 1×10^{-4}M. After incubation, 5-HT was extracted from washed synaptosomes by suspension in 0.4 N PCA and measured by liquid scintillation counting. Protein was measured by the method of Lowry *et al.* (15).

Results

The effect of lithium on the change in forebrain 5-hydroxyindole concentrations induced by raphe stimulation.

The effect of lithium and chlorimipramine on the forebrain concentration of 5-HT and 5-HIAA in unstimulated animals is shown in Table 11.4. It can be seen that lithium had no effect on 5-HT but significantly increased the concentration of 5-HIAA. Similarly chlorimipramine had no significant effect on the forebrain concentration of 5-HT in either group but significantly reduced the 5-HIAA concentration in both the lithium and control groups.

Table 11.4. The effect of lithium and of chlorimipramine on the forebrain concentration of 5-HT and 5-HIAA (ng/g wet weight)

	5-HT concentration (ng/g)		5-HIAA concentration (ng/g)	
	Control	Lithium	Control	Lithium
Saline	614 ± 67	562 ± 42	334 ± 17	374 ± 13*
CMH	537 ± 56	572 ± 38	294 ± 12	279 ± 10
Difference	-77 ± 95	+10 ± 42	-40 ± 17	95 ± 9
p	NS	NS	p<0.05	p<0.001

Results are expressed as the mean ± SEM of nine animals and analysed by the paired t test. (*indicates significant difference between lithium and control animals p < 0.01)

The changes in forebrain 5-hydroxyindoles induced by raphe stimulation in controls and lithium treated animals is shown in Table 11.5. It can be

Table 11.5. The effect of chlorimipramine (CMI) (5 mg/kg i.p.) on the changes in forebrain 5-HT and 5-HIAA concentration induced by raphe stimulation in control animals and in animals which had received 10 day lithium treatment

	Change in 5-HT conc. (ng/g)		Change in 5-HIAA conc. (ng/g)	
	Control	Lithium	Control	Lithium
Saline	+44 ± 53	+71 ± 50	+93 ± 12	+98 ± 21
CMI	+116 ± 59	-42 ± 51	-16 ± 15	+78 ± 74
Difference	+72 ± 99	-109 ± 20	-113 ± 48	-20 ± 22
p	NS	p 0.001	p 0.05	NS

The results are expressed as the mean change ± SEM of nine pairs of animals in each group and analysed by the paired t test (+ and - indicate increases and decreases respectively in 5-hydroxyindole concentration following raphe stimulation).

seen from Table 11.5 that raphe stimulation increased slightly but not significantly the concentration of 5-HT and increased significantly the concentration of 5-HIAA in both the control ($p < 0.001$) and lithium ($p < 0.01$) treated groups. Chlorimipramine had no effect on the change in 5-HT induced by raphe stimulation in the control group but significantly reduced that seen in the lithium group. The increase in 5-HIAA induced by raphe stimulation was completely abolished by chlorimipramine in the control group whereas in the lithium treated group, chlorimipramine failed to reduce significantly the response to stimulation.

The effect of lithium and chlorimipramine on 5-HT uptake into synaptosomes.

The effect of treatment with chlorimipramine on the uptake of 5-HT by synaptosomes prepared from rats treated for 10 days with saline or lithium is shown in Table 11.6. It can be seen that treatment with chlorimipramine significantly reduced the uptake of 5-HT in both the control and lithium treated groups. Furthermore, the degree of inhibition was similar in both groups.

Table 11.6. The effect of chlorimipramine (5 mg/kg/i.p.) on the uptake of 5-HT by synaptosomes prepared from control rats and rats treated with lithium for 10 days

	5-HPT uptake (pmol/mg protein)	
	Saline	Chlorimipramine
Control	15.057 ± 0.624	12.699 ± 0.703*
Lithium	14.369 ± 0.549	11.631 ± 0.724**

The results are expressed as the mean ± SEM of 9 rats. The effect of chlorimipramine is analysed by the Student's t test (* $p<0.05$, ** $p<0.001$)

The results of the study in which the effect of chlorimipramine *in vitro* on the uptake of 5-HT was examined in the presence or absence of lithium is shown in Table 11.7. The uptake of 5-HT was significantly reduced by chlorimipramine in both the presence and absence of lithium. Again the degree to which chlorimipramine reduced the uptake of 5-HT was similar whether lithium was present or absent from the incubation medium.

Table 11.7. The effect of chlorimipramine in vitro (4×10^{-7}M) on the synaptosomal uptake of 5-HT in the presence or absence of lithium in the incubation medium

	5-HT uptake (pmol/mg protein)	
	No chlorimipramine	Chlorimipramine
Control	15.091 ± 1.237	6.801 ± 0.481*
Lithium (2.5×10^{-8}M)	15.228 ± 1.358	6.288 ± 0.469*
Control	11.939 ± 1.455	5.227 ± 0.514*
Lithium (3.3×10^{-8}M)	13.006 ± 1.126	5.633 ± 0.789*

Results are expressed as the mean ± SEM of 10 animals. The effect of chlorimipramine is analysed by the Student's test. (* $p<0.001$)

Discussion

Neither lithium nor chlorimipramine had any effect on the concentration of 5-HT in the forebrain of animals which had not received raphe stimulation. Both drugs did, however, affect the concentration of 5-HIAA. Lithium increased the 5-HIAA concentration, and chlorimipramine reduced it in both the lithium treated and control groups of animals.

An increase in 5-HIAA concentration following acute lithium treatment has been previously observed and interpreted as being due to an increase in the synthesis and turnover of 5-HT (25,26). Treatment with lithium for 10 days or more appears to have little effect on turnover (26,27), and it has been suggested that the increase in 5-HIAA following 10 day treatment may be related to a possible impairment of the 5-HT storage mechanism within nerve terminals (6,7).

As mentioned previously, the reduction in 5-HIAA concentration following chlorimipramine treatment has been interpreted as being due to the inhibition of 5-HT uptake denying extraneuronally released 5-HT access to intracellular MAO. It does not appear to be related to a change in synthesis or turnover (4). Increasing the activity of 5-HT neurones by stimulation of the nucleus raphe medianus should therefore enhance the effect of chlorimipramine on the concentration of 5-HIAA (4,28). This was the case in the control group of animals where the increase in 5-HIAA by raphe stimulation was completely abolished by chlorimipramine. However in the lithium group, the increase in 5-HIAA following raphe stimulation was unaffected by chlorimipramine. The difference observed between the two groups may indicate that in the lithium treated group, the 5-HIAA produced by stimulation is derived from 5-HT which remained predominantly within the intracellular compartment, or that lithium was antagonizing the inhibition of 5-HT uptake by chlorimipramine. If the latter were the case, released 5-HT would still be able to gain access to intracellular MAO.

In order to investigate the second possibility, the interaction between lithium and chlorimipramine on synaptosomal uptake of 5-HT was examined. Both treatment with lithium and the addition of lithium to synaptosomal suspensions *in vitro* had no apparent effect on the ability of chlorimipramine to inhibit 5-HT uptake into synaptosomes. The small extent to which uptake was inhibited by prior treatment with chlorimipramine was probably due to loss of the drug during the extraction of the synaptosomes (29).

It would appear therefore that the increase in 5-HIAA produced by raphe stimulation in the lithium treated animals may well be derived from the metabolism of 5-HT which remains within the intracellular compartment. Within the nerve terminal it is believed that stored 5-HT is protected from deamination while free cytoplasmic 5-HT can be metabolized by monoamine oxidase (1). It can be suggested therefore that lithium interferes with stimulus-release coupling in such a way that 5-HT is released from the storage sites into the cytoplasm rather than the synaptic cleft. Such an effect would require lithium to interfere with the location of the transmitter store within the nerve terminal membrane.

A further point of interest from this study is the fact that chlorimipramine was able to reduce the resting concentration of 5-HIAA in lithium treated animals but not that produced by stimulation. This may indicate that the proposed effect of lithium on 5-HT is only manifest during periods in which the 5-HT neurones are highly active.

The relationship between the possible effect of lithium on the storage of 5-HT discussed previously and the proposed effect of lithium on stimulus-release coupling has yet to be determined.

ACKNOWLEDGEMENT

I should like to express my gratitude to Dr M.H.T. Roberts for his helpful advice on the preparation of the paper, and to Miss Patricia Dummer for typing the manuscript.

References

1. Moir, A.T.B. and Eccleston, D. (1968). *J. Neurochem.,* **15,** 1093
2. Aghajanian, G.K., Rosecrans, J.A. and Sheard, M.H. (1967). *Science,* **156,** 402
3. Kostowski, W.E., Giacolone, E., Garattini, S. and Valzelli, L. (1969). *Eur. J. Pharmacol.,* **7,** *170*
4. Collard, K.J. and Roberts, M.H.T. (1974). *Eur. J. Pharmacol.,* **29,** 154
5. Himwich, H.E. and Alpers, H.S. (1970). *Ann. Rev. Pharmacol.,* **10,** 313
6. Collard, K.J. and Roberts, M.H.T. (1975). *Br. J. Pharmacol.,* **55,** 268P
7. Collard, K.J. and Roberts, M.H.T. (1977). *Neuropharmacology,* (In press)
8. Schildkraut, J.J., Schanberg, S.M. and Kopin, I.J. (1966). *Life Sci,* **5,** 1479
9. Schildkraut, J.J., Logue, M.A. and Dodge, G.A. (1969). *Psychopharmacology,* **14,** 135
10. Lapin, I.P. and Oxenkrug, G.F. (1969). *N. Eng. J. Med.* **281,** 218
11. Grey, K.F. and Pletscher, A. (1961). *J. Neurochem.,* **6,** 239
12. Kurokawa, M., Sakamoto, T. and Kato, M. (1965). *Biochim. Biophys. Acta,* **94,** 307
13. Wadja, I.J., Manigault, I., Hudick, J.P. and Lajtha, A (1973).*J. Neurochem.,* **21,** 1385
14. De Robertis, E., Pellegrino de Iraldi, A., Rodriguez de Lores Arnaiz, G. and Zieher, L.M. (1965). *Life Sci.,* **4,** 193
15. Lowry, O.H., Rosebrough, N.J., Farr, A.L. and Randall, R.J. (1951). *J. Biol. Chem.,* **193,** 265
16. Harada, M. and Nagatsu, T. (1973). *Anal. Biochem.,* **56,** 283
17. DeFeudis, D.V. (1972) *Brain Res.,* **43,** 686
18. Tamir, H. and Huang T-Y. L. (1974) *Life Sci.,* **14,** 83
19. Tamir, H. and Rapport, M. (1976). *Res. Commun. Chem. Pathol. Pharmacol.,* **13,** 225
20. Collard, K.J. (1976). *Br. J. Pharmacol.,* **57,** 446P
21. Quat, W.B. (1968). *Am. J. Physiol.,* **215,** 1448

21. Quat, W.B. (1968). Difference in circadian rhythms in 5-hydroxy-tryptamine according to brain region. *Am. J. Physiol.,* **215,** 1448
22. Okada, F. (1971). *Life Sci.,* **10,** 77
23. Hery, F., Rouer, E. and Glowinski, J. (1972). *Brain Res.,* **43,** 445
24. Schacht, U. and Heptner, W. (1974). *Biochem. Pharmacol.,* **23,** 3413
25. Poitou, P., Guerinot, F. and Bohuon, C. (1974). *Psychopharmacology,* **38,** 75
26. Knapp, S. and Mandell, A.J. (1973). *Science,* **180,** 645
27. Samanin, R., Ghezzi, D. and Garattini, S. (1972). *Eur. J. Pharmacol.,* **20,** 281
28. Bliss, E.L. and Ailion, J. (1970). *Brain Res.,* **24,** 305
29. Hunt, P.F., Kannengeisser, M.H. and Raynaud, J.P. (1975). *Biochem. Pharmacol.,* **24,** 681

12

Lithium Effects on Carbohydrate Metabolism

J. H. LAZARUS

INTRODUCTION

The fact that many patients receiving lithium gain weight (1,2) has led to suggestions that lithium has an effect on carbohydrate metabolism. Although no unitary action of lithium on carbohydrate metabolism has been defined several changes have been described as a result of observations in humans and in animals (3-5).

Studies of glucose tolerance in patients taking lithium have shown that blood glucose can be unchanged or increased, and oral glucose tolerance has been found to be increased or decreased (6-8); glucose utilization after intravenous glucose loading was also increased in one study (9). In many of these human studies changes in the parameters of carbohydrate metabolism have been only slight and interpretation has been made more difficult because of methodological problems as well as lack of control data concerning insulin and glucose levels in psychiatric patients not taking lithium or any other drugs.

More definitive information is available from animal experiments. Studies using rat hemidiaphragm incubations have demonstrated that the lithium ion increases the uptake of glucose into the muscle as well as increasing its utilization (10-15). In the in vitro experiments, where it was noted that lithium had effects on glucose uptake into diaphragm, an increase in glycogen synthesis and concentration at different times after lithium administration was also observed (13-15). *In vivo* experiments in which rats were injected intraperitoneally with lithium ions also resulted in an increase in glycogen deposition and in glycogen synthesis in the diagphragm (16). However, data on liver glycogen distribution after lithium administration *in vivo* are contradictory. For example, in one study (17) an increase in rat liver glycogen was found whereas the converse has been reported in experiments involving shorter times of exposure to lithium (18). The mechanism of these effects of lithium action are not understood but attention has been paid to the many effects of lithium on enzymes concerned in carbohydrate metabolism (5).

In view of the discrepancies noted in the effect of lithium on liver glycogen concentration it seemed important to investigate some variables which might affect this action. Similarly, previous data have demonstrated that lithium can cause an inhibition of insulin release in isolated pieces of rat pancreas and an increase in insulin release under other conditions (4). This prompted the present studies on insulin and glucose levels in human volunteers.

MATERIALS AND METHODS

Animal studies

63 female Wistar rats weres studied. They were divided into three groups according to weight. Animals in group A weighed 90-110 g, those in group B 130-150 g and those in group C 175-195 g. The animals were fed a normal laboratory diet with water ad lib. All experiments were performed in the morning and food was withdrawn during this time. The appropriate dose oif lithium chloride (Alnar) was made up to an injection volume of 1.0 ml with deionised water, and physiological saline was used as the control injection. All injections were administered intraperitoneally. Animals were killed 3 h after injection by a blow on the head. Venous blood was obtained from the jugular veins; the liver and the skeletal muscle from the hind leg was removed and placed in ice-cold physiological saline. Serum lithium was estimated by flame photometry. Liver and muscle glycogen was estimated as follows: 1 g of tissue was homogenised in 10 ml physiological saline. Sodium acetate buffer (pH 4.8) was prepared containing the glycogen debranching enzymes, 50 micrograms/ml glucosidase and 100 micrograms/ml amylo-alpha-1, 4-alpha-1, 6-glucosidase (EC 3.2.1). Incubation of 100 microlitres homogenate and 50 microlitres buffer was carried out at 30 °C for 60 min. Glucose was then estimated by the hexokinase method (19) and tissue glycogen expressed as mg/g wet tissue wt. N-terminal plasma glucagon (total plasma

glucagon) was measured by radioimmunoassay (20) in pooled plasma samples from each dose range.

Human studies

Six normal healthy male volunteers aged 24-40 were studied. All were within 10% of ideal body weight as judged by life insurance tables and had no present or past history of endocrine or metabolic disorder.

After an overnight fast, intravenous canulae were inserted into both antecubital veins and the subject was allowed to rest for 20-30 min. The canulae were kept patent by a slow infusion of normal saline. Glucose (0.5 g/kg body wt) was administered rapidly (over 2 min) intravenously at time 0 through one canula which was then removed. Blood samples were taken from the other canula at -10, 0, 3, 5, 7, 10, 15, 30, 45, 60, 90 and 120 min. At this time, 20 mg/kg body wt. tolbutamide was given intravenously and blood sampling continued at 123, 125, 127, 130, 135, 150, 165 and 180 min. Samples were analysed for glucose and insulin (21).

Following the control experiment all subjects took lithium carbonate B.P. 250 mg twice or three times a day for one week such that serum lithium levels (checked on the 5th day) were within the therapeutic range (0.5-1.5 mmol/l).

At the end of 7 days treatment the study was repeated in an identical way. The morning dose of lithium was taken about 1 h before starting the repeat study.

RESULTS

Animal study

Serum lithium varied between 0.2 and 0.4 mmol/l following the 200 micromoles dose, 0.6-1.8 mmol/l following the 500 micromoles injection and between 1.9 and 2.3 mmol/l at higher dose levels of injected lithium chloride. The effect of injected LiCl on liver glycogen levels in the different groups is shown in Table 12.1.

In all groups there was a significant fall of liver glycogen concentration 3 h after injection of 500 micromoles of LiCl as compared to the control group. In groups A and B a dose of 200 micromoles LiCl also produced a substantial fall in liver glycogen.

When a higher dose of LiCl was injected (1000 micromoles) liver glycogen levels in groups A and B did not differ from the control values and were significantly higher than those found after a dose of 500 micromoles. In contrast, liver glycogen was significantly lowered in

Table 12.1. Lithium effects on liver glycogen and plasma glucagon

Animals	Dose of lithium chloride (micromoles)	Dose of lithium chloride (micromoles/kg body wt)	Liver glycogen (mg/g wet liver wt)		Plasma glucagon (pg/ml)
	0		18.5 ± 0.4	(8)	150
Group A	200	2.0	13.0	(2)	180
(90-110 g)	500	5.0	7.8 ± 2.0 d	(8)	200
	1000	10.0	18.9 ± 0.8	(8)	340
	0		24.9 ± 0.3	(6)	220
Group B	200	1.43	14.8 ± 0.4	(3)	140
(130-150 g)	500	3.56	15.2 ± 1.3 c	(6)	160
	1000	7.1	23.9 ± 2.3	(4)	110
	0		24.8 ± 2.2	(6)	1040
Group C	200	—	—		—
(175-195 g)	500	2.7	18.6 ± 1.8 a	(6)	140
	1000	5.4	16.8 ± 2.3 b	(6)	200

Liver glycogen (mg/g wet liver wt) 3 h after intraperitoneal injection of varying doses of lithium chloride to rats of different weights. Values are shown as mean ± 1 SE. Numbers in brackets refer to number of rats used.
p values refer to significant differences in liver glycogen from control values.
— = not studied.
Differences in plasma glucagon of more than 18 pg/ml are significant at a level of $p < 0.05$.
a $p < 0.05$; b $p < 0.025$; c $p < 0.005$; d $p < 0.0025$.

the heaviest animals following 1000 micromoles of LiCl and was not different from the level found after injection fo 500 micromoles LiCl. When the results were expressed in relation to the dose of administered LiCl per kg body wt the reduction in liver glycogen observed in this group was still present.

Skeletal muscle glycogen levels were not related to body weight. Mean muscle glycogen was 2.40 mg/g wet muscle wt ± 0.37 (SE) in animals given control injections of saline. Following 500 micromoles of LiCl mean muscle glycogen rose significantly ($p < 0.0125$) to 4.40 ± 0.23 mg/g wet muscle wt. A further significant rise in this value to 5.40 ± 0.32 was noted in animals receiving 1000 micromoles LiCl ($p < 0.0125$).

Apart from a high level of 1040 pg/ml seen in the control animals in group C, plasma glucagon levels ranged between 100 and 340 pg/ml (Table 12.1). There was no correlation between plasma glucagon and either liver glycogen or the percentage fall in liver glycogen in any of the groups or for all the groups taken together.

Human study

Figures 12.1 and 12.2 show the mean values for plasma glucose and insulin before and after lithium administration. The mean fasting basal plasma glucose concentrations were not significantly different; there was no significant difference between the glucose values observed in response to i.v. glucose (up to 120 min) although there was a tendency to reduced levels while on lithium. In contrast, blood glucose was significantly lower in the subjects while on lithium in response to tolbutamide injection (123-180 min). During this period the mean blood glucose was at least 20% lower than the mean value before lithium and at 135 min and 150 min it fell by 40% and 44% of control values respectively (Figure 12.3).

Mean insulin concentrations, although higher (Figure 12.2), were not significantly so. Analysis of individual subjects showed, however, that in three there were highly significant rises in insulin levels between 123 and 150 min ($p < 0.001$ by paired t test). In two subjects there was a fall in insulin levels and in one there was no change. In the two subjects who had an insulin fall the blood sugars also were lower during this time compared

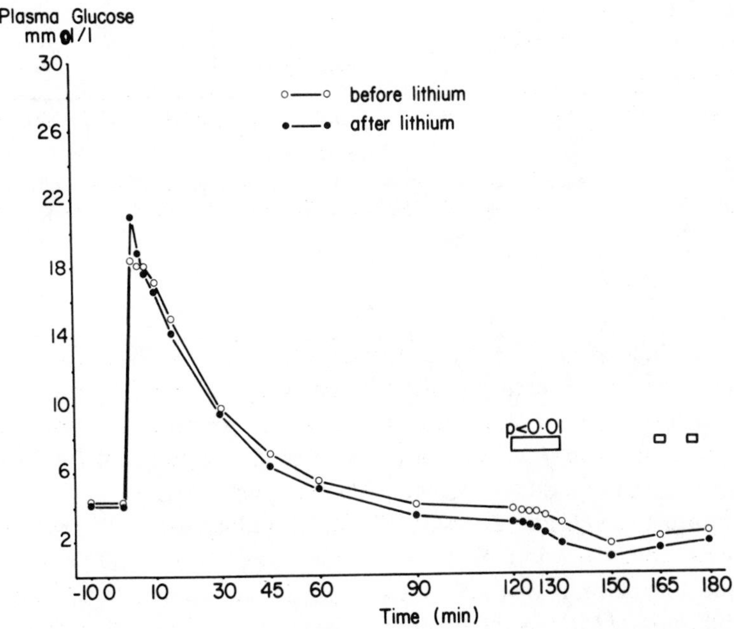

Figure 12.1. Plasma glucose concentrations (mmol/l) during intravenous glucose, tolbutamide tolerance test. Arrows indicate time of administration of glucose and tolbutamide. Standard errors are not shown because of scale. Boxes indicate significant differences between values before and after lithium.

to values in the control study. The effect of these changes was to increase insulin/glucose ratios in all subjects and this is reflected by a mean rise of up to 121% at 135 min and 152% at 150 min (Figure 12.3) of control values.

There was no significant change in body weight, serum electrolytes, cholesterol or triglyceride concentrations during the study.

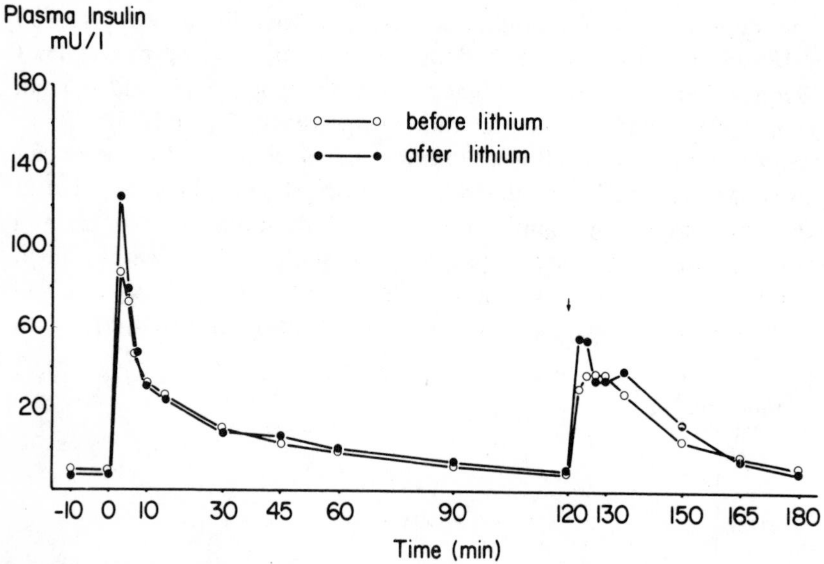

Figure 12.2. Plasma insulin concentrations (mU/l) during intravenous glucose, tolbutamide tolerance test. Arrow shows time of tolubtamide injection. Standard errors not shown because of scale.

DISCUSSION

Acute administration of 500 micromoles LiCl led to a significant fall in liver glycogen in all three groups of animals in 3 h. Similar results were found in 100 g rats 5 h after receiving 200-600 micromoles LiCl by Plenge *et al.* (16). Mellerup *et al.* (22) also documented a significant fall in liver glycogen in similar animals receiving 900 micromoles LiCl.

In contrast Krulik and Zvolsky (17) found an increase in liver glycogen following administration of LiCl (1-2 mmol/kg/day) to 170 g rats for 10 days. Furthermore, in the present study an administered dose of 1000 micromoles LiCl in the two lighter groups of animals did not lead to a fall in liver glycogen whereas a pronounced decrease was noted with this dose by Plenge *et al.* (16) in animals of similar weight. The time difference

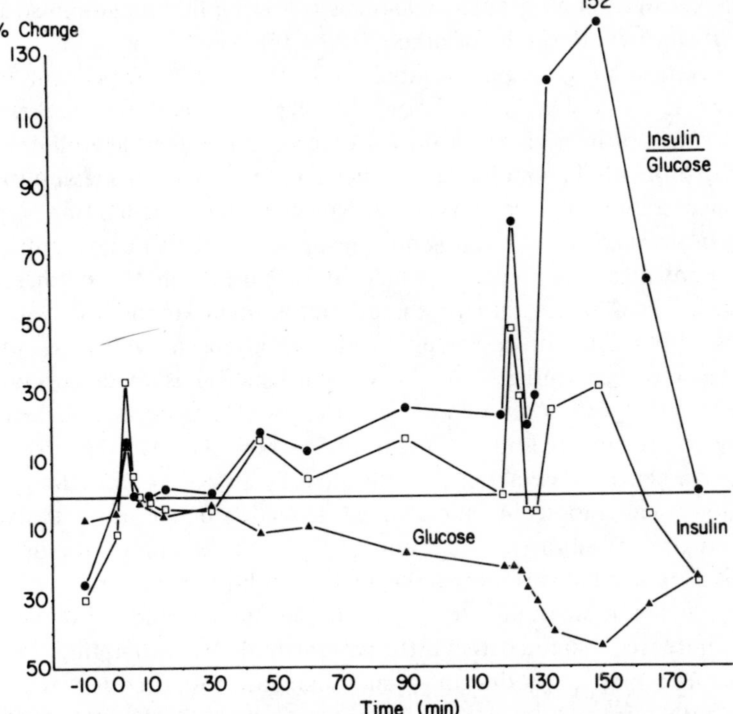

Figure 12.3. Percentage change in plasma glucose (▲), plasma insulin (□) and insulin: glucose ratios (●) after one week of lithium administration during intravenous glucose, tolbutamide tolerance test. The horizontal line indicates 0% and values below this indicate negative changes.

is unlikely to explain this as these authors found a similar fall in liver glycogen 3 h after administration of 900 micromoles LiCl.

The percentage fall of liver glycogen was not related to total body weight. However, the possibility remains that the reduction in hepatic glycogen concentration is related to total liver weight as this was not measured. Mellerup *et al.* (22) found that total glucagon like activity was increased in the plasma after lithium administration and suggested that this (together with an increase in liver phosphorylase activity) accounted for the observed decrease in liver glycogen.

The values of plasma N-terminal reactive glucagon (total glucagon-like activity) found in the present study tended to decrease following lithium administration in groups B and C although this decrease was not statistically significant. Thus, no definite relationship between plasma glucagon and liver glycogen has been found in this study. The rise in muscle glycogen in all groups of animals following lithium administration is in agreement with results of others (13,14,16).

The control of glycogen metabolism in the liver is dependent on a complex series of regulatory enzymatic steps (23) and this makes the measurement of liver glycogen only a crude end point in determining the effect of lithium. The major factor that controls glycogen metabolism is the concentration of phosphorylase a, which catalyses the limiting step of glycogen breakdown. Lithium is not known to affect this enzyme directly but is known to affect factors which are important in the synthesis of glycogen. Thus lithium inhibits the enzyme protein kinase (24) which in turn is responsible for removing the active glycogen synthetase which promotes glycogen synthesis. As the whole mechanism is under the control of cyclic AMP lithium may also affect it by its effects on this nucleotide. Clearly, more investigation is required to show whether the effect of lithium on glycogen metabolism is mediated by an action on cyclic AMP, an action via alterations in cation milieu, an action on enzyme activity, or a combination of all three. The results of this study emphasize the importance of experimental variables in the analysis of lithium effects.

The glucose toblutamide test used in the human study provides an opportunity to examine two different methods of promoting insulin release. The first, a routine intravenous glucose tolerance test was not significantly affected by lithium administration. Lithium did cause a significant fall in plasma glucose during tolbutamide infusion despite the fact that not all subjects showed a significant rise in insulin secretion. The insulin secretion is dependent in part on the ambient glucose concentration at the start of the tolbutamide infusion and variation in this may have altered the results. A separate tolbutamide test was not practical in this study. Nevertheless a dramatic increase in insulin/glucose ratios was noted and an overall increase in insulin secretion is strongly suggested.

While the precise details of insulin secretion have not been defined the process is known to be dependent on the ambient concentration of cyclic AMP, glucose and calcium ions in the pancreatic islets (25).

In addition it has been suggested that the actual mechanics of insulin release are dependent on the intracellular integrity of the microtubules and microfilaments (26). There is evidence that disruption of microfilaments leads to an increase in insulin secretion rate in pancreatic B cells (27). Direct effects of lithium on microtubules in the pancreas have not been demonstrated but other tissues have been examined in this respect. For example, in the thyroid gland, disruption of microtubules is known to cause an inhibition of thyroid hormone secretion (28). Lithium also inhibits thyroid hormone secretion (29) and recent evidence suggests that this effect is mediated by microtubular disruption (30). Thus the fact that lithium has opposite effects on hormone secretion from two glands may be explained, at least in part, by its action on microtubules. Further investigation is required into the effect of lithium on the role of calcium in microtubular function in view of the importance of the latter in hormone secretory processes.

Lithium, then, appears slightly to stimulate insulin secretion in the human as measured over a short time period. A study to assess the potential value of this cation in the management of maturity onset diabetes mellitus is now required.

ACKNOWLEDGEMENTS

I thank Dr R.H. Greenwood for collaboration in the human studies. I am grateful to Dr K.D. Buchanan for assay of plasma glucagon and to Dr S. Luzio for the plasma insulin measurements.

References

1. Kerry, R.J., Liebling, L.I. and Owen, G. (1970). *Acta Psychiat. Scand.*, **46**, 238
2. Mellerup, E.T., Thomsen, H.G., Bjorum, N. and Rafaelsen, O.J. (1972). *Acta Psychiat. Scand.*, **48**, 332
3. Mellerup, E.T., Plenge, P. and Rafaelsen, O.J. (1974). *Dan. Med. Bull.*, **21**, 88
4. Mellerup, E.T. and Rafaelsen, O.J. (1974). In: J.R. Boissier, H. Hippius and P. Pichot (eds.) *Neuropsychopharmacology* pp. 617-620. (Amsterdam: Excerpta Medica)
5. Mellerup, E.T. and Rafaelsen, O.J. (1975). In: F.N. Johnson (ed.) *Lithium Research and Therapy* pp. 381-389. (London: Academic Press)
6. Van der Velde, C.D. and Gordon, M.W. (1969). *Arch. Gen. Psychiat.*, **21**, 478
7. Shopsin, B., Stern, S. and Gershon, S. (1972). *Arch. Gen. Psychiat.*, **26**, 566
8. Vendsborg, P.B., Mellerup, E.T. and Rafaelsen, O.J. (1973). *Acta Psychiat. Scand.*, **49**, 97
9. Heninger, G.R., Mueller, P.S. (1970). *Arch. Gen. Psychiat.*, **23**, 310
10. Bhattacharya, G. (1959). *Nature,* **183**, 324
11. Bhattacharya, G. (1961). *Biochem, J.*, **79**, 369
12. Bhattacharya, G. (1964). *Biochim. Biophys. Acta.*, **93**, 644
13. Clausen, T. (1968). *Biochim. Biophys, Acta.*, **150**, 66
14. Haugaard, E.S., Serlick, E. and Haugaard, N. (1973). *Biochem. Pharmacol.*, **22**, 1023
15. Haugaard, E.S., Frazer, A., Mendels, J. and Haugaard, N. (1975). *Biochem. Pharacol.*, **24**, 1187
16. Plenge, P., Mellerup, E.T. and Rafaelsen, O.J. (1970). *J. Psychiat. Res.*, **8**, 29
17. Krulik, R. and Zvolsky, P. (1970). *Activ. Nerv. Suppl.*, **12**, 279
18. Plenge, P., Mellerup, E.T. and Rafaelsen, O.J. (1969). *Lancet,* **ii**, 1012
19. Sleia, M.W. (1969). In: H.U. Bergmeyer (ed) *Methods of Enzymatic Analysis,* pp. 117-123. (New York: Academic Press)
20. Buchanan, K.D. (1973). In: *Studies on the pancreatic-enteric hormones. Ph.D. Thesis,* Queens University of Belfast
21. Hales, C.N., Randle, P.J. (1963). *Biochem. J.*, **88**, 137

22. Mellerup, E.T., Thomsen, H.G., Plenge, P. and Rafaelsen, O.J. (1970). *J. Psychiat. Res.,* **8,** 37
23. Hers, H.G. (1976). *Ann. Rev. Biochem.,* **45,** 167
24. Horn, R.A., Walaas, O. and Walaas, E. (1973). *Biochim. Biophys. Acta,* **313,** 296
25. Cerasi, E. and Luft, R. (1976). In: R. Luft (ed.) *Insulin,* pp. 109-137
26. Gepts, W. and Pipeleers, D. (1976). In: R. Luft (ed.) *Insulin,* pp. 7-52
27. Orci, L., Gabbay, K.H. and Malaisse, W.J. (1972). *Science,* **175,** 1128
28. Wolff, J. and Bhattacharyya, B. (1975). *Ann. N.Y. Acad. Sci.,* **253,** 763
29. Spaulding, S.W., Burrow, G.N. Bermudez, F. and Himmelhoch, J.M. (1972). *J. Clin. Endocrinol. Metab.,* **35,** 905
30. Bhattacharyya, B. and Wolff, J. (1976). *Biochem. Biophys. Res. Comm.,* **73,** 383

13

Lithium Effects on Rat Brain Glucose Metabolism in Long-Term Lithium-Treated Rats

P. PLENGE

INTRODUCTION

In reports on different aspects of pharmacological effects of lithium in rats, e.g. on kidney water re-absorption, brain dopamine and brain serotonin metabolism (1-3) it can be seen that the effect of lithium is dependent on, or enhanced by, peak values in the body lithium concentration produced by injection of lithium, in contrast to administration of lithium via the food. Also, in manic-depressive patients receiving lithium treatment some pharmacological effects seems to be connected with the increase in serum lithium concentration following the intake of the daily dose of lithium (4). This holds true for the decrease in serum phosphate concentration (5) and the increase in glucose tolerance (6) following the intake of a normal dose of lithium in patients on prophylactic lithium treatment.

In the present study the concentration and turnover of different brain metabolites was measured in long term lithium treated rats. By investigating the parameters at different times after the administration of lithium, results were found which indicated that most of the effects of lithium on the above-mentioned parameters were dependent on the changes of lithium concentration, rather than on the absolute concentration of lithium in the brain.

METHODS

Experimental procedure

Female Wistar rats, weighing about 100 g at the start of the experiment were used. They were injected intraperitoneally once daily for 15 days in the morning with 400 micromoles of either NaCl or LiCl. The rats had free access to food and to 50 mM NaCl as drinking solution. Using this procedure the lithium treated rats increased their weight more than the control rats did: average weight increases from the four experiments were: control rats 3.76 g/day, lithium treated rats 4.37 g/day, $p < 0.001$, paired t-test, two tailed.

Analysis

The two cerebral hemispheres were used for analysis of glucose, glucose-6-phosphate, fructose-1.6-diphosphate, lactate, 6-phosphogluconate, malate, citrate, alpha-ketoglutarate, glutamate and glycogen (7). The specific activities of glucose, glutamate and glycogen were determined as previously described (8). Blood was taken from the frozen heart and the concentration and specific activity of blood glucose were determined (8).

Brain and serum lithium concentrations were determined in a separate experiment, using atomic absorption spectrophotometry.

The significances of the differences between the means were determined using Student's t test (two tailed).

RESULTS

The concentration of lithium in brain and serum, 1 to 8 hours after the injection of lithium in rats treated with one daily injection of 400 micromoles of lithium is seen in Figure 13.1. It is seen that brain lithium concentration varied between 0.3 mmol/kg 24 hours after the injection, to a maximum of about 0.8 mmol/kg about 6 hours after the injection. The serum lithium concentration varied between 0.15 mmol/l and 2.3 mmol/l respectively 24 hours and 1 hour after the injection of lithium.

The concentration of the different brain metabolites 1, 2, 4 and 8 hours after the injection of lithium are shown in Table 13.1. As a general picture it is seen that, for most of the metabolites, the deviations from control level are most marked 1 and 2 hours after the injection; after 4, and especially after 8 hours the lithium effect is wearing off.

The specific activities of the different metabolites and the total amount of radioactivity in the brains were expressed relative to the specific activity

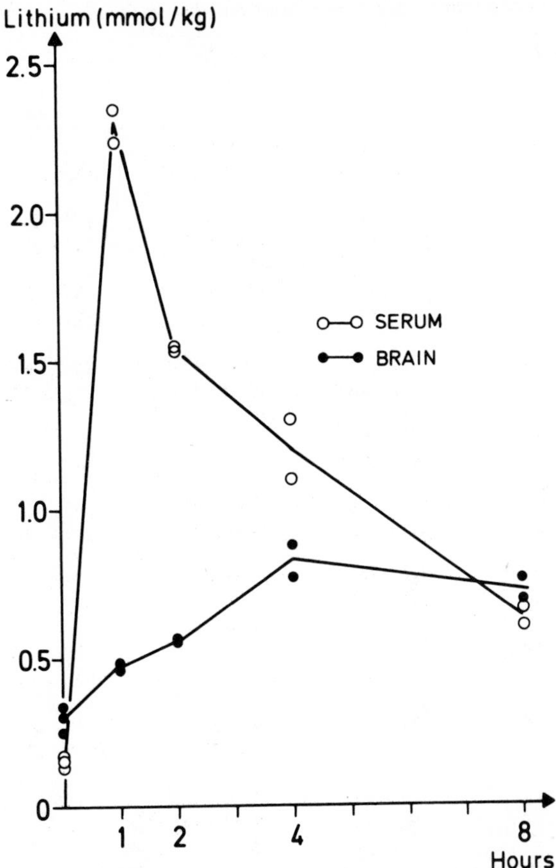

Figure 13.1. Lithium concentration in blood and brain in long-term lithium treated rats, 1-8 hours after the last intraperitoneal injection of 400 micromoles of LiCl. 2-3 rats at each point.

of the blood glucose, thus correcting for variability in uptake of radioactive glucose from the peritoneal cavity in the individual rats.

The total amount of radioactivity in the brains relative to the specific activity of blood glucose is shown in Figure 13.2. It can be seen that lithium increased the uptake of radioactive glucose in the brain, 4 minutes after the injection of radioactive glucose, 1, 2, 4, and 8 hours after the injection of lithium.

Figure 13.3 presents the specific activity of brain glycogen relative to the specific activity of blood glucose. Lithium decreased the relative specific activity of glycogen, 1, 2 and 4 hours after the injection, with a return to control values 8 hours after the injection of lithium. The total amount of

Table 13.1. Concentrations of different brain metabolites in long-term lithium treated rats

Brain metabolite	Treatment	Time since last injection			
		1 hour	2 hours	4 hours	8 hours
Glucose	Na	1186 ± 186	1200 ± 150	961 ± 159	1450 ± 242
	Li	1690 ± 246[d]	1540 ± 240[d]	1065 ± 104[d]	1463 ± 249
Glucose-6-P	Na	138 ± 21	120 ± 14	137 ± 25	147 ± 14
	Li	158 ± 19[c]	130 ± 17[a]	145 ± 21	163 ± 16[c]
Fructose-1,6-P2	Na	135 ± 21	133 ± 13	155 ± 12	121 ± 17
	Li	143 ± 19	146 ± 15[b]	173 ± 20[b]	121 ± 19
Lactate	Na	1944 ± 177	2900 ± 400	2662 ± 493	2785 ± 449
	Li	1796 ± 186[b]	2820 ± 430	2727 ± 482	2834 ± 307
6-P-Gluconate	Na	23.8 ± 1.8	10.4 ± 1.2	27.8 ± 3.9	11.7 ± 1.1
	Li	25.6 ± 1.5[d]	11.7 ± 0.9[c]	29.3 ± 3.3	12.0 ± 1.0
Glycogen	Na	2940 ± 230	2920 ± 200	2930 ± 255	2840 ± 210
	Li	3420 ± 240[d]	3360 ± 270[d]	3670 ± 363[d]	3010 ± 250[b]
Citrate	Na	411 ± 73	291 ± 34	374 ± 91	436 ± 69
	Li	363 ± 44[a]	315 ± 31[a]	395 ± 99	403 ± 87
Alpha-keto-Glutarate	Na	55.1 ± 10.8	—	72.6 ± 8.2	55.5 ± 9.1
	Li	65.4 ± 9.3[c]	—	65.5 ± 10.6[a]	57.9 ± 11.0
Malate	Na	473 ± 36	534 ± 21	548 ± 24	369 ± 17
	Li	471 ± 27	512 ± 29[b]	539 ± 29	384 ± 15[c]
Glutamate	Na	13141 ± 339	13300 ± 408	13630 ± 342	13785 ± 353
	Li	13069 ± 546	12650 ± 348[d]	13470 ± 267	14062 ± 257[c]

Concentrations expressed as nmol/g brain w.w. ± SD (15 to 20 rats involved in each mean score).
Treatments consisted of 400 micromoles NaCl or LiCl.
a: $p < 0.05$; b: $p < 0.025$; c: $p < 0.01$; d: $p < 0.001$.

radioactive glucose being incorporated into brain glycogen, 12 minutes after the injection of radioactive glucose and 1, 2, 4 and 8 hours after the injection of lithium is seen in Table 13.2. The table shows that lithium decreased the turn-over of glycogen 1 and 2 hours after the injection of lithium, with a return to normal 4 hours after the injection.

The specific activity of brain glutamate relative to the specific activity of blood glucose is seen in Figure 13.4. Lithium was found to decrease the turnover of glutamate 1 and 2 hours after the injection. In contrast to this, it is seen that lithium increased the turnover of glutamate 4 hours after the injection with a return to control turnover 8 hours after the injection of lithium.

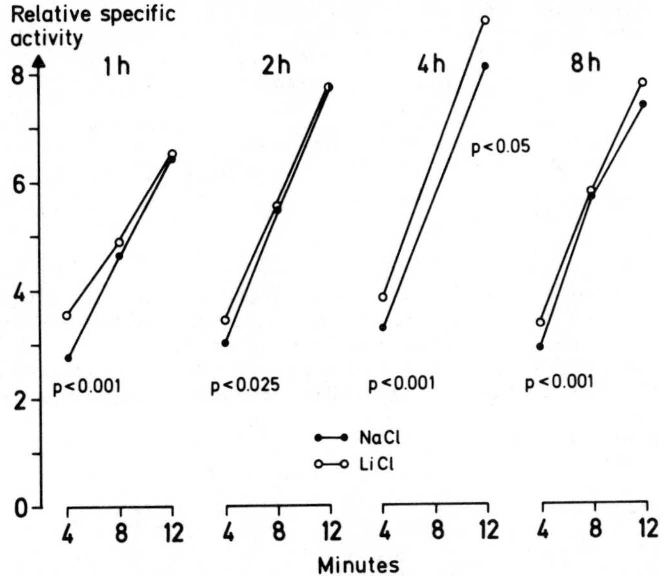

Figure 13.2. Total radioactivity in brain perchloric acid extract relative to a specific activity of 10 000 DPM/micromol blood glucose in long-term lithium treated rats. The rats were killed by rapid freezing 1-8 hours after the last intraperitoneal injection of 400 micromoles LiCl and 4-12 minutes after injection of radioactive glucose. 4-7 rats at each point.

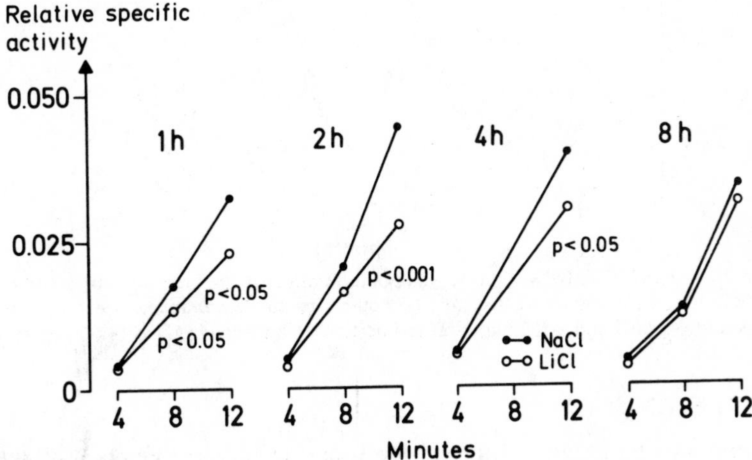

Figure 13.3. Specific activity of brain glycogen relative to the specific activity of blood glucose in long-term lithium treated rats, 1-8 hours after the last intraperitoneal injection of 400 micromoles LiCl and 4-12 minutes after injection of radioactive glucose. 4-7 rats at each point.

Table 13.2. Incorporation of radioactive glucose in rat brain glycogen

	DPM in glycogen/g brian w.w. ± SD Time since last injection			
	1 hour	2 hours	4 hours	8 hours
Control	950 ± 184	1237 ± 220	1125 ± 167	936 ± 206
Lithium	715 ± 154	955 ± 161	1132 ± 246	919 ± 251
p	< 0.05	< 0.025	n.s.	n.s

Incorporation of radioactive glucose in rat brain glycogen 12 minutes after intraperitoneal injection of 10 microCi U-^{14}C D-glucose. The rats were injected once daily for 16 days with 400 micromoles of NaCl or LiCl and frozen in liquid nitrogen 1-8 hours after the last injection. Radioactivity is expressed as DPM in glycogen/g brain w.w. ± SD relative to a specific activity of blood glucose of 10 000 DPM/micromol glucose. 4-5 rats in each group

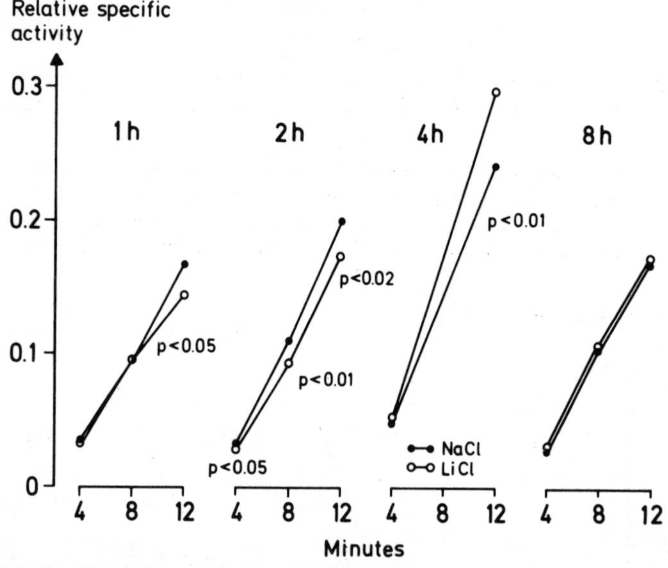

Figure 13.4. Specific activity of brain glutamate relative to the specific activity of blood glucose in long-term lithium treated rats, 1-8 hours after the last intraperitoneal injection of 400 micromoles LiCl and 4-12 minutes after injection of radioactive glucose. 4-7 rats at each point.

DISCUSSION

Lithium has, in *in vitro* studies, been found to increase glucose uptake in isolated rat muscle (9). In experiments with acute administration of a large dose of lithium to rats (8) lithium was found to increase both the uptake and the concentration of glucose in brain. From Figure 13.2 it is seen that lithium also increased the uptake of glucose in the rat brain in long-term treated rats during the first few hours after the daily injection of lithium.

This corresponds well with the results seen in Table 13.1, where lithium was found to increase brain glucose concentration.

The well-known effect of lithium on tissue glycogen concentration was also found in the present experiment, and by the use of radioactive glucose and a time-response curve it has been possible to elucidate the mechanism of the lithium effect further. In Table 13.1 it is seen that lithium increased the concentration of glycogen, and in Figure 13.3 it is seen that the labeling of glycogen was decreased from 1 to 4 hours after the administration of lithium. In table 13.2 there is calculated the amount of radioactive glucose which, in the first 12 minutes after the injection of radioactive glucose, is incorporated in brain glycogen. The table shows that only 1 and 2 hours after the injection of lithium the turnover of brain glycogen was decreased with a normalization 4 hours after the injection of lithium, even though the concentration of glycogen at that time was increased about 30% above control level. These findings together could be taken to indicate that lithium affects glycogen metabolism by inhibiting the breakdown of glycogen.

Brain glutamate was found to be affected by lithium. Table 13.1 and Figure 13.4 show that both the concentration and the turnover of glutamate varied as a function of time after the administration of lithium. Both concentration and turnover of glutamate was found to be decreased 2 hours after the injection of lithium. Four hours after the injection of lithium the glutamate concentration had normalized, but the turnover was increased, and 8 hours after the injection the glutamate concentration was increased and the turnover normalized. The results seem to indicate that lithium inhibits the turnover of glutamate and that, when the lithium concentration stabilizes, the organism counteracts and abolishes the lithium inhibition via homeostatic regulatory mechanisms.

If the effect of lithium on glutamate metabolism is compared with the concentration of lithium in the brain (Figure 13.1) at the different time intervals investigated, another aspect of the lithium effects appears. Lithium only decreases the turnover of glutamate in the period when the concentration of lithium in the brain is increasing: metabolic regulatory mechanisms counteract and abolish the lithium inhibition as soon as the brain lithium concentration is stabilized at its peak concentration. This is illustrated by the increased turnover at 4 hours after lithium administration to re-establish the glutamate concentration, and the "overshoot" at 8 hours after lithium administration, where the glutamate concentration is increased above control level.

The same type of picture is seen in the lithium effect on brain glycogen metabolism; also, the concentration of the other brain metabolites (Table 13.1) indicates that for most of the metabolites the lithium effect is most marked shortly after the injection of lithium, the effect disappearing 8 hours after the injection — at a time when the brain lithium concentration is almost at its highest value.

Similar effects of lithium on other parameters have, as mentioned earlier, been described both in human and in animal studies. The question of whether the therapeutic effect of lithium is in some way connected to the changes in brain and body lithium concentrations which follow the administration of normal lithium preparations, cannot be answered by this investigation, but patients can be treated with good result (4) with a one dose schedule, where the whole 24-hour dose of lithium is administered at bedtime. This treatment schedule gives a change in serum lithium concentration from a peak value of about 1 3 mmol/l to a lowest value of about 0.4 mmol/l (10), and as previously reported (5) some of the blood parameters which were measured were found to follow a pattern similar to the one seen in the present investigation, i.e. changes occurred in the period, where the lithium concentration was increasing.

Such results might tentatively suggest that administration of lithium every second or third day would possibly be sufficient to maintain the prophylactic effect of lithium.

A report (11) showing that electroconvulsive therapy administered with regular time intervals of several weeks can have a prophylactic effect against recurrent depressive episodes similarly indicates that continuous treatment is not necessary in all cases, when a prophylactic effect against manic-depressive episodes is wanted.

References

1. Olesen, O.V., Schou, M. and Thomsen, K. (1976). *Neuropsychobiology,* **2**, 134
2. Stefanini, E., Argiolas, A., Gessa, G.L. and Fadda, F. (1976). *J. Neurochem.,* **27**, 1237
3. Knapp, S. and Mandell, A.J. (1975). *J. Pharmacol. Exp. Ther.,* **193**, 812
4. Bech, P., Vendsborg, P.B. and Rafaelsen, O.J. (1976). *Acta Psychiat. Scand.,* **53**, 70
5. Mellerup, E.T., Lauritsen, B.J., Dam, H. and Rafaelsen, O.J. (1976). *Acta Psychiat. Scand.,* **53**, 360
6. Vendsborg, P.B. (1977). (To be published)
7. Lowry, O.H. and Passoneau, J.V. (1972). *A Flexible System of Enzymatic Analysis.* (New Yor: Academic Press)
8. Plenge, P. (1976). *Int, Pharmacopsychiat.,* **11**, 84
9. Kohn, P.G. and Clausen, T. (1972). *Biochim. Biophys. Acta.,* **225**, 798
10. Lauritsen, B.J., Mellerup, E., Rasmussen, S. and Wildschiødtz, G. (To be published)
11. Stevenson, T.H. and Georghegan, J.J. (1951). *Am. J. Psychiat.,* **107**, 743

14

Lithium and Glucose Tolerance

P. VENDSBORG

INTRODUCTION

That lithium increases glucose uptake in muscle tissue in vitro has been found in several investigations (1-5). Also, an increased incorporation of carbon-14 labelled glucose in glycogen was found both *in vitro* and *in vivo.* Blood sugar level has been found to change after lithium administration to animals (6), but not to humans (7-9). That lithium after all increases glucose uptake into tissues in humans is indicated by the fact that serum inorganic phosphate decreases after an oral lithium load (7). That phosphate uptake is in fact secondary to glucose uptake is known regarding the effect of insulin and has also been shown *in vitro* for lithium (10). It is therefore supposed that lithium administration causes an increase in glucose uptake which is weaker, or has another mechanism, than that caused by insulin. This enables the homeostatic mechanisms in the organism to maintain an unchanged blood glucose level.

Another way of showing that lithium does increase glucose uptake in humans is by measuring the effect of lithium in a situation where the glucose disposal rate is maximal so that an extra effect of lithium can be seen. The administration of an acute glucose load could be such a situation.

Van der Velde and Gordon (11) have shown that lithium does in fact increase oral glucose tolerance. We have shown that intravenous glucose tolerance is increased the day after the first doses (8), whereas no change was seen after long term treatment (9). Some investigators have been unable to find any influence of lithium on glucose tolerance (12), whilst others (13) found that lithium decreased glucose tolerance.

In an attempt to clear up the discrepancies we have made further investigations in humans and have elaborated an animal model.

HUMAN STUDIES

In order to find out how the glucose tolerance changes with the length of the treatment we have measured it before and during lithium administration.

The patients were diagnosed as manic depressives who had all, except one, recovered from a depressive phase. They were thereafter started on prophylactic lithium treatment. Glucose tolerance tests were performed before, and 1 day, 5-8 days, 2-4 weeks, 2-4 months and more than half a year after the treatment was started. We used the intravenous glucose tolerance test with a fixed load of 25 g of glucose. The filling blood glucose values were plotted on semilogarithmic paper and as the reaction is of 1st order formed a straight line. The slope of the line is an expression of the rate of glucose disposal and was expressed as the K value according to Conard (14). The glucose tolerance tests were performed in the morning between 9 and 10 a.m. The patients received the full lithium dose in the evening, i.e. about 12 hours before the test.

Table 14.1 shows the mean K values at the different times during the treatment. We found again that the glucose disposal rate was increased the day after the treatment was started. Thereafter came a fall in K values and some weeks after the start the mean K values were not significantly different from the starting value. A secondary rise in K values was seen which was significant after half a year.

In order to see whether the glucose tolerance was increased in connection with the increase in lithium concentration which takes place each day in the hours after the lithium administration, a test was made 2 hours after the medicine was taken. As the K value normally varies during the day the test was performed in the morning at the usual time. A small dose of lithium was given in the evening, so that it would compensate for the fall during the night and lithium concentration in the morning would be equal to the evening concentration. The patients were the same ones who had participated in the abovementioned investigation. The test was always made the day after a usual test had taken place and at a time when the patients had been on lithium treatment for several months.

Table 14.2. shows the mean K values on the two consecutive days. It is seen that the glucose disposal rate is greater 2 hours after lithium administration than 12 hours after.

Table 14.1. K values during lithium treatment in humans

Time	K value	p value
Before	1.0 ± 0.1 (19)	—
1st morning	1.6 ± 0.2 (19)	0.001
5th to 8th day	1.5 ± 0.2 (16)	0.02
2nd to 4th week	1.2 ± 0.2 (9)	NS
2nd to 4th month	1.6 ± 0.3 (8)	NS
More than ½ year	1.6 ± 0.3 (10)	0.05

Mean ± SEM. Number of experiments in parentheses. Paired t test was used

Table 14.2. K values after lithium administration in long term treated patients

Time after lithium administration	K value
12 hours	1.6 ± 0.3 (10)
2 hours	2.4 ± 0.5 (10)
	$p < 0.05$

Mean ± SEM. Number of experiments in parentheses Paired t test was used

The human experiments show that lithium initially in the treatment does increase glucose disposal rate, and also 12 hours after its administration. Later, this effect disappeared at 12 hours, but was still present 2 hours after lithium administration. The finding of increased glucose tolerance after more than half a year of lithium treatment is not in accordance with our previous findings. The reason for this discrepancy could be that the patients in this investigation are manic depressive patients who were started on lithium after a depressive period. Two factors which are known to decrease glucose tolerance could therefore give a low initial value. First, they could still be in a slightly depressive state (15), second they were in a stress situation because they were hospitalized. These two factors disappeared during the investigation. The very low mean K value in the first glucose tolerance test when compared with normally found values is in accordance with this. In our previous investigation (9) the patients were not manic depressive and they were in the same situation regarding hospitalization at both glucose tolerance tests.

ANIMAL STUDIES

An animal model for intravenous glucose tolerance tests was elaborated.

Rats were anaesthetized and a small plastic catheter inserted into the jugular vein on the one side and into the carotid artery on the other side. Injections of 2 microlitres of 50% glucose per gram rat body weight were made into the jugular vein in 60 seconds. Blood samples were drawn from the artery at 3 min intervals during 24 minutes. K values were calculated as in the human experiments. The rats weighed about 200 g.

Figure 14.1 shows the variations in glucose tolerance at varying times after lithium administration. The dose administered was 800 micromoles subcutaneously given in the loose tissue at the back of the neck. It is seen that the glucose tolerance during the first 3 hours after the lithium injection was higher than the control animals given sodium although the difference only reached statistical significance at 3 hours. After 5 hours no significant difference was seen. The rats were fasted for 24 hours.

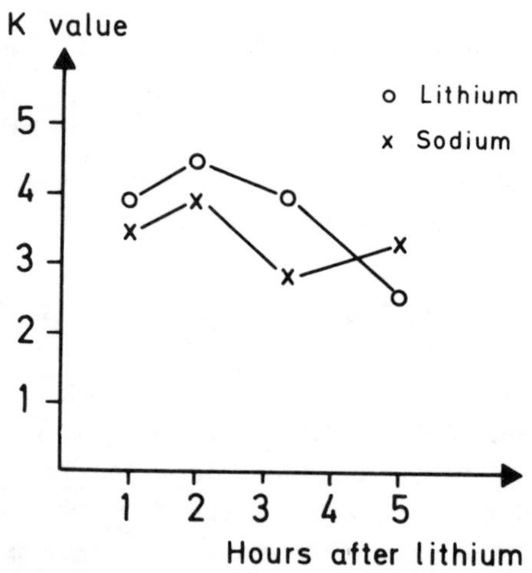

Figure 14.1. Glucose tolerance (expressed as K values) at intervals after lithium administration

Table 14.3 shows the glucose disposal rate after long and short term lithium administration. The administration of 400 micromoles of lithium subcutaneously does increase the K value significantly at 2 hours. Long term lithium administration, where the last dose was given 18-24 hours before the glucose tolerance test, also increased the tolerance, although not significantly. An extra dose 2 hours before the glucose tolerance test resulted in a significant difference between lithium and control rats. The results presented here, although preliminary, show that under certain conditions lithium increases glucose tolerance in rats. The effect varied with the interval between administration of lithium and the glucose tolerance test.

Table 14.3. K values after acute and long term lithium treatment in rats

Lithium administration	K value		p value
	Sodium chloride	Lithium chloride	
2 hours before glucose tolerance test	3.6 ± 0.3 (15)	4.6 ± 0.3 (13)	< 0.02
long term treated	4.1 ± 0.4 (14)	5.1 ± 0.3 (15)	NS
long term + 2 hours before	4.3 ± 0.3 (10)	5.3 ± 0.2 (10)	< 0.02

Mean ± SEM
Number of experiments in parentheses.

In Figure 14.1 it is seen that the glucose tolerance varies in the control animals. This could be a reaction to the hormonal changes caused by the stress or pain following the injection. It could also be diurnal variation, as all the animals were injected in the morning and the glucose tolerance test performed during the day, the 5-hour test therefore always in the afternoon.

The long term treated control rats seem to have a higher K value than the control rats in the acute experiments. A stress factor could also be responsible here. The long term treated animals, used to being handled and injected, were clearly more calm both after the injection with drug and, maybe more importantly, after the anaesthetic barbiturate which was given shortly before the glucose tolerance test.

Both the animal and human experiments seem to show without doubt that lithium in the intact organism can increase glucose disposal rate. On the other hand, the experiments also indicate why the effect does not show up in all experimental designs.

References

1. Bhattacharya, G. (1959). *Nature,* **183,** 324
2. Bhattacharya, G. (1961). *Biochem. J.,* **79,** 369
3. Bhattacharya, G. (1964), *Biochim. Biophys. Acta.,* **93,** 644
4. Clausen, T. (1968). *Chim. Biophys. Acta.,* **150,** 56
5. Clausen, T. (1968). *Biochim. Biophys. Acta,* **150,** 66
6. Plenge, P., Mellerup, E.T. and Rafaelsen, O.J. (1970). *J. Psychiat. Res.,* **8,** 29
7. Vendsborg, P.B., Mellerup, E.T. and Rafaelsen, O.J. (1973). *Acta Psychiat. Scand.,* **49,** 97

8. Vendsborg, P.B. and Rafaelsen, O.J. (1973). *Acta Psychiat. Scand.*, **49**, 601
9. Vendsborg, P.B. and Prytz, S. (1976). *Acta Psychiat. Scand.*, **53**, 64
10. Plenge, P., Mellerup, E.T. and Rafaelsen, O.J. (1971). *Int. Pharmacopsychiat.*, **6**, 52
11. Van der Velde, C.D. and Gordon, M.W. (1969). *Arch. Gen. Psychiat.*, **21**, 478
12. Heninger, G.R. and Mueller, P.S. (1970). *Arch. Gen. Psychiat.*, **23**, 310
13. Shopsin, B., Stern, S. and Gershon, S. (1972). *Arch. Gen. Psychiat.*, **26**, 566
14. Conard, V. (1975). *Acta Gastro-ent. Belg.*, **18**, 727
15. Mueller, P.S., Heninger, G.R. and McDonald, R.K. (1969). *Arch. Gen. Psychiat.*, **21**, 470

15

Influence of Lithium on Hormonal Stimulation of Adenylate Cyclase

A. GEISLER, R. KLYSNER and P. THAMS

INTRODUCTION

In spite of intensive research the mechanism of action of lithium (Li) in manic-depressive psychosis is still obscure. One line of research focuses on the possibility that Li exerts its effects by inhibiting hormonal stimulation of the membrane-bound enzyme adenylate cyclase (AC), which converts ATP to cyclic AMP. This effect of Li can be demonstrated during conventional use of Li, since in Li-treated patients the epinephrine-induced rise in plasma cyclic AMP was inhibited (1), as well as the accumulation of cyclic AMP in the platelets in response to prostaglandins (2). Similarly, in Li-treated rats ADH-stimulated urinary cyclic AMP excretion was reduced, an effect which was correlated to the polyuria caused by Li (3).

In *in vitro* experiments, especially with broken cell preparations, high concentrations of Li are often necessary to inhibit AC, whereas in studies using intact cell preparations low (about 2 mM) concentrations of Li inhibited the rise of cyclic AMP, e.g. brain slices (4), retina (5) and renal medulla (6). Furthermore, it has been shown that the inhibitory effect of Li on cyclic AMP accumulation in an intact cell preparation (skeletal muscle) was related to the intracellular concentration of Li (7).

The effect of Li on AC is selective, since only hormone-stimulated enzyme activities are inhibited leaving basal and fluoride-stimulated activities unaffected. Studies of the influence of Li on AC may therefore contribute to elucidate the regulatory mechanisms of this enzyme, which plays a central role in mediating the hormone-receptor interaction into intracellular events. For such studies the fat cell is suitable, because one catalytic subunit is connected via an intermediary component termed a transducer with several specific hormone receptors, allowing experiments concerning the localization of the action of Li on AC.

From a clinical point of view it is noteworthy that Li and neuroleptics have one therapeutic effect in common, i.e. the antimanic action. As it has been suggested that neuroleptics exert their effects by blocking dopamine receptors connected with AC (8), it may be relevant to study the effect of Li on this enzyme.

METHODS

Fat cells were prepared from epididymal fat from male Wistar rats (150-200 g) (9). The isolated cells were incubated in Krebs-Ringer-HEPES buffer for 1 hour at 37°C with or without Li before addition of hormones. The reaction was stopped after 5 min by adding TCA, and after ether extraction and lyophilization, cyclic AMP was measured.

Homogenates containing dopamine-sensitive AC were prepared from various brain regions (10). After 1 hour of preincubation in the presence of drugs as indicated the reaction was initiated by adding ATP.

In both tissue preparations cyclic AMP was determined in unpurified samples by a competitive protein binding method previously described (11).

RESULTS

Experiments with fat cells

When fat cells were preincubated with increasing concentrations of Li a dose-dependent inhibition of cyclic AMP accumulation after stimulation with 0.1 microM norepinephrine was demonstrated. This inhibition was statistically significant and maximal after 1 hour of preincubation at a concentration of 15 mM of Li ($p < 0.001$).

The type of the Li-induced inhibition of cyclic AMP formation was investigated by performing dose-response curves for norepinephrine with and without 15 mM of Li (Figure 15.1). These results indicate that the inhibition by Li was of a mainly non-competitive type. However, the inhibitory effect was not purely non-competitive as it decreased with increasing concentrations of hormones, but could not be abolished.

Stimulation of AC by glucagon was likewise inhibited by Li.

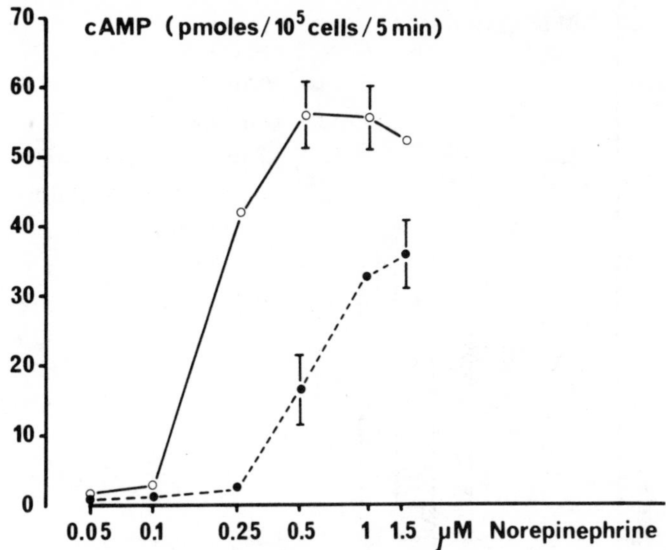

Figure 15.1. Dose-response curves of norepinephrine with (•------•) and without (o———o) lithium (15 mM) in rat fat cells.

In other experiments the effects of Li (40 mM) and the beta-adrenergic blocking agent propranolol (0.3 microg/ml) alone and in combination on the norepinephrine-induced cyclic AMP accumulation were studied. As shown in Figure 15.2, Li reduced the cyclic AMP accumulation to 73% of that observed in control samples, whereas propranolol decreased the accumulation to 80%. However, by combining the drugs, the cyclic AMP accumulation was reduced to 33% of the accumulation of cyclic AMP in the controls, i.e. the combined effect of the two drugs was more than additive.

By directly adding the individual inhibitory effects of Li and propranolol only a total inhibition of 53% of controls was obtained. This synergistic effect of Li and propranol has been observed repeatedly and suggests a more complex effect of Li on hormone-stimulated cyclic AMP accumulation in fat cells than a pure non-competitive type of inhibition.

Experiments with brain homogenates

In these experiments broken cell preparations were used for measurement of AC activity (10).

It has been demonstrated that this AC is sensitive to stimulation by dopamine in a dose-dependent manner with half-maximal stimulation

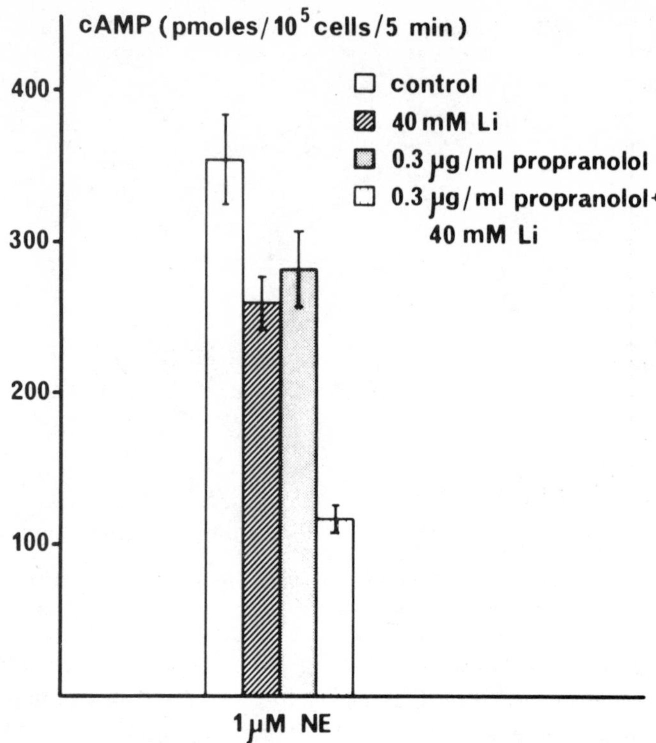

Figure 15.2. Effect of lithium and propranolol alone and in combination on cyclic AMP accumulation in rat fat cells.

obtained at a concentration of 10 microM of dopamine, whereas other catecholamines are less potent. The dopaminergic specificity of this enzyme has been further characterized using various dopaminergic agonists (12).

The AC activity in response to dopamine in homogenates from rat olfactory tubercle was significantly inhibited by 5 mM of Li, whereas basal and fluoride-stimulated enzyme activities were un-affected. (Table 15.1).

Similar results were obtained with enzyme preparations from rat striatum and limbic cortex. In other experiments an inhibitory effect of 2 mM of Li could also be demonstrated.

In striatal homogenates the inhibitory effect of Li (20 mM) on dopamine-sensitive AC was found to be of a purely non-competitive type. In contrast, in this tissue it was found that the potent neuroleptic drug, alpha-flupenthixol, inhibited the dopamine-activated enzyme in a competitive manner. Furthermore, it was demonstrated that the inhibitory effects of Li and alpha-flupenthixol were additive (Table 15.2).

Table 15.1. Influence of lithium on adenylate cyclase from rat olfactory tubercle

	Basal activity	NaF 1×10^{-2} M	Dopamine* 2×10^{-5} M	Dopamine* 1×10^{-3} M
NaCl 5 mM	3.2 ± 0.4	45.0 ± 4.1	2.1 ± 0.4	5.8 ± 0.8
LiCl 5 mM	4.2 ± 0.6	36.0 ± 3.9	0.7 ± 0.3 **	3.5 ± 0.3**

Results are expressed as pmoles cyclic AMP formed/2 mg tissue/2.5 min
*Increase of basal enzyme activity
Means ± SEM (n = 8-12)
**$p < 0.05$ in comparison with NaCl

Table 15.2. Effect of lithium and alpha-flupenthixol on striatal adenylate cyclase activity

	Activity in presence of dopamine 1 × 10-3 M*	Percentage inhibition of stimulation above basal activity**
Control	8.6 ± 0.19	0
Lithium (10 mM)	7.4 ± 0.19	29
Alpha-flupenthixol (5×10^{-8} M)	7.4 ± 0.17	29
Lithium (10 mM) + alpha-flupenthixol (5×10^{-8} M)	5.9 ± 0.20	64

*Expressed as pmoles cyclic AmP formed/6 min/0.2 mg tissue; means ± SEM (n = 5-6)
**Basal enzyme activity in absence and presence of the drugs was 4.4 ± 0.05 pmoles cyclic AMP/6 min/0.2 mg tissue.

DISCUSSION

It has been shown in several studies that Li has an inhibitory effect on AC from various tissues (13) including brain (4). One aspect of investigations concerning this action of Li may be aimed at elucidating the mechanism by which Li modifies the activity of AC. In this way Li may be used as a tool for examining the processes involved in activation of AC, especially the regulatory role of other cations. While certain studies (3,6) indicate that one side effect, i.e. polyuria, is — at least in part — associated with alterations in the cyclic AMP metabolism, it should be emphasized that conclusions with respect to the therapeutic action of Li based on our present knowledge of its effects on the cyclic AMP system can, at the best, be considered suggestive.

The results presented here formed part of our studies concerning the mode of action of Li on AC activity. The observations on brain homogenates that basal and fluoride-stimulated enzyme activities — representing activity of only the catalytical subunit — were unaffected by Li, indicate a non-involvement of this subunit in Li-induced inhibition. In accordance with the findings of other investigators (13), only the hormone-activated AC was inhibited by Li, thus leaving the possibilities that the hormone-receptor interaction and the transducer function may be the targets for Li.

The type of inhibition by Li demonstrated on AC activity in brain homogenates was clear-cut non-competitive, an observation only partially confirmed by studies on intact fat cells. This non-competitive inhibition indicates a site of action of Li different from the specific hormone receptor, which is blocked in a competitive way by neuroleptic drugs. Consequently Li may modify the transfer of the stimulus to the catalytical subunit induced by hormone binding, i.e. at the level of the transducer, the structure of which is largely unknown.

The effect of Li on AC can be antagonized by magnesium (13) lending support to the idea that Li may interfere with magnesium-sensitive sites participating in regulation of the enzyme activity. In this connection it may be speculated that the magnesium site located to the transducer component that has been observed by Roy (14) may be involved in the action of Li on AC. Of course, it is also possible that Li may alter the function of AC by influencing other regulatory sites.

Thus, the mixed type of inhibition by Li on cyclic AMP accumulation in fat cells and the synergistic effect of Li and propranolol may indicate a modifying action of Li on receptor activation by hormones (15).

The combination of Li and alpha-flupenthixol had an additive inhibitory effect on stıiatal AC, an effect that may be related to the clinical observations that combined treatment of mania with Li and neuroleptic drugs as haloperidol may occasionally lead to dyskinesias (16). However, the question whether the common effect of these two types of psychotropic drugs on dopamine-sensitive AC is of relevance for their antimanic properties remains to be answered.

ACKNOWLEDGEMENT

This investigation was supported by grants from P. Carl Petersens Fond to Arne Geisler.

References

1. Ebstein, R.P., Belmaker, R.H., Grunhaus, L. and Rimon, R. (1976). *Nature,* **259**, 411
2. Murphy, D.L., Donelly, C. and Moskowitz, J. (1973). *Clin. Pharmac. Ther.,* **14**, 810

3. Christensen, S. and Geisler, A. (1977). *Acta Pharmacol. Toxicol.*, **40**, 447
4. Forn, J. and Valdecasas, F.G. (1971). *Biochem. Pharmacol.*, **20**, 2773
5. Schorderet, M. (1977). *Biochem. Pharmacol.*, **26**, 167
6. Beck, N. and Kim, K.S. (1975). *Endocrinology,* **96**, 744
7. Frazer, A., Haugaard, E.S., Mendels, J. and Haugaard, N. (1975). *Biochem. Pharmacol.*, **24**, 2273
8. Clement-Cormier, Y.C., Kebabian, J.W. and Petzold, G.L. (1974). *Proc. Nat. Acad. Sci.* USA, *71,* 1113
9. Schwabe, U. and Ebert, R. (1972). *Naunyn-Schmiedeberg's Arch. Pharmacol.*, **274**, *287*
10. Kebabian, J.W., Petzold, G.L. and Greengard, P. (1972). *Proc. Nat. Acad. Sci.*, USA, **69**, 2145
11. Geisler, A., Klysner, R., Thams, P. and Christensen, S. (1977). *Acta Pharmacol. Toxicol.*, **40**, 356
12. Klysner, R. and Geisler, A. (In preparation)
13. Forn, J. (1975). In: F.N. Johnson (ed.) *Lithium Research and Therapy,* pp. 485-497 (New York: Academic Press)
14. Roy, C. (1976). *J. Supramol. Struct.*, **4**, 289
15. Thams, P. and Geisler, A. (To be published)
16. Loudon, J.B. and Waring, H. (1976). *Lancet,* **ii**, 1088

16

Irreversible Effects of Lithium Administration on Transport Processes in Erythrocytes and Platelets

K. MARTIN

INTRODUCTION

A study of manic depressive patients revealed that the administration of lithium significantly reduces the uptake of choline by erythrocytes; during the first six weeks of treatment the influx of choline is reduced to about half. Later it falls to around 10% of the control value (1). This inhibition appears to be an irreversible effect of lithium: it is independent of the prescence of lithium in the extracellular or intracellular water and when a patient is taken off lithium the activity of the transport system returns to normal only at the rate at which erythrocytes are removed from the circulation and replaced by new cells (2). Before investigating the possibility that lithium inhibits in a similar way choline transport in the CNS, the experiments reported in this chapter were carried out to establish whether or not the erythrocytes from various species differ in their response to lithium.

The surprising observation that the inhibition of choline transport following lithium administration is apparently irreversible suggested that it might be interesting to find out to what extent other effects of lithium on transport processes depend on the continued presence of lithium. Platelets from patients on lithium are readily available and it is known that the administration of lithium leads to a stimulation of 5-HT uptake by these cells (3,4). In some preliminary experiments the 5-HT uptake by platelets from normal subjects, depressed patients not on lithium and depressed patients on lithium was measured in the absence and presence of external lithium.

METHODS

Choline influx into erythrocytes was measured as described previously (1,2).

5-HT uptake by platelets was measured using a slightly modified version of the cellophan tube method (5); a preliminary dialysis of the platelet rich plasma (PRP) against a large volume of Krebs buffer reduced the lithium concentration in the PRP (when this was obtained from a patient on lithium) to less than 5% of the original value.

RESULTS AND DISCUSSION

Experiments with human erythrocytes had shown that incubating these cells *in vitro* for 2 hours with 2 mM lithium reduced the capacity of the transport system by about 20%; no further inhibition resulted from either higher lithium concentrations or longer incubation periods. When erythrocytes from various species were incubated with 2 mM lithium for 2 hours it became clear that the choline transport system is significantly inhibited only in humans and monkeys, not effected in many species and increased in the rat (Table 16.1).

Table 16.1. Choline influx (initial rate) into erythrocytes from various species following pre-incubation (2 hours, 37°C) with 2 mM lithium

Species	Choline transport n mole/(1 cells)/min		Effect of pre-incubation with 2 mM Li
	Na	Li	Li/Na
Human (20)	45 ± 10	32 ± 8	0.73
Monkey (Rhesus) (1)	20.7 ± 1.5	17.6 ± 2	0.85
Monkey (Patas) (2)	53.4 ± 4.1	48 ± 4	0.90
Pig (2)	2.98 ± 0.5	2.97 ± 0.3	1.00
Dog (3)	6.96 ± 0.53	7.2 ± 0.59	1.03
Cat (3)	5.37 ± 0.2	5.84 ± 0.3	1.08
Rabbit (6)	34.8 ± 6.1	32.9 ± 4.2	0.94
Rat (15)	17.7 ± 3.9	24.8 ± 3.6	1.40

As with human erythrocytes, increasing the concentration of lithium or the length of the incubation period had no effect. Since in man the prolonged administration of lithium results in a much more pronounced inhibition of choline transport than can be produced by *in vitro* exposure of erythrocytes to the ion, lithium was administered to rats and monkeys. The rats were killed after 3-5 weeks; their plasma lithium levels varied between 0.2 and 0.3 mmol/l and choline influx into the erythrocytes was increased by about 50%. Choline influx was measured using lithium free buffer but the possibility that the increased influx resulted from the presence of lithium in the intracellular water was not investigated.

In monkeys, where the inhibition resulting from *in vitro* exposure of erythrocytes to lithium was similar to that found with human red cells, the administration of lithium produced a progressive reduction in the capacity of transport system (Figure 16.1).

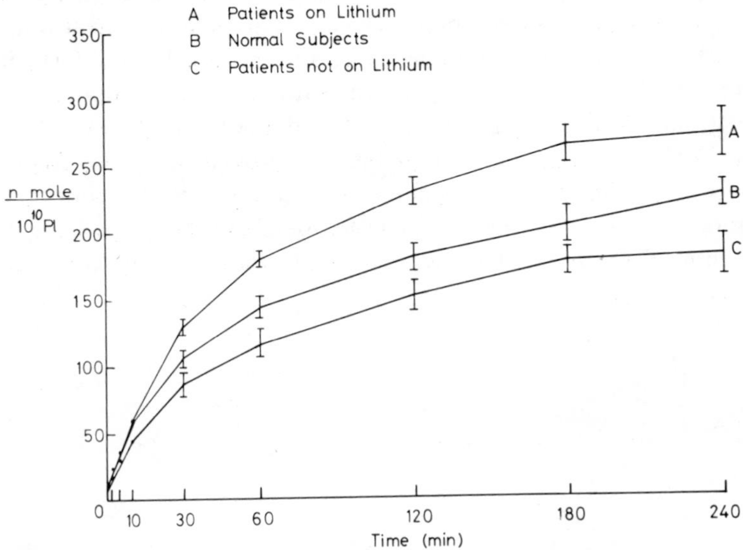

Figure 16.1. The uptake of choline by erythrocytes following the daily administration of lithium to two Patas monkeys. Choline uptake is expressed as the ratio of intracellular over extracellular concentration of choline after 10 min incubation with 1 microM carbon-14-choline.

The initial dosing schedule — 100 mg lithium a day to a Patas monkey weighing between 10 and 11 kg — resulted in very low plasma levels which were nevertheless effective in producing some inhibition of choline transport. The dose of lithium was subsequently increased and the rate of choline influx during the following weeks fell to levels that are considerably below the control rate and also well below the rate found following prolonged *in vitro* exposure of the cells to lithium.

The fact that the plasma levels of lithium increased during the period of treatment makes it difficult to distinguish between the effect of lithium concentration on the one hand and that of prolonged presence of lithium in the body on the other. However, the time course of this progressive inhibition of choline transport is very similar to that found in patients with constant lithium levels, suggesting that it is the result of the prolonged presence of lithium.

These data suggest that the monkey is probably a better experimental animal than the rat for an investigation of the question: does lithium inhibit choline transport not only in erythrocytes but also in the CNS of manic depressive patients?

Preliminary experiments designed to investigate the mechanism of action by which lithium affects 5-HT uptake by platelets confirmed that lithium increases the rate of uptake when administered to patients but has no effect on platelets from normal subjects when added to the incubation medium (3,4,6). It could also be shown that reducing the lithium level in the PRP obtained from patients on lithium did not alter the rate of 5-HT uptake, indicating that the stimulation is independent of the continued presence of lithium in the external medium. Our results also confirm that the rate of 5-HT uptake by platelets obtained from patients with endogenous depression is less than that found with platelets from normal subjects (7) (Figure 16.2).

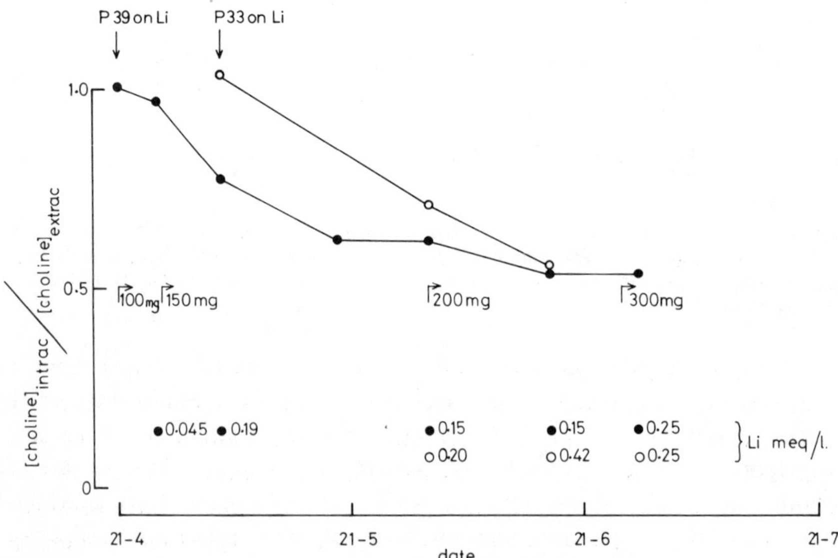

Figure 16.2. Uptake of 5-HT by platelets; uptake was measured using the cellophan tube method and 10 microM 5-HT in the external medium.

When lithium is administered to these patients the rate of 5-HT uptake is increased above normal. A meaningful interpretation of these data is possible only after it has been investigated to what extent the stored radioactivity represents 5-HT and to what extent it represents metabolites.

References

1. Lee, G., Lingsch, C., Lyle, P.T. and Martin, K. (1974). *Br. J. Clin. Pharmacol.,* **1**, 365
2. Lingsch, C. and Martin, K. (1976). *Brit. J. Pharmacol.,* **57**, 323
3. Murphy, D.L., Colburn, R.W., Davis, J.M. and Bunney, Jr., W.E. (1969). *Life Sci.,* **8**, 1187
4. Murphy, D.L., Colburn, R.W., Davis, J.M. and Bunney, Jr., W.E. (1970). *Am. J. Psychiat.,* **127**, 339
5. Born, G.V.R. and Gilson, R.E. (1959). *J. Physiol.,* **146**, 472
6. Born, G.V.R., Grignani, G. and Martin, K. (In preparation)
7. Hallstrom, C.O.S., Rees, W.L., Pare, C.M.B., Trenchard, A. and Turner, P. (1976). *Postgrad. Med. J.,* **52**, (Suppl. 3), 40

17

Effects of Lithium on Sodium Transport Across Membranes

D. A. T. DICK, G. J. NAYLOR and E. G. DICK

ACTION OF Li ON Na-K EXCHANGE PUMP

There are four main actions of Li on the Na pump which are already known

1. Internal Li can be transferred outwards by the pump at approximately 10% of the rate of Na transfer (1).

2. External Li can partly substitute for K in activating outward transfer of Na by the pump (2).

3. Li can partially substitute for Na or K in activating Na-K-Mg ATPase (3).

4. Li can substitute for internal Na in stimulating the production of further pumping sites (4).

We shall keep these in mind in investigating and attempting to interpret the action of Li in normal subjects and patients suffering from depressive illness. Since the effect of lithium appears to be different in manic depressive patients and in normal subjects, it is necessary first to consider variations in sodium transport in patients and in normal subjects.

RELATION BETWEEN MOOD AND Na-K EXCHANGE PUMP IN MANIC DEPRESSIVE ILLNESS

There is some evidence of a general change in Na transport in body cells during depressive illness, e.g. residual (mainly intracellular) Na falls on recovery from depressive illness (5). In our work we have, however, studied only red cells from depressed patients on the assumption that these may give at least some indication of changes taking place in other cells. After the initial finding that erythrocyte Na concentration probably falls on recovery from a depressive illness, further studies were made on the associated changes in Na pump activity. Thus, in a group of female psychotic depressives (both unipolar and bipolar), during recovery from the depressed state there were significant changes in the erythrocytes, reduction in intracellular Na ($p < 0.01$) and increase in Na-K ATPase activity ($p < 0.0125$) although the increase in ouabain-sensitive K influx was not significant (6). When the actual changes of mood (improvement scored positively) which occurred during recovery (assessed independently by the nursing staff) were correlated with the accompanying changes of Na pump activity, significant correlations were obtained (Figure 17.1). No significant changes or correlations of Na pump activity were found in a group of neurotic depressives.

In a study of 23 female patients suffering from manic depressive psychosis (manic type), a significant increase in ouabain-sensitive K influx of red cells was found on recovery from the mania ($p < 0.001$) although no significant change was found in Na concentration or Na-K ATPase (7). However, when the initial severity of the mania (equal to the change on recovery since final scores were zero), was correlated with the change in erythrocyte Na-K ATPase on recovery, a significant correlation was obtained ($n = 14$, $rho = +0.669$, $p < 0.02$) (improvement scored positively). This apparent change in Na pump activity is similar to that found on recovery from depression and suggests that biochemically mania is similar to, and not opposite to, depression.

An investigation of the relation between Na pump activity and the severity of depressive illness was made in a group of 11 mentally defective patients (8). These were divided into more severe and less severe groups according to two different criteria.

1. The more severe group had 20 or more weeks ill per annum and the less severe 19 or less.

2. The more severe group had six or more episodes of illness per annum and the less severe five or less.

The groupings were not exactly the same according to the two criteria. However, by either method of grouping the more severe patients had a significantly lower erythrocyte Na-K ATPase level (Table 17.1). The severity of depressive illness again appears to be correlated with pump activity.

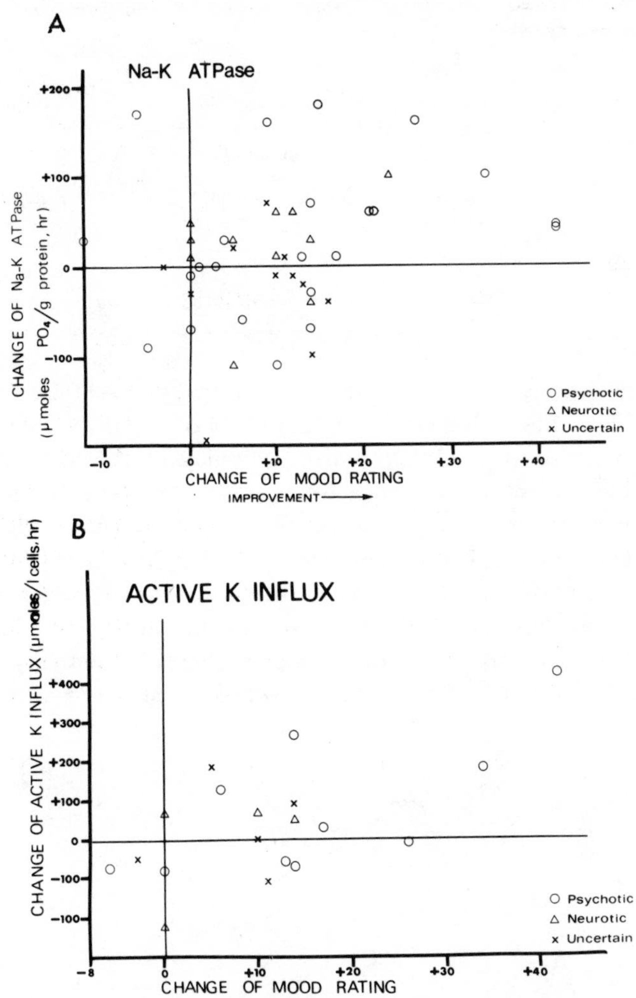

Figure 17.1. Recovery from manic depressive illness in psychotic and neurotic groups of patients. Relation between change of mood and change of (A) Na-K ATPase and (B) ouabain-sensitive (active) potassium influx.

A further investigation of the relation between depression and Na pump activity was made in a group of four mental defectives with short-cycle manic-depressive psychosis, undergoing mood fluctuations with cycles between 4 and 9 weeks long (9). In studies lasting approximately 6 months, i.e. 4 to 5 cycles, correlations were found between the patient's mood and Na-K ATPase measurements in red cells. In two patients, mood and ATPase correlated negatively in phase with each other (data for Patient 2

Table 17.1. Na-K ATPase levels in erythrocytes of patients suffering from manic depressive psychosis, grouped by severity

	Less severe	More severe	Significance of difference (p)
	(mmol PO_4/l RBC, h)		
By episodes of illness	0.696 SD 0.240	0.401 SD 0.162	< 0.025
By number of weeks ill	0.678 SD 0.267	0.424 SD 0.159	< 0.05

are illustrated in Figure 17.2); in one patient mood and ATPase correlated again negatively but with a lag of 14 days (27% of cycle) (ATPase lagging behind mood); in the fourth patient mood and ATPase correlated positively but almost exactly out of phase (44% of cycle) with each other, a situation somewhat similar to correlating negatively and in phase as in the first two patients. The erythrocyte Na and ATP concentrations and some parameters of Na pump activity correlated with the cycles of mood in some patients but not in others. There was thus again some indication of correlation between the mood of manic depressive patients and the activity of the red cell Na pump. It must be noted that since the concept of

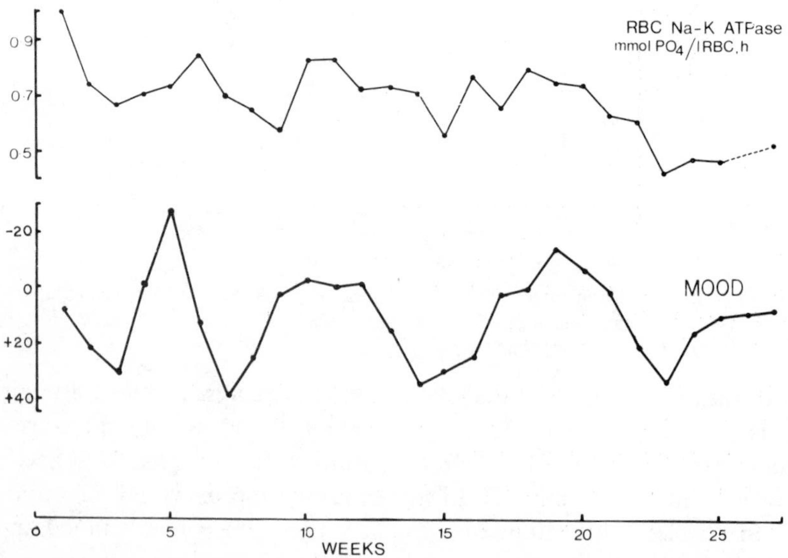

Figure 17.2. Relation between mood and erythrocyte Na-K ATPase in one short cycle manic depressive patient studied over a period of 6 months.

improvement is not applicable to cyclic illness, mania has been scored positive and depression negative. Thus it is difficult to relate the sign of the correlation obtained to that found in the depressive and manic groups.

RELATION BETWEEN MOOD AND Na-K EXCHANGE PUMP IN NORMAL SUBJECTS

A relation between mood and the Na-K exchange pump was suggested by some findings in three normal subjects (unpublished results). In all cases Na-K ATPase levels in red cells correlated positively with mood estimated by a self-assessment system and only compared with biochemical data at the end of the 12-week experiment). As seen from the data shown in Table 17.2, Na-K ATPase activity correlated positively with mood in all three subjects, while ouabain-sensitive K influx and the flux sodium ATPase ratio (see Conclusion) correlated negatively. The fact that Na-K ATPase and ouabain-sensitive K influx correlated with mood in opposite senses is so far unexplained.

A further feature of Na-K exchange pump data is their correlation with age in female subjects. Figure 17.3 shows that erythrocyte Na concentration increases with age while Na-K ATPase decreases; the changes are highly significant ($p < 0.0005$) in both cases) (70). No similar changes with age are found in males. From the data it is not possible to decide whether the change in females occurs suddenly at the menopause or is a gradual change with age.

Table 17.2. Correlations between mood rating and erythrocyte Na-K exchange pump activity in normal subjects

Subject	Na-K ATPase		Ouabain-sensitive K influx		Flux sodium ATPase ratio*	
	n	rho	n	rho	n	rho
1	12	+0.158	12	-0.630	12	-0.385
2	12	+0.367	12	-0.235	12	-0.339
3	10	+0.735	10	-0.574	10	-0.774
Mean	28	+0.43	28	-0.49	28	-0.50
p	<0.02		<0.01		<0.01	

* see Conclusion
rho is Spearman's rank correlation coefficient

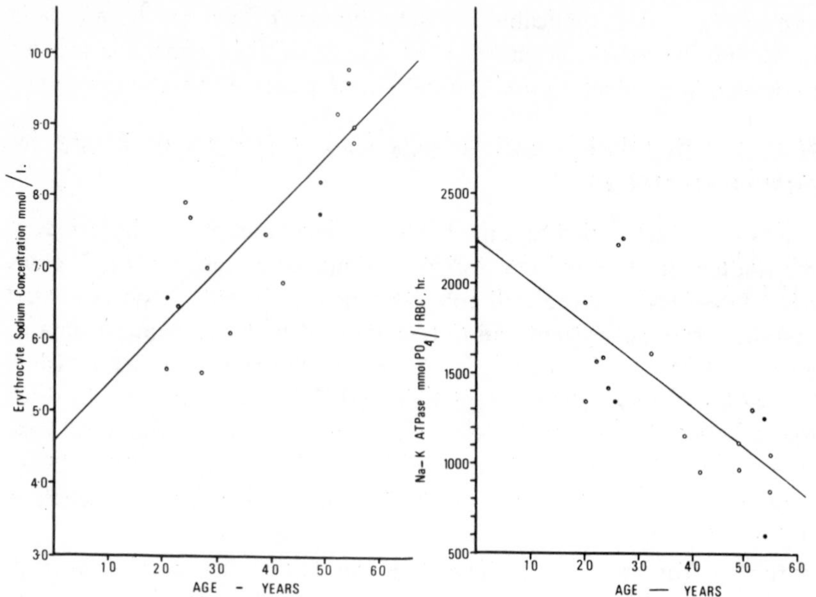

Figure 17.3. Relation between age of normal female subjects and (left) erythrocyte sodium concentration and (right) Na-K ATPase.

EFFECTS OF Li ON Na-K EXCHANGE PUMP IN MANIC DEPRESSIVE ILLNESS

The effect of Li treatment was tested in a group of 10 patients in a double blind cross over trial (11). Measurements of erythrocyte Na concentration, Na-K ATPase, and ouabain-sensitive K influx were made twice before and twice after the çross-over date. Five patients received placebo first and Li second, and 5 Li first and placebo second. The mean values of the measurement on and off Li are shown in Table 17.3. A significant change occurred only in Na-K ATPase which increased when on Li therapy. This finding suggests that Li has a stimulatory effect on the Na pump in depressive patients. Whether this effect is correlated with the improvement of the illness was the subject of a follow up study on the same group of patients.

The patients were divided into responders to Li therapy who had a decrease in the number of episodes of illness while on Li therapy and non-responders who had no decrease or an increase. Responders had a lower erythrocyte Na-K ATPase than non-responders when off Li (Table 17.4); this difference was significant ($p < 0.002$) (8). When the increase in Na-K ATPase brought about by Li therapy was examined, it was found that responders had a significantly greater increase than non-responders;

Table 17.3. Effect of lithium on Na-K exchange pump of erythrocytes. During Li treatment, plasma level was 0.77 ± 0.11 mM and erythrocyte level was 0.62 ± 0.14 mM (n = 10)

	During placebo treatment	During lithium treatment	Significance of difference (p)
Na concentration (mM)	6.17 SD 0.28	6.40 SD 0.28	NS
Na-K ATPase (mmol PO4/l RBC,h)	0.600 SD 0.069	0.831 SD 0.066	< 0.01
Ouabain-sensitive K influx (mmol/l RBC,h)	1.53 SD 0.053	1.63 SD 0.052	NS

again the difference was significant ($p < 0.01$). Thus patients who respond to Li therapy have a lower erythrocyte Na-K ATPase when off Li than those who do not and they experience a greater rise in Na-K ATPase during the response.

Table 17.4. Na-K ATPase in erythrocytes of depressive patients and response to Li treatment.

	ATPase when off Li	Change in ATPase with Li treatment
	(mmol PO_4/l RBC,h)	
Responders	0.36 ± 0.08	+0.44 ± 0.20
Non-responders	0.73 ± 0.21	+0.049 ± 0.20
Significance of difference (p)	<0.02	<0.01

EFFECTS OF Li ON Na-K EXCHANGE PUMP IN NORMAL HUMAN SUBJECTS AND IN ANIMALS

The effect of Li therapy was tried in a group of 11 normal human subjects who took 1 g of Li carbonate daily for 14 days. Erythrocyte measurements made before and at the end of Li treatment are shown in Table 17.5 (12). It is seen that unlike manic depressive patients, normal subjects showed no increase of Na-K ATPase; indeed there is a significant *decrease* ($p < 0.005$) in ouabain-sensitive K influx. It appears therefore that there is a difference between the effect of Li on the erythrocyte Na pump in manic depressive and normal human subjects.

In a study of Li treatment in rats, a group of 16 animals was given Li carbonate in the diet and a similar control group given normal diet (12). After 2 weeks the animals were killed, blood collected and erythrocyte Na-K ATPase estimated. The mean and standard deviation for the Li-treated group was 3.95 ± 1.13 mmol PO_4/1 RBC, h and for the control group 4.03 ± 1.08 mmol and PO_4/ RBC, h. There was no significant difference between the two groups. Li thus appears to have no effect on the erythrocyte Na pump in normal rats.

Table 17.5. Effect of Li treatment on erythrocyte measurements in normal subjects

	Before Li	After Li	Significance of change (p)
Na concentration (mmol/l RBC)	7.8 ±0.4	7.7 ±0.4	NS
Na-K ATPase (mmol PO_4/l RBC,h)	1.64±0.12	1.65±0.10	NS
Ouabain-sensitive K influx (mmol/l RBC,h)	1.57±0.04	1.41±0.02	<0.005

CONCLUSION

One of the main problems in drawing conclusions from these studies is a puzzling variability of correlation or lack of correlation between the three different measures of Na-K exchange pump activity. These are summarized in Table 17.6 (12).

Of course there is no difficulty in envisaging two possible correlations between Na concentration and Na-K ATPase. If changes of Na concentration are the result of changes in ATPase a negative correlation might be expected; on the other hand if changes of ATPase result from changes in Na concentration (13) then a positive correlation would be expected. Similarly it is possible to envisage Na concentration as either the cause of or the result of the level of ouabain-sensitive K influx and thus either positively or negatively correlated with it. It is more difficult to explain the lack of correlation (or negative correlation) between Na-K ATPase and ouabain-sensitive K influx although it must be remembered that while the latter is measured in the living erythrocyte and is thus affected by the internal Na concentration, the former is measured on erythrocyte membranes in a standard incubation medium and is

Table 17.6. Significance of correlations between biochemical measurements in erythrocytes

	Na concentration and Na-K ATPase	Na concentration and ouabain-sensitive K influx	Na-K ATPase and ouabain-sensitive K influx
Normals	0	+	0
Recovered manic depressives	+	0	0
Short cycle manic depressives	+	—	0
Depressives illness—recovered	0	—	0
Manic illness—recovered	0	—	0

\+ = significant positive correlation ($p < 0.05$)
– = Significant negative correlation ($p < 0.05$)
0 = no significant correlation

independent of Na concentration; lack of correlation between Na-K ATPase and ouabain-sensitive K influx may thus be due to variations in erythrocyte Na concentration. In some cases an attempt has been made to overcome this problem by calculating an empirical factor combining the various measures of pump activity, the so-called 'flux sodium ATPase ratio or (oubain-sensitive K influx)/(Na concentration) × (Na-K ATPase). In some cases this ratio has provided useful correlations which may be of predictive value in the prognosis and treatment by Li of depressive illness (8). However, the fundamental problem of why the correlations between the biochemical measures of pump activity should vary as they do between normal subjects and different types of depressive patients is still unsolved.

In spite of these difficulties, the many measures of Na-K exchange pump activity which have been made in manic depressive illness do show a general correlation between pump activity and the clinical state of the patient both without and with Li treatment. Li has been shown to increase erythrocyte Na-K ATPase in manic depressive patients at the same time as it produces an improvement in clinical state. However, Li appears to affect the erythrocyte Na-K pump in patients in a manner different from its effect in normal subjects.

ACKNOWLEDGEMENT

This work was supported by a grant from the Scottish Hospitals Endowment Research Trust.

References

1. Keynes, R.D. and Swan, R.C. (1955). *J. Physiol.,* **147**, 626
2. Beaugé, L. (1975).' *J. Physiol.,* **246**, 397
3. Skou, J.C. (1960). *Biochim. Biophys. Acta,* **42**, 6
4. Boardman, L.J., Hume, S.P., Lamb, J.F. and Polson, J. (1975). *J. Physiol.,* **244**, 677
5. Coppen, A. and Shaw, D.M. (1963). *Brit. Med. J.,* **2**, 1439
6. Naylor, G.J., Dick, D.A.T., Dick, E.G., Le Poidevin, D. and Whyte, S.F. (1973). *Psychol. Med.,* **3**, 502
7. Naylor, G.J., Dick, D.A.T., Dick, E.G., Worrall, E.P., Peet. M., Dick, P. and Boardman, L.J. (1976). *Psychol. Med.,* **6**, 659
8. Naylor, G.J., Dick, D.A.T. and Dick, E.G. (1976). *Psychol. Med.,* **6**, 257
9. Naylor, G.J., Reid, A.H., Dick, D.A.T. and Dick, E.G. (1976). *Brit. J. Psychiat.,* **128**, 169
10. Naylor, G.J., Dick, D.A.T., Worrall, E.P., Dick, E.G., Dick, P. and Boardman, L. (1977). *Gerontology,* **23**, 256
11. Naylor, G.J., Dick, D.A.T., Dick, E.G and Moody, J.P. (1974). *Pschopharmacologia,* **37**, 81
12. Naylor, G.J., Smith, A., Boardman, L.J., Dick, D.A.T., Dick, E.G. and Dick, P. (1977). *Psychol. Med.,* (In press)
13. Boardman, L., Huett, M., Lamb, J.F., Newton, J.P. and Polson, J.M. (1974). *J. Physiol.,* **241**, 771

18

Lithium Regulation of Membrane ATPases

A. I. M. GLEN

INTRODUCTION

More than one person in every thousand of the population of Edinburgh now takes lithium on a long term basis for treatment of affective disorder. It is a solemn thought, and we have no reason to suspect that this is an unduly high figure in comparison with other centres. It is apparently necessary to eat this potentially toxic element continuously in order to stop the attacks, and for a number of years I have been asking myself why this should be. It might be explained in two ways:

1. The illness presents episodically, but the underlying biochemical lesion is continuously present and lithium has a continuous effect upon it;
2. The illness presents episodically, the underlying biochemical lesion is also episodic and lithium, although continuously administered, expresses a therapeutic effect on the biochemical lesion episodically.

In an earlier communication (1) the view was taken that both conditions were present, i.e. that there was a continuing biochemical lesion which predisposed to the episodic illness, but that there was also an acute biochemical change associated with the episode and that lithium acted therapeutically on both the acute episodic lesion and also on the predisposing cause. We suggested that the K^+-like effect of lithium could have a stimulating effect on Na/K ATPase (the sodium pump) episodically during the illness only, but that there was also a continuing effect of lithium on Mg ATPase. We were unable at that time to separate in clinical investigations the illness effect on ATPases from a lithium effect on ATPases and in laboratory experiments to separate the action on Na/K ATPase from the action on Mg ATPase. I should like to present now the results of a number of studies which may elucidate the problem and emphasise the importance of orientation (sidedness) of presentation of lithium at the membranous interface, in the red blood cell and at the synapse. This work was undertaken in the laboratories of the Medical Research Council Brain Metabolism Unit in Edinburgh, in collaboration with a number of colleagues, but the bulk of the work was done by Drs John Hesketh and Bill Reading.

WHY ATPases?

Hypotheses to account for the aetiology of affective illness have centred on the involvement of electrolytes (2) or catecholamines (3) or both (receptor sensitivity) (4). While many of the early clinical studies of electrolyte metabolism have been equivocal, it is difficult to escape from the fact that a substantial number of reports have suggested a disorder of sodium transport at least as an accompaniment of affective illness. If this is accepted, the question becomes one of the effect of the illness on membrane ATPases and the interaction of these ATPases on transmitter release and reuptake. The current fashionable theories to account for this interaction are those of Berle and Pushkin (5) in which it is postulated that as a result of the energy provided by a magnesium ATPase activation there is fusion of actin and myosin-like protein at the nerve ending with the resultant expulsion of transmitter into the synaptic cleft. The alternative to the vesicular explosion hypothesis is the position taken by Vizi (6) in which Na/K ATPase is seen as controlling *inhibition* of transmitter release, i.e. *activation* of Na/K ATPase is said to *stop* transmitter release and *inactivation* of Na/K ATPase by an inflow of potassium to allow the transmitter to escape. In either of these situations one might expect an illness effect on membrane ATPases to have a profound effect on synaptic transmission. An alternative hypothesis to account for the illness in terms of receptor sensitivity (4) seems likely to involve a Ca-Mg ATPase activation process.

STUDIES TO SUPPORT THE HYPOTHESIS THAT THE EFFECT OF LITHIUM ON ATPases IS DEPENDENT ON ITS ORIENTATION TO ONE OR OTHER SIDE OF THE MEMBRANE

I should like now to describe a number of clinical and laboratory studies on membrane ATPases in man and in animals which I hope may substantiate the hypothesis that the effect of lithium on ATPases in the biological situation depends largely on the orientation or sidedness effect of lithium at that particular time:

1. Studies in man showing an illness effect on ATPase independent of a lithium effect.
2. Experimental studies in animals to demonstrate the importance of orientation (sidedness) in the action of lithium on ATPases.
3. The importance of species differences in understanding the action of lithium.

ATPase activities in depressive illness

Reduction of sodium transport has been described as an accompaniment of depressive illness, either as an inference from isotope exchange studies (2,7,8,9) or directly in the studies of the transfer of Na from blood to CSF. Depression is also associated with reduction in active transport of sodium from saliva (10) and from the erythrocyte (11). Naylor *et al.* (12) found a reduction in potassium entry in erythrocytes from depressive

Table 18.1. Specific activities of ATPase in erythrocyte membranes prepared from blood of ill, untreated depressive patients and from control subjects.

	Na/K ATPase activity	Mg ATPase activity	Ca/Mg ATPase activity	Age	Sex
Controls	342 ± 42 (10)	347 ± 41 (10)	940 ± 99 (10)	41 ± 4 (10)	4 male 6 female
Depressive patients	217 ± 47 [a] (21)	279 ± 23 (21)	894 ± 61 (19)	46 ± 4 (21)	8 male 13 female
Depressive patients (age and sex matched)	199 ± 33 [b] (10)	313 ± 27 (10)	902 ± 72 (10)		
Unipolar depressive patients	156 ± 31 [c] (9)	256 ± 45 (9)	819 ± 115 (7)	50 ± 5 (9)	1 male 8 female
Bipolar depressive patients	263 ± 42 (12)	294 ± 23 (12)	937 ± 74 (12)	42 ± 5 (12)	7 male 5 female

Results are shown for a group of ill, untreated depressive patients, a portion of the group matched for age and sex and the same patients divided into unipolar and bipolar depressive groups according to diagnosis. Specific activities are expressed as nmol Pi/h/mg protein and values given are means ± SEM with number of subjects in brackets. The mean age (years) ± SEM and sex composition of each group is also shown. Age and sex-matched groups were compared using a two-tailed paired t test, a $p < 0.025$. Other groups were compared using a two-tailed Student's t test, b: $p < 0.05$, c: $p < 0.005$ compared to controls.

patients associated with reduction in Na/K ATPase during the depressive phase and this increased on recovery from the illness. We have also shown in our laboratories that the membrane Na/K ATPase activity is significantly reduced in the depressive phase of the illness (13) (Table 18.1).

The effect of lithium on erythrocyte membrane ATPases

Naylor *et al.* (14) reported that lithium increased activity of Na/K ATPase in the erythrocyte membrane of depressed patients but it was difficult to determine whether the effect was due to recovery from the illness or to a direct pharmacological effect of lithium. Hesketh (15) has examined the effect of lithium on membrane ATPases at 2 to 4 weeks and at one year (15) (Tables 18.2, 18.3, and 18.4). There was a significant increase in Mg ATPase and Ca ATPase. The changes in Na/K ATPase in relation to lithium could not be clearly established. Patients who were continued on

Table 18.2. Specific activities of ATPases in erythrocyte membranes prepared from blood of a group of ill, untreated depressive patients and a group of patients who had received lithium treatment for at least 1 year.

	Untreated patients	Treated patients (total group)	Lithium-recovered patients	Lithium-failed patients
Na/K ATPase activity	217 ± 137 (21)	223 ± 91 (14)	248 ± 95 (9)	179 ± 65 (5)
Mg ATPase activity	279 ± 107 (21)	350 ± 113[a] (14)	331 ± 130 (9)	384 ± 66[a] (5)
Ca + Mg ATPase activity	894 ± 280 (19)	841 ± 281 (14)	768 ± 298 (9)	975 ± 183 (5)
Ca ATPase activity	618 ± 211 (19)	490 ± 190[a] (14)	437 ± 189[b] (9)	585 ± 151 (5)
Age	46 ± 16 (21)	50 ± 16 (14)	47 ± 17 (9)	54 ± 11 (5)
Sex	8 male 13 female	6 male 8 female	3 male 6 female	3 male 2 female

The lithium-treated group was also divided into those patients who had recovered and those who were ill (lithium-failed). Values given are means ± standard deviations with the number of subjects in parentheses. The age and sex composition of the groups is also given; age in years (mean ± SD). Groups were compared using a student's t test. a: $p < 0.01$, b: $p < 0.05$ compared to the untreated group lithium and who were rated as 'lithium failures' were found to have an increase in Mg ATPase without the changes in Ca ATPase and the Na/K ATPase was not increased. The question arises from these experiments

Table 18.3. Specific activities of ATPases in erythrocyte membranes prepared from blood of depressive patients while ill and untreated and from the same patients after 9-12 months lithium treatment.

	untreated	lithium-treated
Na/K ATPase	185 ± 80	273 ± 80 [b]
Mg ATPase	303 ± 113	439 ± 203 [a]
Ca + Mg ATPase	785 ± 258	1191 ± 292 [b]
Ca ATPase	483 ± 175	751 ± 183 [b]

Activities are expressed as nmol P_i/hr/mg protein. Values given are means ± SD from 9 patients. Groups were compared using a two-tailed paired t test, a: $p < 0.01$, b: $p < 0.005$

showing alterations in erythrocyte membrane ATPases as to the origin of the changes in specific activity in non-nucleated cells. We have established that significant changes can take place over a period of three to four weeks at a time when such a change could not be interpreted as arising from a turnover of the red cell population. Since there is no protein synthesis in the red cell membrane (15), we have examined the membrane fragments with regard to the binding of ions. Using sensitive methods of flameless atomic absorption spectrophotometry we could not detect lithium in the preparation. However, we were able to detect both calcium and magnesium in erythrocyte membranes which were prepared in a similar way to those in which we had measured ATPase activity. We could find no significant difference between controls and lithium-treated membranes with regard to magnesium binding but there was a significant increase in binding of calcium in the lithium-treated membranes (16) (Tables 18.5 and 18.6).

Animal studies which demonstrate the importance of sidedness or orientation in regard to the action of lithium on ATPases

In the red cell membranes it is clear that Na/K ATPase is activated from the K-sensitive (outward facing) side of the membrane. Similarly the Mg ATPase and Ca ATPase is activated from the inward facing side of the membrane. Alteration in the distribution of lithium across the red cell would clearly influence the proportion of Na/K activation and Ca^{++}

and Mg^{++} activation. Mendel and his colleagues have suggested that the clinical response to lithium is related to the internal concentration of lithium within the red cell (17). In a peripheral cell with a slow turnover of energy systems this is clearly not important but in the neuron these changes can clearly become critical. We have examined the importance of orientation with regard to the entry of Na into the cerebrospinal fluid as effected by lithium on the blood facing side of the choroid plexus and on the CSF side. Amidsen and Schou (18) could not demonstrate any effect of lithium on the transfer of Na from blood to brain, but here lithium was given as a single intraperitoneal injection. In the experiments in our labori-tories lithium was presented at the CSF side of the choroid plexus by vent-riculocisternal perfusion and here it was found that there was an increase in the rapid phase (blood CSF) of entry of Na (19). Lithium presented at this side also increased the CSF sécretion rate which would be in keeping with increased Na entry. On the other hand lithium presented on the blood side inhibited Na entry and slowed CSF secretion (Tables 18.7, 18.8 and 18.9) (20).

Table 18.4. Specific activites of a ATPases in erythrocyte membranes prepared from blood of a group of depressive patients while ill and untreated and from the same patients after 2-4 weeks of lithium treatment.

	untreated	lithium-treated
Na/K ATPase	318 ± 167 (6)	319 ± 86 (6)
Mg ATPase	255 ± 93 (6)	364 ± 86* (6)
Ca + Mg ATPase	969 ± 192 (5)	888 ± 226* (5)
Ca ATPase	683 ± 150 (5)	559 ± 162 (5)

Two patients also received electroconvulsive shock treatment during this period. Activities are expressed as nmol P_i /hr/mg protein. Values given are means ± SD with number of subjects in parentheses. Groups were compared using a two-tailed paired t test, *$p < 0.05$

The importance of species differences in determining the action of lithium

Lee *et al.* (21) and Lingsch and Martin (22) found that choline transport into the human erythrocyte was markedly diminished by treatment with lithium. Further, when lithium was stopped the inhibition of choline transport persisted for some weeks, even months. These authors were

Table 18.5. Effect of lithium on magnesium binding to human red cell membrane

Red cell membranes		Red blood cells	
Control	Patient	Control	Patient
13.70	18.38	5.53	4.96
15.43	21.74	3.18	5.45
19.44	15.53	5.05	3.87
14.14	19.82	9.36	5.43
13.48	14.19	5.55	4.88
9.09	12.50	3.71	5.89
16.04	22.21	4.87	5.13
19.63	23.03	4.05	6.24
17.55	14.98		5.18
16.33	16.06		
10.42			
15.10			
15.03 ± 3.18	17.84 ± 3.71	5.16 ± 1.90	5.22 ± 0.67
N.S.		N.S.	

Results are expressed as nmol/mg protein in the case of the membranes and for the whole red blood cells as mmol/l red cells. Mean values are given together with the SD.

Table 18.6. Effect of lithium on calcium binding to human red cell membrane

Red cell membranes		Red blood cells	
Control	Patient	Control	Patient
8.16	10.49	0.83	0.20
5.21	5.20	1.37	0.25
5.99	12.48	0.28	0.23
5.09	8.69	0.60	0.11
4.29	6.85	0.11	0.34
2.64	6.91	0.11	0.88
3.20	4.91	0.13	0.66
4.39	7.25	0.13	0.25
			0.13
4.87 ± 1.71	7.84 ± 2.59	0.45 ± 0.46	0.34 ± 0.26
$p < 0.025$		N.S.	

Results are expressed as nmol/mg protein in the case of the membranes and for the whole red blood cells as mmol/l red cells. Mean values are given together with the standard deviations.

unable, however, to obtain this effect in the rat erythrocyte. It is of interest that Hesketh (15) found that the plasma/cell distribution of lithium in the rat was different from that in man, a much larger proportion of lithium being found as an intracellular ion. In this connection Hesketh also found that, in rats given lithium chronically in diet, there was little activation of Mg ATPase in the red cell membrane in contradiction to that in man given similar weight-for-weight doses over a similar period of time. The inference again is that the orientation or sidedness in the effects of lithium are of considerable importance in determining ATPase activation in the red cell. Schless and his co-workers (23) have shown that lithium distribution in high K^+ and low K^+ sheep red cells is determined by the characteristics of the cell membrane and have further suggested that on the basis of twin studies in man the lithium distribution may be genetically controlled. It remains to be seen how this relates to the illness.

Action of lithium in the rat brain

Reading *et al.* (24) found that rats given lithium by intraperitoneal injection showed an inhibition of Na/K ATPase in the whole synaptosomal preparation followed by activation of Mg ATPase and Mg/Ca ATPase at the second week. However, these rats showed marked weight loss and other evidence of toxicity despite the fact that their plasma lithium levels were of the order of 0.4 mmol/l. When the animals were given access to a salt lick the effect on Mg ATPase was minimal. Hesketh (15) carried out similar experiments but in this case the rats were given lithium in diet. Hesketh was also able to make up preparations rich in synaptic vesicles. Again he found evidence of Mg ATPase activation but the effect was not so striking as when the rats were given lithium by intraperitoneal injection without the salt lick. The inference here is again of a species difference, i.e. the action of lithium in the rat appears to be related to a marked sodium diuresis which is not found in man.

Interaction of ATPase with transmitter systems

I have suggested that a reduction of the activity of Na/K ATPase is associated with the depressive phase of affective illness and have emphasised the importance of the distribution of lithium across the membrane in determining its action. The effect of these changes of ATPase activity on transmitter release and reuptake in brain can only be inferred in man. Vizi (6), however, in a series of experiments, has shown that different experimental conditions known to lead to inhibition of Na/K ATPase can promote acetylcholine release from nerve terminals. Vizi (25) has also shown that lithium increases resting release of acetylcholine and inhibits stimulated release. The effect of lithium in preventing recurrence of affective illness points, in my view, to a continuous effect on an intermittent membranous lesion and for this reason I have stressed the importance of the sidedness effect of lithium. At present we can only infer these effects in brain; further progress may depend on the development of new methods for determining sub-cellular ion distribution.

Table 18.7. The effects of potassium-free perfusion, and potassium-free perfusion in the presence of 1mM lithium, on Na^{24} entry into CSF and brain and upon CSF secretion rate.

	CSF Secretion rate (micro litres/min)	Fast component of Na^{24} entry into CSF $\frac{\text{cpm/ml CSF}}{\text{cpm/ml plasma}}$	Slow component of Na^{24} entry into CSF $\frac{\text{cpm/ml CSF}}{\text{cpm/ml plasma}}$ per 30 min	Na^{24} entry into brain $\frac{\text{cpm/g wet brain}}{\text{cpm/ml plasma}}$
Controls (2.98 mM K in perfusion fluid)	10.8 ± 1.7 (6)	0.122 ± 0.032 (11)	0.039 ± 0.024 (11)	0.079 ± 0.006 (6)
K-free perfusion	9.5 ± 2.3^{a} (14)	0.109 ± 0.019^{b} (13)	0.044 ± 0.029 (13)	0.088 ± 0.011 (10)
K-free $+ Li^{+}$ perfusion	12.2 ± 3.3^{a} (10)	0.152 ± 0.039^{b} (9)	0.033 ± 0.028 (9)	0.078 ± 0.010 (7)

Values represent means ± S.D. with the number of estimations in brackets. Statistical comparisons were done using a Student's t test and the significances shown are for differences between K^{+} free perfusion in the absence and presence of lithium,
a: $p < 0.05$; b: $p < 0.005$.

Table 18.8. The effects of 1 mM lithium present in the perfusing fluid Na^{24} entry into CSF, into brain and upon CSF secretion rate

	CSF Secretion rate (micro litres/min)	Fast component of Na^{24} entry into CSF $\frac{\text{cpm/ml CSF}}{\text{cpm/ml plasma}}$	Slow compnent of Na^{24} entry into CSF $\frac{\text{cpm/ml CSF}}{\text{cpm/ml plasma}}$ per 30 min	Na^{24} entry into brain $\frac{\text{cpm/g wet brain}}{\text{cpm/ml plasma}}$
Controls	10.8 ± 1.7 (6)	0.122 ± 0.032 (11)	0.039 ± 0.024 (11)	0.079 ± 0.006 (6)
+1 mM Li^{+} in perfusion fluid	13.8 ± 2.9 (7)	$0.158 \pm 0.031^{*}$ (7)	0.035 ± 0.028 (7)	0.084 ± 0.013 (7)

Values represent means ± S.D. with the number of estimations in brackets. Statistical comparisons were done using a Student's t test.
*$p < 0.05$

ACKNOWLEDGEMENTS

I should like to thank the authors concerned for permission to reproduce tables from published papers, the editor of the Journal of Neurochemistry for permission to reproduce tables 18.1, 18.7, 18.8 and 18.9 and my secretary for her help.

Table 18.9. The effects of 0.6-1.2 mM lithium in plasmá on CSF secretion rateand Na^{24} entry into CSF and brain

	CSF Secretion rate (micro litres/min)	Fast component of Na^{24} entry into CSF cpm/ml/CSF / cpm/ml plasma	Slow component of Na^{24} entry into CSF cpm/ml CSF / cpm/ml plasma per 30 min	Na^{24} entry into brain cpm/g wet brain / cpm/ml plasma
Control	10.8 ± 1.7 (6)	0.122 ± 0.032 (11)	0.039 ± 0.024 (6)	0.079 ± 0.006 (6)
0.6-1.2 mM	6.51 ± 1.7[b] (8)	0.069 ± 0.029[a] (3)	.040 ± 0.012 (3)	0.080 ± 0.021 (4)

Statistical comparisons used a Student's t test
a: $p < 0.05$; b: $p < 0.001$

References

1. Glen, A.I.M. and Reading, H.W. (1973). *The Lancet,* **ii**, 1239
2. Coppen, A. (1967). *Br. J. Psychiat.* **113**, 1237
3. Ashcroft, G.W., Eccleston, D., Knight, F. MacDougall, E.J. and Waddell, J.L. (1965). *J. Psychosom. Res.,* **9**, 129
4. MRC Brain Metabolism Unit (1972). *The Lancet,* **ii**, 573
5. Berl, S., puszkin, S. and Nicklas, W.J. (1973). *Science,* **179**, 441
6. Vizi, E.S. (1977). *J. Physiol.,* **267**, 261
7. Coppen, A. and Shaw, D.M. (1963). *Brit. Med. J.,* **ii**, 1439
8. Baer, S.L., Platman, S.R. and Fieve, R.R. (1970). *Arch. Gen. Psychiat.,* **22**, 108
9. Carroll, B.J. (1972). In: Davies, B., Carroll, B.J. and Mowbray, R.M. (eds.) *Depressive Illness: Some Research Studies,* pp. 247-257. (Springfield, Illinois: C.C. Thomas)
10. Glen, A.I.M., Ongley, G.C. and Robinson, K. (1969). *Nature,* **221**, 565
11. Hakim-Neaverson, M., Spiegel, D.A. and Lewis, W.C. (1974). *Life Sci.,* **15**, 1739
12. Naylor, G.J., Dick, D.A.T., Dick, E.G., Le Poidevin, D. and Whyte, S.F. (1973). *Psychol. Med.,* **3**, 502
13. Hesketh, J., Glen, A.I.M. and Reading, H.W. (1977). *J. Neurochem.,* **28**, 1401
14. Naylor, G.J., Dick, D.A.T., Dick, E.G. and Moody, J.P. (1974). *Psychopharmacologia,* **37**, 81
15. Hesketh, J.E. (1976). Ph.D. Thesis, University of Edinburgh
16. Glen, A.I.M., Loudon, J.B., McGovern, A.J. and Wilson, H. (In preparation)
17. Mendels, J. (1975). In: Johnson, F.N. (ed.) *Lithium Research and Therapy* pp. 43-62. (London: Academic Press)
18. Amdisen, A. and Schou, M. (1969). *Psychopharmacologia,* **12**, 236
19. Glen, A.I.M. and Hesketh, J.E. (1975). *J. Physiol.,* **252**, 83
20. Hesketh, J.E. (1977). *J. Neurochem.,* **28**, 597
21. Lee, G., Lingsch, C., Lyle, P.T. and Martin, K. (1974). *Br. J. Clin. Pharmac.,* **1**, 365
22. Lingsch, C. and Martin, K. (1976). *Br. J. Pharmac.,* **57**, 323
23. Schless, A.P., Frazer, A., Mendels, J., Pandey, G.N. and Theodiorides, V.J. (1975). *Arch. Gen. Psych.* **32**, 337
24. Reading, H.W., Dewar, A.J. and Kinloch, N. (1975). *Biochem. Soc. Trans.,* **2**, 507
25. Vizi, E.S. (1975). In: Johnson, F.N. (ed.) *Lithium Research and Therapy.* pp. 291-410. (London: Academic Press)

19

The Effects of Lithium on Calcium and Magnesium Metabolism

C. CHRISTIANSEN, P. C. BAASTRUP and I. TRANSBØL

INTRODUCTION

In the last decade some reports have indicated that lithium has an effect on serum levels of calcium and magnesium (1-4), but the results from these studies are conflicting. Recently, a few investigators have postulated decreased bone calcium in lithium treated rats (3-5) and man (6), but Hennemann and Zimmerberg (4) were unable to verify these findings.

In the last few years we have demonstrated that the measurement of bone mineral content (BMC) in the forearm by photon absorptiometry is highly correlated to total bone calcium in well-defined large groups of patients with moderate osteopenia (7,8).

Since the studies concerning the effect of lithium on calcium and magnesium metabolism seem conflicting, and since most investigations have dealt with the initial phase of lithium treatment, we report here a study in a large group of outpatients on lithium maintenance treatment, in which photon absorptiometry was used to evaluate BMC. Furthermore the biochemical indices of bone metabolism were determined to compare the biochemical and the bone status in such patients.

PATIENTS

96 long term lithium-treated manic depressive outpatients, who attended the lithium clinic at Glostrup Hospital took part in the first investigation. 13 manic depressive patients who were admitted to the psychiatric department at Glostrup Hospital took part in the second study. They were

seven men and six women aged 21-65 years (mean 45 years). None had been treated with any psychopharmacological drugs.

Two groups of control subjects were studied. Group I (146) served as controls for the measurement of bone mineral content (BMC). Group II (194) served as controls for the measurement of serum calcium, magnesium and proteins. From this latter group a subpopulation of 99 controls were drawn as controls for the measurement of serum PTH, alkaline phosphatases and phosphate.

METHODS

BMC was measured as described by Christiansen and Rødbro (8). Serum PTH was measured by radioimmunoassay using a double-antibody technique. To diminish the possible importance of inter-assay variation, the PTH levels were measured blind in series containing samples from both patients and controls. Serum calcium, magnesium and lithium were determined by atomic absorption spectrophotometry (Perkin Elmer 403). The serum levels of calcium and magnesium were corrected to a constant serum protein level (9). Serum proteins, alkaline phosphatases, and phosphate were measured routinely in our laboratory.

In the second study the BMC and the biochemical parameters were determined at time t_0; thereafter the patients were treated with lithium orally (mean dose 28 mmol/day, range 13-47). The BMC and the biochemical parameters were determined 1 month (t_1), 2 months (t_2), and 3 months (t_3) after lithium treatment was started.

Student's t test for paired differences was used for evaluation of the effect of treatment, and Student's t test for averages was used for comparison with normal subjects.

RESULTS

The first study

The mean values ± SEM for the measured parameters are given in Table 19.1.

As a group, the 96 lithium-treated patients had BMC values lower than the normal mean (93% of the normal value): 16% had BMC values lower than the mean minus 2 SD of their corresponding control grup. A highly significant increase in PTH ($p < 0.001$) was found in the lithium-treated patients whether calculated from raw data or after logarithmic transformation. 14 of the patients had serum PTH levels above the normal range (mean ±2 SD). The mean serum calcium and magnesium levels in the patients were higher than in the controls ($p < 0.001$), while the serum levels of alkaline phosphatases, phosphate and proteins were virtually of the same order in the patients and the controls.

Table 19.1. Significance of difference between BMC and serum levels of biochemical parameters in lithium-treated patients and their controls (Study 1)

	Lithium-treated patients			Control subjects			Significance of difference from normal mean
	n	mean	SEM	n	mean	SEM	
BMC(%)	96	93	1.6	146	100	1.3	$p < 0.001$
Serum PTH (micro g/l)	96	0.30	0.01	99	0.22	0.01	$p < 0.001$
Serum calcium* (mg/l)	96	100.7	0.4	194	98.9	0.2	$p < 0.001$
Serum magnesium* (mg/l)	96	22.4	0.2	194	20.3	0.1	$p < 0.001$
Serum alkaline phosphatases (K.A.u./100 ml)	96	5.8	0.2	99	5.7	0.2	NS
Serum phosphate (mg/l)	96	33.1	0.5	99	34.3	0.4	NS
Serum proteins (mg/l)	96	74.0	0.5	194	75.1	0.3	NS

NS = Not significant
* Protein corrected (9)

Table 19.2. Bone mineral content (BMC), PTH, calcium, and magnesium in patients and controls (Study 2)

	Manic depressive patients Mean ± 1 SD	Normals Mean ± 1 SD	Significance of difference
BMC (per cent of corresponding normal mean)	96.2 ± 14.7	100 ± 16.3	NS
Serum PTH (micro.g/l)	0.31 ± 0.06	0.34 ± 0.07	NS
Serum calcium (mmol/l)	2.46 ± 0.08	2.47 ± 0.07	NS
Serum magnesium (mmol/l)	0.86 ± 0.07	0.83 ± 0.05	NS

The second study

The results are given in Table 19.2 and Figure 19.1. The salient features are as follows: the mean values for all the four measured parameters (BMC, serum-PTH, serum calcium and serum magnesium) were not significantly different from the normal mean at time t_0 (before lithium treatment).

After lithium therapy was instituted, a highly significant increase in all three biochemical parameters was observed, and a moderate but significant decrease in BMC was found.

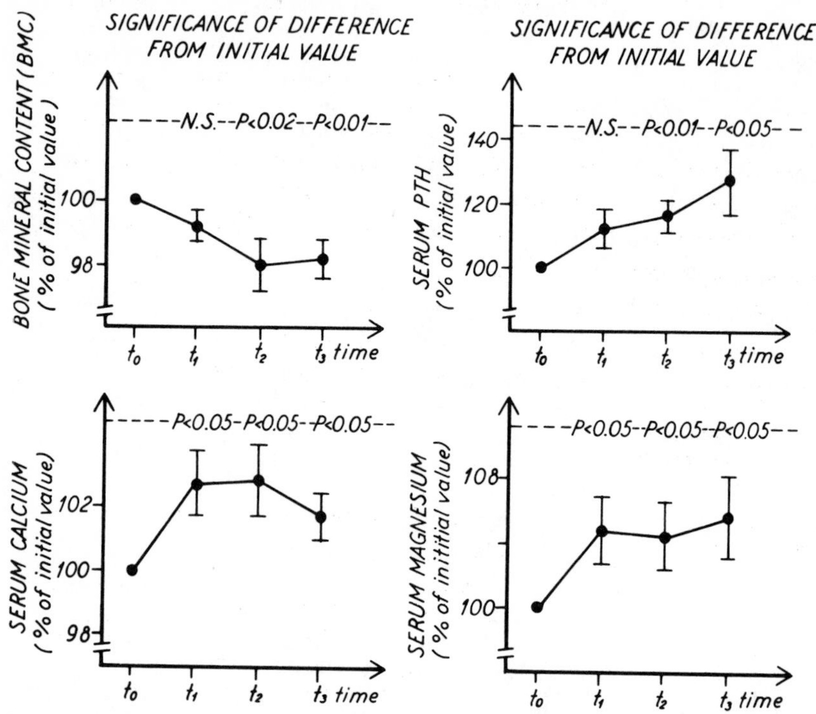

Figure 19.1. Mean values of BMC, PTH, calcium, and magnesium (per cent of initial value) as a function of time during treatment with lithium in 13 manic depressive patients. Each point on chart represents mean ± 1 SE of mean.

DISCUSSION

These studies elucidate two important points regarding the disturbed mineral metabolism in lithium treated patients: lithium — and not the underlying disease — is the true cause; and the mineral metabolism disturbances develop quite early after institution of lithium therapy.

The increased serum levels of PTH and calcium are characteristic of the feed-back anomaly observed in primary hyperparathyroidism. Furthermore, a tendency towards hypermagnesaemia is seen in hyperparathyroid patients with a modest degree of hypercalcaemia (10). The observations on the effects of lithium upon urinary calcium in man are scanty (11), but reveal a decreased excretion consistent with the known action of parathyroid hormone upon the tubular reabsorption of calcium.

Lithium may, in one way or another, increase the threshold levels of serum calcium necessary for complete suppression of parathyroid hormone secretion. In this manner a resetting of the calciostat is created resembling the 'set-point error', which has been proposed in genuine hyperparathyroidism (12).

Until now the disturbances in calcium and magnesium metabolism in lithium treated patients appear to have had little clinical relevance.

ACKNOWLEDGEMENT

This study has been supported by grants from the Danish Medical Research Council; the Danish Hospital Foundation for Medical Research, Region of Copenhagen, Faroe Islands and Greenland; F.L. Smidth & Co. Foundation.

References

1. Fizel, D., Coppen, A. and Marks, V. (1969). *Br. J. Psychiat.*, **115**, 1375
2. Mellerup, E.T., Plenge, R., Ziegler, R. and Rafaelsen, O.J. (1970). *Int. Pharmacopsychiat.*, **5**, 25f
3. Birch, N.J. and Jenner, F.A. (1973). *Br. J. Pharmacol.*, **47**, 586
4. Henneman, D. and Zimmerberg, J.J. (1974). *Endocrinology*, **94**, 915
5. Birch, N.J. and Hullin, R.P. (1972). *Life Sci.*, **11**, 1095
6. Hullin, R.P. and Nordin, B.E.C. (1975). (Personal commumication)
7. Christiansen, C., Rødbro, P. and Lund, M. (1973). *Br. Med. J.*, **4**, 695
8. Christiansen, C. and Rødbro, P. (1975). *Scand. J. Clin. Lab. Invest.*, **35**, 425
9. Christiansen, C., Naestoft, J., Hvidberg, E.F., Larsen, N.E. and Petersen, B. (1975). *Clin. Chim. Acta*, **62**, 65
10. King, R.G. and Stanbury, S.W. (1970). *Clin. Sci. Mol. Med.*, **39**, 281
11. Björum, N., Hornum, I., Mellerup, E.T., Plenge, P.K. and Rafaelsen, O.J. (1975). *Lancet*, **i**, 1243
12. Murray, T.M., Peacock, M., Powel, D., Monchick, J.M. and Potts Jr., J.T. (1972). *Clin. Endocrinol*, **1**, 235

20

Lithium Effects on Serum Magnesium and Calcium in Manic Depressive Psychosis

V. SRINIVASAN, S. PARVATHI DEVI and A. VENKOBA RAO

INTRODUCTION

The use of lithium salts in the treatment of mania was first reported by Cade (1). The prophylactic action of lithium salts against both manic and depressive states was later confirmed (2). The mechanism underlying the therapeutic effects of lithium on the clinical state of such patients remains largely obscure. Lithium has been shown to affect nerve excitation, synaptic transmission and neuronal metabolism (3).

Alterations in electrolyte distributions in affective disorders are pointed out as a consequence of genetic defects of the enzymatic capacity of the adenosine triphosphatase (ATPase) activated pump mechanism (4). Cade (5) reported raised plasma magnesium levels in depressives both before and after recovery from illness. Considerably low serum magnesium levels in depressives which rose significantly on recovery from illness have been observed by Frizel *et al.* (6) and Carney *et al.* (7). Significant difference in the mean serum magnesium and calcium concentrations in manic depressives before and after clinical treatment was not noted by Naylor *et al.* (8).

An increase in serum magnesium has been found when lithium is administered either to animals or to man acutely as well as chronically (9-13). Hennemann and Zimmerberg (14) did not find any change in serum magnesium level after lithium. Chronic administration of lithium to rats as well as to man was found to evoke increase of serum calcium (10,12). Aronoff *et al.* (9) and Vendsborg *et al.* (15) did not find any change in the serum calcium level after lithium administration. Carman and co-workers (16) have suggested that the antidepressant action of lithium might be related to increase in serum calcium or serum magnesium.

MATERIALS AND METHOD

The effects of lithium carbonate on total serum magnesium and total serum calcium in manic depressives have been studied to attempt an understanding of the therapeutic efficacy of lithium on the 'milieu interieur'. Eleven male and six female patients with the mean age of 37.4, diagnosed as affective disorder (M:10 D:7) (ICD 296) formed the material for the present study. Of the seventeen patients, ten had manic or hypomanic symptoms of high intensity and frequency. Seven were depressive at the time of consultation. The patients received lithium carbonate in doses varying from 450 to 1250 mg/day. Serum lithium estimations were made, its concentration being maintained in the range (0.4-1.0 mmol/l). Patients were rated serially with the Hamilton rating scale for depression (17) and the Beigel manic rating scale for mania (18). Fasting blood samples were obtained from these patients at 8.00 a.m. during the pre-treatment period and 7, 14, 30 and 60 days after lithium treatment. Total serum magnesium was estimated by Neill and Neely's method (19) and total serum calcium by Clark and Collip's modification of the Kramer-Tisdall method (19). Statistical analysis of the data was made using Student's t test.

RESULTS

1. A significant increase of total serum magnesium in manic depressives occurred on recovery following lithium.
2. A significant increase in the mean total serum magnesium was observed 60 days following lithium treatment ($p < 0.001$). The pretreatment mean serum magnesium level was 1.66 ± 0.14 mmol/l which rose to 1.86 ± 0.12 at the end of 60 days.
3. No change in serum total calcium was noted after lithium therapy.
4. The mean total serum calcium did not alter significantly with lithium treatment. The pretreatment serum mean calcium level was 5.21 ± 0.31 mmol/l and 60 days following lithium treatment the level was 5.29 ± 0.21 mmol/l.
5. The pretreatment total manic score was in the range of 110-210 (157 mean) and 24-46 (34.2 mean) after therapy.
6. The pretreatment Hamilton Depression Rating Quotient of the seven depressive subjects was in the range of 0.24-0.38 (0.32 mean). The score was 0.02-0.10 (0.07 mean) after 60 days of lithium treatment.

A decrease in both the intensity and frequency of manic symptoms has been noted in ten subjects who had either mania or hypomania after 60 days of lithium treatment.

Table 20.1. Mean values for serum magnesium and calcium levels (mmol/l) and Beigel's manic rating and Hamilton depression rating scores.

Content	No. of sub-jects	Pretreatment phases	Number of days after lithium treatment			
			7 days	14 days	30 days	60 days
Total magnesium (mean ± SD)	(17)	1.66 ± 0.14	1.55 ± 0.14	1.66 ± 0.16	1.66 ± 0.10	1.86* ± 0.12
Total calcium (mean ± SD)	(17)	5.21 ± 0.31	5.30 ± 0.22	5.36 ± 0.16	5.34 ± 0.14	5.29 ± 0.19
Total manic score: mean and range	(10)	157.0 (110-210)	132.2 (80-188)	114.2 (76-164)	76.8 (64-102)	34.2 (24-46)
Total Hamilton rating quotient and range	(7)	0.32 (0.24-38)	0.24 (0.20-0.32)	0.22 (0.18-0.28)	0.19 (0.16-20)	0.07 (0.02-10)

*The increase is significant at p = 0.001
(Pre-treatment vs. recovery)

DISCUSSION

An increase of total serum magnesium in all subjects has been observed after 60 days of lithium treatment, suggesting thereby a common pathophysiology which may perhaps underlie both depressive and manic episodes.

Magnesium is the second highly prevalent cation in intracellular fluids. It is essential for the activity of several enzyme systems and plays an important role in neurochemical transmission (20,21). Magnesium deficiency manifests with signs of neuromuscular dysfunction, hyper-irritability and psychotic behaviour (22,23). Hypomagnesaemia, is associated clinically with states of neuronal hyperexcitability while hypermagnesaemia has a sedative or depressant effect (24). An unstable state of the central nervous system, i.e. hyper-excitability, has been reported to underlie both manic and depressive behaviour (25,26). Neuronal excitability is intimately linked with the relative concentration of ions across the cell membrane (27).

Magnesium is essential for the stabilization of the electrochemical equilibrium across axonal membranes. It is necessary for the storage of the neurotransmitter in the intracellular storage granules. It antagonizes the calcium-dependent extraneuronal release of the adrenergic neurotransmitter substance (28). The re-uptake of the neurotransmitter substance into the presynaptic neuron is driven by the adenosine triphosphatase (ATPase) activated pump mechanism which in turn is dependent upon an adequate concentration of magnesium ion. A relative deficiency of magnesium ion in the central nervous system might serve as a trigger for the onset of manic depressive psychosis. Lithium improves and restores the clinical condition, probably by mobilizing magnesium from its reservoir and reinforcing it at the cellular level in the central nervous system.

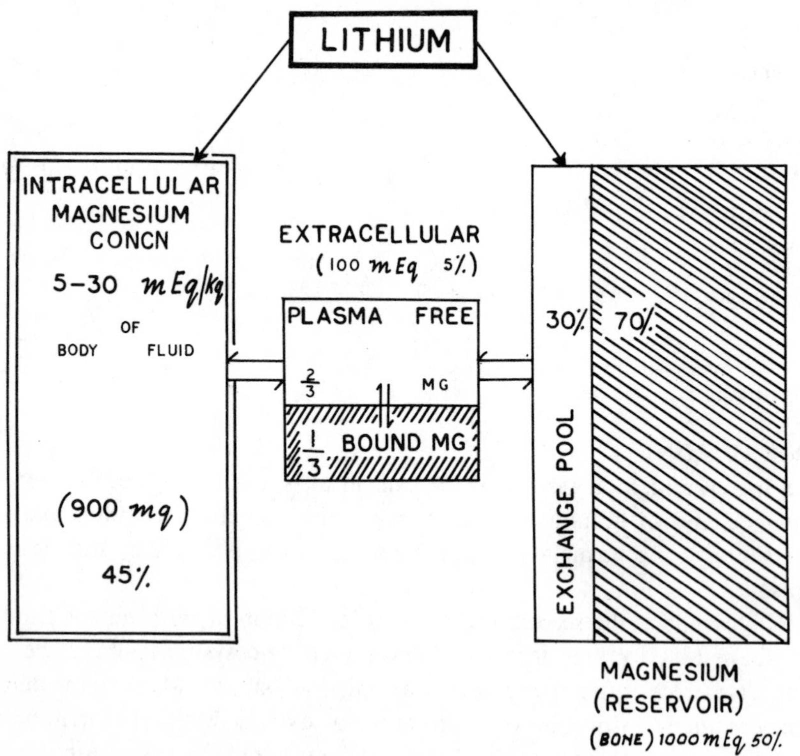

Figure 20.1. Distribution of magnesium in the human body and probable site of action of lithium in manic depressives.

Sinced ionized magnesium is really a physiologically active entity, total serum magnesium concentration may be taken as an index of magnesium turnover. Free magnesium in plasma is in equilibrium with magnesium bound to plasma proteins and an exchange of magnesium between plasma, the intercellular compartment and bone which is the main magnesium reservoir, prevails (21). The measurement of serum total magnesium thus becomes meaningful in assessing plasma ionic magnesium activity in plasma.

SUMMARY AND CONCLUSION

An increase of serum total magnesium concentration has been observed in manic depressives with lithium treatment. Serum total calcium did not change significantly with lithium treatment. A deficiency of magnesium at the cellular level in the central nervous system has been thought as the probable cause for both manic and depressive episodes. Lithium may restore the clinical magnesium from its storage depots, supplementing central nervous cellular levels with it.

ACKNOWLEDGEMENTS

The authors thank the Dean, Madurai Medical College, Madurai and the Director of Medical Education, Government of Tamilnadu, Madras, for their kind permission to publish these findings. Dr. M. Prakash Appaya and Dr. V. R. Vivekananthan, Postgraduate Department of Psychiatry and Mr. N. Nammalvar, Clinical Psychologist are thanked for their assistance.

References

1. Cade, J.F.J. (1949). *Med. J. Aust.*, **36**, 349
2. Baastrup, P.C. and Schou, M. (1967). *Arch. Gen. Psychiat.*, **16**, 162
3. Singer, I. and Rotenberg, D. (1973). *N. Engl. J. Med.*, **289**, 254
4. Nelson, R.W. and Cohen, J.L. (1976). *Am. J. Hosp. Pharm.*, **33**, 658
5. Cade, J.F.J. (1964). *Med. J. Aust.*, **51**, 195
6. Frizel, D., Coppen, A. and Mark, V. (1969). *Br. J. Psychiat.*, **115**, 1375
7. Carney, M.W.P., Sheffield, B.F. and Sebastian, J. (1973). *Br. J. Psychiat.*, **122**, 427
8. Naylor, G.J., Fleming, L.W., Stewart, E.W., McNamee, H.B. and D.Le Poidevin (1972). *Br. J. Psychiat.*, **120**, 583
9. Arnoff, M.S., Events, R.G. and Durell, J. (1971). *J. Psychiat. Res.*, **8**, 139
10. Andreoli, V.M., Villani, F. and Brambilla, G. (1972). *Psychopharmacologia*, **25**, 77
11. Birch, N.J. and Jenner, F.A. (1973). *Br. J. Pharmacol.* **47**, 586
12. Mellerup, E.T., Plenge, P., Rafaelson, O.J. (1973). *Int. Pharmacopsychiat.*, **8**, 178
13. Mellerup, E.T., Lauritsen, B., Dam, H., and Rafaelson, O.J. (1976). *Acta Psychiat. Scand.*, **53**, 360
14. Henneman, D. and Zimmerberg, J.J. (1974). *Endocrinology*, **94**, 915
15. Vendsborg, P.B., Mellerup, E.T. and Rafaelson, O.J. (1973). *Acta Psychiat. Scand.*, **49**, 97
16. Carman, J.S., Post, R.M., Teplitz, T.A. and Goodwin, F.K. (1974). *Lancet*, **i**, 1243
17. Hamilton, M. (1960). *J. Neurol. Neurosurg. Psychiat.*, **23**, 56
18. Beigel, A., Murthy, D.L. and Bunney, W.E. Jr. (1971). *Arch. Gen. Psychiat.*, **25**, 256

19. Oser, B.L. (1971). *Hawk's Physiological Chemistry* (New York: McGraw Hill Publishing Co.)
20. Livingston, D.M. and Wacker, W.E.C. (1971). *Triangle,* **10,** 169
21. Shills, M.E. (1969) *Medicine,* **48,** 61
22. Wacker, W.E.C. and Parisi, A.F. (1968). *N. Engl. J. Med.,* **278,** 658, 712 and 772
23. Goodman, L.S. and Gilman, A. (1975). *The Pharmacological Basis of Therapeutics.* 5th edn. (New York: McMillan)
24. Wacker W.E.C. and Parisi, A.F. (1968). *N. Engl. J. Med.,* **278,** 658, 712 and 772
25. Shills, M.E. (1969). *Medicine* **48,** 61
26. Daly, R.M. and Gold, G. (1976). *N. Y. State J. Med.,* **76,** 188
27. Whybrow, P.C. and Mendels, J. (1969). *Am J. Psychiat.,* **125,** 1491
28. Dubrovsky, B. and Dongier, M. (1974). Paper delivered at a symposium held at St. Mary's Hospital, Montreal, June 1974
29. Hodgkin, A.L. (1958). *Proc. R. Soc.(Biol).,* **148,** 1
30. Rubin, R.P. (1970). *Pharmacol Rev.,* **22,** 389

21

Serum Potassium Levels During Lithium Therapy of Manic Depressive Psychosis

N. HARIHARASUBRAMANIAN, S. PARVATHI DEVI
and A. VENKOBA RAO

INTRODUCTION

Disturbances of electrolyte metabolism are among the many biochemical abnormalities reported in affective disorders (1-3). An influence of lithium on ionic balance is one possible mechanism which may underly its therapeutic actions (4). Changes in body sodium, potassium, calcium and magnesium induced by lithium have been investigated (5-9). In this chapter a study of changes in serum potassium levels occurring with lithium therapy of manic depressive psychosis is presented.

MATERIALS AND METHOD

25 patients (17M:8F) diagnosed as manic depressive psychosis (ICD 296) attending the Lithium Clinic at the Department of Psychiatry, Government Erskine Hospital, Madurai, India, formed the subjects for the study. Their ages ranged from 17 to 56 years. At the time of commencement of treatment, ten were in the hypomanic or manic phase and fifteen in the depressive phase.

The patients had been attending the clinic as outpatients; some of them needed in-patient care when symptoms became aggravated. The functioning of the clinic and observations analysed therein are presented in Chapter 38.

Pre-treatment blood samples were drawn and patients were administered lithium tablets at 450-1200 mg/day in divided doses. The patients were reviewed at weekly intervals for a month; then at 2 to 3 weekly intervals thereafter and later at longer intervals. At each review, clinical and psychometric assessment of progress was done; serum lithium levels were estimated and the lithium dosage adjusted to keep the levels between 0.61 and 1.2 mmol/l. Serum potassium levels at different periods of treatment were compared with the initial pre-treatment levels and the statistical significance of observations was analysed, using Student's test.

RESULTS

1. The mean pre-treatment value of serum potassium from all the subjects was 4.27 ± 0.33 mmol/l and was within the accepted normal range of 3.5-5.5 mmol/l.

2. A significant increase in serum potassium, within physiological limits, was observed at 30, 60 and 90 days of treatment, when remission set in.

3. A return of the levels towards the pre-treatment values was noted beyond 120 days of therapy.

4. In five patients who relapsed during treatment, serum potassium at the time of occurrence of relapses was higher than at the time of remission.

Table 21.1. Serum potassium levels in manic depressive psychosis

Days of therapy	Serum potassium (mmol/l)	Level of significance with respect to pre-treatment levels	
		t*	p
Pre-treatment	4.27 ± 0.33 (25)		
7	4.47 ± 0.37 (19)	0.3	NS
14	4.74 ± 0.35 (15)	2.33	0.05
30	4.76 ± 0.46 (14)	4.25	0.001
60	4.7 ± 0.22 (13)	2.4	0.05
90	4.7 ± 0.28 (10)	2.68	0.01
120	4.43 ± 0.47 (10)	1.35	NS
150	4.38 ± 0.29 (10)	0.5	NS
180	4.4 ± 0.23 (5)	0.3	NS
240	4.33 ± 0.17 (5)	0.5	NS
300	4.4 ± 0.13 (5)	1.08	NS
Occurrence of relapses	5.39 ± 0.21 (10)	4.25	0.001

Values = Mean ± SD (number of readings)
*Student's t test
p = Probability levels
NS = Not significant

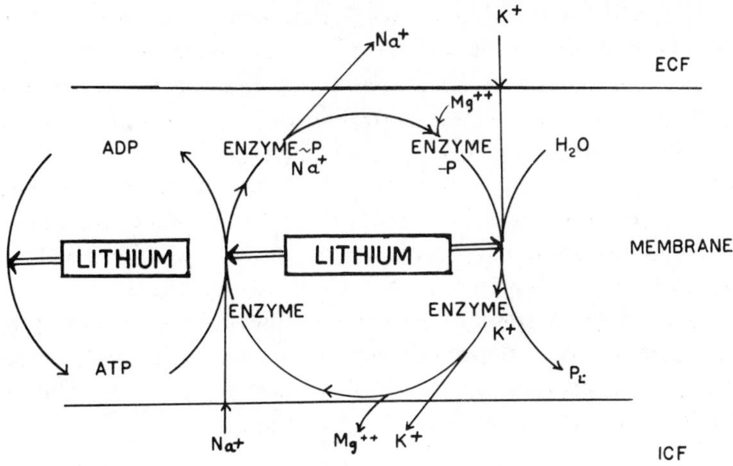

Figure 21.1. The Na,K-ATPase system and the action of lithium

DISCUSSION

Plasma levels of potassium are maintained constant within narrow physiological limits through:

1. An active transport of potassium into cells, involving Na^+,K^+-ATPase;

2. Regulation of renal secretion and loss of potassium by aldosterone and acid-base status of the body.

Lithium, as it enters the cells, disturbs the electrochemical equilibrium across the cell membrane and increases potassium-conductance (10). This results in a loss of potassium into the extracellular fluid (11) and consequently hyperkalemia.

Intracellularly, lithium replaces sodium, which is fixed to the intracellular enzyme-site of Na^+,K^+-ATPase during phosphorylation of the enzyme (12). It forms stable complexes with ADP (13). Lithium-ADP complex, while partly restoring the ATPase activity, retards potassium transport into cells, a process which requires dephosphorylation of the enzyme, with potassium getting fixed at the external site of the enzyme (12). Lithium competes with potassium for the external site and also inhibits the linked uptake of potassium and chloride (14).

Increase in extracellular potassium activates ATPase from outside, while intracellular lithium checks the functioning of the enzyme. This balanced action helps in stabilization of membrane functions and consequently nerve excitation and impulse transmission. Observations of a defective

Na^+, K^+-ATPase function in manic depressive psychosis (15,16) and of excessive activation of the enzyme by catecholamines in stress situations (17) are of relevant interest. Extracellular potassium regulates neural excitability through inducing a state of depolarization, as is well known of the phenomenon of spreading cortical depression (18).

Hyperkalemia is a stimulus for aldosterone secretion. Increase in aldosterone secretion and stimulation of activity in zone glomerulosa with lithium administration have been shown (19,20). Aldosterone tends to restore the serum potassium towards the pre-treatment levels.

If lithium fails to stabilize excitability, uncontrolled neural function which is manifest as a relapse of symptoms, is accompanied by release of potassium from neurons, further raising plasma potassium. This would explain the high levels noted at the time of relapses.

CONCLUSIONS

Lithium administration induces a physiological hyperkalemia, at the time of remission from illness. The increase in serum potassium appears to be a consequence of action of lithium on cell membranes. While remission is maintained, the raised levels tend to return to the pre-treatment state.

References

1. Baer, L., Platman, S.R. and Fieve, R.R. (1970). *Arch. Gen. Psychiat.,* **22**, 108
2. Shaw, D.M. (1966). *Br. Med. J.,* **2**, 262
3. Frizel, D., Coppen, A. and Mark, V. (1969). *Br. J. Psychiat.,* **115**, 1375
4. Schou, M. (1973). *Biochem. Soc. Trans.,* **1**, 81
5. Coppen, A. and Shaw, D.M. (1967). *Lancet,* **ii**, 805
6. Aronoff, M.S., Events, R.G. and Durall, J. (1971). *J. Psychiat. Res.,* **8**, 139
7. Shaw, D.M. (1973). *Biochem. Soc. Trans.,* **1**, 78
8. Mellerup, E.T., Lauritsen, B., Dam, H. and Rafaelsen, O.J. (1976). *Acta. Psychiat. Scand.,* **58**, 360
9. Saran, B.M. and Russell, G.F.M. (1976). *Psychol. Med.,* **6**, 381
10. Partridge, L.D. and Thomas, R.C. (1974). *Nature,* **249**, 578
11. Giacobini, E. (1969). *Acta. Psychiat. Scand. Suppl.,* **207**, 85
12. Nakao, M. (1974). *Life Sci.,* **15**, 1849
13. Lazarus, L.H. and Kitron, N. (1974). *Lancet* **ii**, 225
14. Kjeldsen, C.S., Lund-Andersen, H. and Hertz, L. (1973). *Biochem. Soc. Trans.,* **1**, 111
15. Dick, D.A.T., Naylor, G.J., Dick, E.G. and Moody, J.P. (1974). *Biochem. Soc. Trans.,* **2**, 505
16. Hokin-Naeverson, M., Spiegel, D.A. and Lewis, W.C. (1974). *Life Sci.,* **15**, 1739
17. Grafstein, B. (1956). *J. Neurophysiol.,* **19**, 154
18. Chappuis, A., Enz, A. and Iwangoff, P. (1975). *Triangle,* **14**, 93
19. Murphy, D.L., Goodwin, F.K., and Bunney, W.E. Jr. (1969). *Lancet,* **ii**, 48
20. Parvathi Devi, S., Venkoba Rao, A., Hariharasubramanian, N. and Srinivasan, V. (1973). *Ind. J. Psychiat.,* **15**, 250

Part IV:
Physiological Effects of Lithium

Introduction

Whatever the biochemical effects of lithium may be, it seems clear that certain organs in the body are likely to be more susceptible than others to the actions of lithium.

The problems of measuring the levels of lithium in body tissues are lucidly outlined by Dr Bond in Chapter 22 in which he also gives details of an interesting technique for assessing lithium levels in the brain, an organ which, on *a priori* grounds, might be expected to be vitally involved in the psychiatrically important effects of lithium. Another facet of the problem of determining brain levels of lithium is dealt with by Dr Wraae (Chapter 23) who examines the pharmacokinetics of lithium with particular reference to brain, cerebrospinal fluid and blood serum.

When lithium enters the brain it has effects which are manifested by changes in brain electrical activity. In Chapter 24, Professor Zerbi and his colleagues examine some aspects of the EEG concomitants of lithium therapy.

Lithium has long been known to have actions at the level of the endocrine system, particularly involving the thyroid gland. An exciting development of this line of investigation is described by Dr Parvathi Devi in Chapter 25; here the effects of lithium on the pineal gland are explored. The pineal has been a relatively little understood organ and has not, hitherto, been assigned a role of any importance in the control of psychopathological states, but its involvement in serotonin metabolism and Dr. Parvathi Devi's demonstration that pineal-adrenocortical functions are significantly modified by lithium, may herald a reappraisal of the status of this curious organ.

The interface between endocrine effects and fundamental biochemical changes is illustrated by Dr Horrobin and his colleagues (Chapter 26): they suggest that lithium may induce a blockade of hormone-stimulated prostaglandin biosynthesis without, at the same time, affecting basal synthesis levels. The linking of work on prostaglandins with research into lithium effects is a development of great significance; it also sets our knowledge of the endocrine actions of lithium into a new, and potentially fruitful, context.

Professor Jenner and Dr Eastwood next present a review of the renal effects of lithium. This draws together the threads from many strands of investigation, including work on cyclic AMP. and antidiuretic hormone. In this chapter, reference is made to a few studies in which the suggestion has been made that lithium may induce renal damage; as Jenner and Eastwood say, such reports must be considered with great care. Professor Schou and Dr Birch have some interesting points to make on this issue and these have been included as Addenda to Chapter 27.

The conditions for which lithium is primarily prescribed have a periodic or cyclical nature, and if follows that lithium effects on processes which show periodicity are of potential interest. Dr Mellerup and his colleagues choose a number of body functions showing diurnal rhythms and investigate the effects upon these functions of lithium administration: their findings are presented in Chapter 28.

Not all the effects which lithium produces on body tissues are necessarily related directly to the therapeutic actions of the drug. For example, lithium is known to lead to leukocytosis in the blood and this is generally regarded as peripheral to any psychiatrically important actions which lithium may have. It is, nevertheless, of considerable concern to all who are involved with lithium administration to patients that all effects of lithium which may have a bearing on the patients' well-being should be fully explored. Dr Perez-Cruet, in Chapter 29, examines the effects of lithium on leukocytosis and lymphopenia and advances an interesting hypothesis for the mechanism of such effects.

Another aspect of lithium side effects is taken up by Dr Hsu and Dr Rider in Chapter 30. The administration of lithium to pregnant females is something which has to be viewed with the greatest caution since the picture of the effects which lithium may produce on the offspring of such females is still far from complete—though one should quickly add that the evidence so far is relatively reassuring and no firm information is available to suggest that lithium produces significant effects of a teratogenic nature. Hsu and Rider take a slightly different approach to this question and instead of concentrating on anatomical changes in the offspring of lithium-treated females they examine instead the behavioural and biochemical effects and their findings are, in their own words, intriguing.

In the last analysis, the reason why lithium has attracted so much attention is that it affects the behaviour of certain classes of psychiatric patient, but behavioural studies of lithium action have been surprisingly few. Dr Harrison-Read presents a stimulating account of the way in which behavioural work and biochemical hypothesis may be blended together to produce new insights into the possible mode of action of lithium (Chapter 31).

The different levels of analysis of lithium action, from the molecular to the social psychological level, are reviewed in the final chapter of this section, Chapter 32.

22
Techniques for Analysing Lithium Distribution in Brain

P. A. BOND

Since their introduction into the field of psychotherapy (1) lithium salts have excited much interest and stimulated considerable research. An important aspect of our understanding the mode of action of this drug is the distribution of lithium in the body—especially in the brain, its presumed site of action. Several studies have explored the distribution in various body tissues including whole brain (2-4). These studies have shown that distribution is uneven, with high concentrations in bone and kidney while levels in whole brain are similar to plasma.

This chapter describes the background to, and problems encountered in, a study of the distribution of lithium in rat brain, which was carried out by Drs Brookes, Judd and myself (5). The work stemmed from the intention of Dr Judd to study the effect of lithium on rat behaviour. We felt that, although plasma lithium levels could be used as a guide, those in brain were more relevant. Especially important was the possibility of locally high concentrations in the brain. In most cases, examination of the literature will give all the background information for the proposed study, but in this instance, apart from the paucity of relevant studies, there were other circumstances which persuaded us that we should measure brain lithium levels ourselves. The problems which prompted this decision will be discussed in some detail; some of these are common to most research, while others are peculiar to studies with lithium. Before dealing with the lithium problems, however, two other areas crucial to the study will be discussed. These are, firstly, the method of tissue treatment prior to lithium measurement, and secondly the choice of brain dissection technique. In a previous study of the uptake of gamma-aminobutyric acid into brain slices, a new tissue solubilising agent had been used for radioactive counting. This agent, Soluene-100, was a toluene solution of a quarternary ammonium base (ammonium-1-pyrrolidene dithiocarbamate). Its advantage over such agents as hyamine hydroxide, which had been used previously, was its greater efficiency and capacity for tissue. It seemed opportune to test the suitability of Soluene-100 for atomic absorption spectrometry and use it for the study of brain lithium distribution. Soon after starting this work Jackson and co-workers (6) described the use of Soluene-100 for the measurement of tissue zinc, copper, iron, and manganese by atomic absorption spectrometry, confirming its applicability to this technique. In the event, Soluene-100 proved a very useful agent. It was compared with the standard technique of wet ashing as described by Birch and Jenner (3), based on the procedure of Chang and co-workers (7). The results of estimations of lithium, sodium, and magnesium obtained by the two methods on similarly treated animals were not significantly different. The advantage of the Soluene method over other methods, such as the various wet and dry ashing procedures, lies in its extreme simplicity and the accuracy that ensues when the whole procedure is carried out in a single closed vessel, with additions monitored by weighing. Digestion by Soluene proceeds rapidly and is generally complete overnight at room temperature. Fatty tissues such as brain are especially well dealt with. The tissue solution was diluted with 2-ethoxyethanol to reduce the viscocity sufficiently for passage through the atomizer of the atomic absorption spectrometer. This (usually three-fold) dilution of a 10% tissue solution determined the limits of sensitivity of the method. Apart from lithium, levels of sodium and magnesium were also measured. In the case of magnesium, hydrochloric acid and lanthanum nitrate were added to prevent precipitation and eliminate interference.

The final measurement was by atomic absorption spectrometry using a Hilger-Watt-Atomspek AA2 instrument. With samples of sufficiently low viscocity this final measurement posed few problems apart from minor adjustment to burner height and gas flow rates.

The second problem, namely the choice of dissection technique for rat brain, proved relatively simple. Few methods have been described and that of Glowinski and Iversen (8) with which I had had previous experience seemed ideal for the purpose. It yields seven well defined regions, the smallest of which is still sufficient for lithium measurement. Ebadi and co-workers (9) using the method of Konig and Klippel (10), had 16 regions, though they pooled the tissues from 2-4 brains for each determination. Having decided on a method, a number of brains were dissected by two people until the technique was almost identical and the weights of each region were similar to those published by Glowinski and Iversen (8).

Several problems seem to be peculiar to lithium studies and their many solutions have led to difficulty in sorting out the lithium literature. In this case decisions were guided by the need to match conditions in the projected behavioural study to those for brain lithium distribution. It should be stressed that the work was carried out at the Unit for Metabolic Studies in Psychiatry at Sheffield, under the direction of Professor Jenner. In such a unit, where work on many aspects of lithium research has proceeded over the years, a collective fund of experience grows which is drawn upon, almost unconsciously by individual workers. For example, the choice of animals for the work was guided by previous experience, the CFY strain Wistar rats from Carworth, Europe, were already known to be subject to minimal variation and their reactions to lithium were well established.

The solution of the major problem of how to administer lithium to rats also depended very much on previous experience. Differences in methods of administration have led in the past to great difficulty in comparing results in otherwise similar studies. There are several aspects to this problem, each requiring a decision between several possibilities. Firstly, the form in which lithium is given, usually as the carbonate, chloride or citrate can influence results. For example Morrison and co-workers (11) found differences in absorption rate and plasma levels, between lithium carbonate and chloride given to rats i.p. or orally. In our case lithium chloride was chosen for its good solubility in water. The route of administration is important and has again been subject to many variations from one study to another. Lithium has usually been given by injection i.p. or i.v. or orally by stomach tube, in drinking water or in food, each being subtly different. Our decision to give lithium in the diet was governed partly by experience, but more by the belief that this route has many major advantages and that the few disadvantages could be overcome with practice. The advantages are the relatively steady blood level of lithium, the ease of administration, the lack of disturbance during chronic dosage and the absence of several serious problems associated with some of the other routes. The disadvantages lie mainly in not knowing how much lithium the individual rat will take in and one's reliance on the acceptance of the food by the animal. In practice, very predictable plasma levels are achieved even with animals housed in groups of five or six. For example, Edelfors (12) using Wistar rats for a study of brain lithium distribution, gave lithium chloride at the same concentration in the diet and for a similar duration as in our study. The fact that he found exactly the same plasma level of 0.59 mmol/l is probably fortuitous, though it does emphasize the consistency attainable by this method of dosing. Acceptance of the food was good, with no significant difference in growth rate. A further problem lies in relating dosage in rats to that in man. Therapeutic doses of lithium give human serum levels between 0.8 and 2 mmol/l, in rats such levels are associated with severe toxicity, so that any results obtained with such animals must be suspect, especially in behavioural studies. In our study we did include a series of animals on higher doses of lithium achieving a plasma level of 0.79 mmol/l as opposed to 0.59 mmol/l on the lower dose. These animals gained weight more slowly than normal and had increased fluid intake and output. They looked in poor condition compared with animals on the lower lithium intake. A plasma level of 0·6 mmol/l is close to the upper limit for maintaining rats free of toxicity. The final problem in dosage lies in deciding the frequency and duration of lithium administration. Frequency is of no concern where lithium is given in the diet, but duration is very important, especially when it is remembered that lithium requires quite an appreciable time to exert its therapeutic action. It was decided to measure brain lithium distribution after three time periods 2, 14 and 42 days covering the likely duration of the behavioural study. In the event, the results at these three times was so similar that only the results after 14 days treatment were published (5).

These were the problems encountered and the solutions reached in carrying out the study. The results (Table 22.1) will now be considered and these will be related to other reported work. In our study the concentration of lithium in rat brain was not strikingly different in any of the seven regions examined. Values covered a 1.4 fold range on a diet giving a plasma level of 0.59 mmol/l, and an almost two-fold range when the plasma level was 0.79 mmol/l. The lack of startling regional differences is not unexpected, though on both diets significant differences were detected between certain regions and plasma. On the lower lithium diet these were the low values in pons and medulla, cerebellum, and hypothalamus, whilst higher values in corpus striatum and cortex failed to reach significance. On the higher lithium diet the content of most regions was raised compared with plasma, and significant differences are seen with regions of higher lithium content (such as cortex and corpus striatum) when compared with plasma. A very similar pattern of distribution was

Table 22.1. Rat brain and plasma concentrations of sodium, magnesium and lithium after the administration of a normal diet or diets with added NaCl (30 mmol/kg dry food) LiCl (30 mmol or 45 mmol/kg dry food) for 14 days

	Normal diet	Sodium diet NaCl 30 mmol/kg dry food		Lithium diet LiCl 30 mmol/kg dry food			Lithium diet LiCl 45 mmol/kg dry food
	Na	Na	Mg	Na	Mg	Li	Li
Pons and medula	51.7 0.91 (6)	52.8 0.89 (10)	5.69 0.38 (10)	47.3*** 0.95 (10)	5.03 0.24 (10)	0.49* 0.021 (12)	0.74 0.029 (6)
Cerebellum	52.7 0.96 (6)	51.7 0.79 (10)	5.61 0.24 (10)	48.9*** 1.46 (10)	4.42*** 0.14 (10)	0.46* 0.025 (12)	0.79 0.031 (6)
Hypothalamus	52.8 0.77 (6)	53.1 0.92 (10)	6.11 0.37 (6)	48.7*** 1.68 (10)	4.35 0.40 (6)	0.48* 0.017 (12)	0.63* 0.037 (5)
Hippocampus	52.5 1.10 (6)	52.8 1.46 (10)	5.86 0.37 (6)	52.1 0.92 (10)	4.62*** 0.38 (6)	0.61 0.023 (12)	1.0* 0.047 (6)
Mid-brain	54.7 0.58 (6)	55.1 0.89 (10)	5.28 0.33 (10)	52.6*** 0.85 (10)	4.58 0.20 (10)	0.55 0.021 (12)	0.90* 0.023 (6)
Corpus striatum	51.3 0.96 (6)	51.5 1.61 (10)	7.41 0.36 (6)	49.6 0.85 (10)	4.49*** 0.39 (6)	0.64 0.021 (11)	1.16* 0.051 (5)
Cortex	51.8 0.73 (6)	51.2 0.47 (10)	5.67 0.21 (10)	47.5*** 1.71 (10)	5.03*** 0.14 (10)	0.63 0.022 (12)	1.22* 0.040 (5)
Cortex (19.00h)	—	—	—	—	—	0.52** 0.040 (5)	—
Whole brain	—	—	—	—	—	0.55 0.037 (6)	0.92 0.063 (6)
Plasma	—	—	0.69 0.03 (13)	—	0.90*** 0.03 (12)	0.59 0.020 (12)	0.79 0.031 (6)

Values are expressed as mmol/kg fresh tissue or as mmol/l of plasma and represent the mean (first figure) ± **the SEM (second figure):** the number of observations is in parentheses. All values are from rats killed at 10.00 h unless otherwise stated.

*Significantly different from plasma concentration
**Significantly different from cortex (10.00 h) concentration
***Significantly different from Na diet concentration
} $p < 0\ 05$, t test

seen with both dosage regimes. The effect of lithium on sodium and magnesium levels was also investigated. There was a significant reduction in sodium content of all regions except hippocampus and corpus striatum. The content of magnesium was also reduced in all regions, reaching significance in all but the pons and medulla and midbrain.

While there have been several studies of brain lithium distribution in rodents, monkey and man, only a few of these are directly comparable to our study. Table 22.2 summarizes the results in rats and mice, expressed where possible in relationship to whole brain lithium, to render them more easily comparable and to make more obvious those regions with lithium levels above or below the average. A cursory glance at this table is sufficient to see the problems posed by the use of different dissection techniques. The study of Edelfors (12) resembles ours very closely. His rats, like ours, were given LiCl in the diet at 30 mmol/kg and a plasma level of 0.59 mmol/l (exactly the same as ours) was attained. Most of his results

Table 22.2. Distribution of lithium in the brains of rodents

	Bond *et al.* (5)	Hi *et al.* (13)	Ebadi *et al.* (9)	Edelfors (12)	Messiha (14)
Animal species	Rat	Rat	Rat	Rat	Mouse
Dosage	Chronic	Chronic	Acute	Chronic	Acute
Duration	14 days	18 days	Single	21-35 days	Single
Route	Diet	i.p.	i.v.	diet	i.p.
Salt	LiCl	LiCl	LiCl	LiCl	LiCl
Pons & medulla	0.89	—	0.89	—	—
Cerebellum	0.84	1.0	1.07	0.83*	1.07
Hypothalamus	0.87	—	1.18	1.86	—
Hippocampus	1.11	—	1.29	—	1.19
Midbrain	1.0	—	—	—	—
Corpus striatum	1.16	—	—	—	1.07
Cortex	1.15	1.0	—	1.05	1.12
Thalmus	—	—	1.18	0.73	—
Diencephalon	—	1.0	—	—	0.67
Colliculus	—	—	1.13	—	—
Brain stem	—	0.95	—	—	0.90
Grey matter	—	—	—	0.76	—
White matter	—	—	—	2.71	—
Caudate	—	—	1.75	—	—
Globus pallidus	—	—	1.80	—	—
Putamen	—	—	1.44	—	—
Cerebrum	—	—	1.32	—	—
Whole brain (mmol/kg)	0.55	—	1.22	—	0.67
Plasma (mmol/l)	0.59	—	—	0.59	0.45

Values in brain regions are related to Whole brain lithium, except for Edelfors, 1975 where the relationship is to plasma level
*Plus pons

agree with ours except that the hypothalamus in his study contained over twice as much lithium as in ours. The only other study of brain distribution in rat after chronic (12-18 days) lithium by Ho *et al.* (13) showed no significant difference between the diencephalon, which includes the hypothalamus, and their three other regions. A study in the rat by Ebadi and co-workers (9), in which a single large dose of lithium was given, showed a similar spread and distribution of lithium levels to our own. Messiha (14) reported regional brain levels of lithium in mouse 8 hours after a single dose. The results were strikingly similar to ours and though no separate levels in hypothalamus were reported, the lowest levels were recorded in the diencephalon.

Very few reports have appeared of brain lithium distribution in primates and man. A detailed study of distribution in monkey and one human brain by Spirtes (15) and an earlier one by Francis and Traill (16) are summarized in Table 22.3. Spirtes (15) records the distribution of lithium in

Table 22.3. Distribution of lithium in the brains of monkey and man

	Spirtes (15)	Spirtes (15)	Francis & Traill (16)	
Species	Monkey	Man	Man 1	Man 2
Cerebral grey	—	—	0.6	0.69
Cerebral White	—	—	0.75	0.97
Pons & medulla	0.45	—	1.4	1.86
Cerebellum	0.39	—	0.68	0.86
Hypothalamus anterior	0.46	1.03		
posterior	0.46	0.42		
Hippocampus	0.57	0.88		
Midbrain	0.46	—		
Cortex occipital	0.43	0.87		
frontal	0.36	0.52		
temporal Lobe	0.37	0.22		
sensory	0.46	—		
motor	0.45	—		
Thalamus anterior	0.82	0.76		
posterior	0.56	0.37		
Corpus callosum	0.56	0.51		
Amygdala	0.48	0.42		
Caudate	0.65	1.41		
Substantia nigra	—	0.65		
Globus pallidus	0.41	0.65		
Putamen	0.59	—		
Retrosplenial cingulate gyrus	—	1.73		
Subcallosal cingulate gyrus	—	0.22		
Whole brain (half) (mmol/kg)	0.50	—		
Plasma or serum (mmol/l)	1.0	—	0.25	0.35
Whole blood (mmol/l)	—	—	—	—

Values in brain regions are related to blood level of lithium monkey brain following oral dosage of lithium carbonate for 3-6 weeks. There was a just over a two-fold difference between highest and lowest values, with mean levels of 0.5 mmol/kg very similar to those in our rat study. The plasma level of 1 mmol/l was, however, much higher than in our rats. In the larger species even areas such as hypothalamus could be subdivided. In most cases the several parts of an area were similar, though in some instances there were significant differences within a region; for example between anterior and posterior thalamus (1.5 times) and sensory cortex and cortex tip (1.3 times).

Studies in man have been few and are subject to the problems inherent in all post mortem work. Spirtes (15) reported values from a manic depressive male who died of excess alcohol and Darvon. The lithium level in whole blood was 0.86 mmol/l. The distribution of lithium was different in many respects from that in monkey brain in the same report. The difference between highest and lowest regions was considerable, being nearly eight-fold, and large differences occurred between, for example, anterior and posterior hypothalamus (2.5 times), anterior and posterior thalamus (2 times) and between different parts of the cortex (4 times). Although the pronounced difference within the thalamus was observed also in monkey, those within hypothalamus and cortex were not. An earlier study by Francis and Trail (14) records lithium levels in a much more limited range of areas in two patients. Results in the two patients were comparable and there was a two-fold difference between highest and lowest areas. Comparison of these two human studies is impossible because the brain regions measured have little in common.

To summarize all these results is difficult. There are regional differences in lithium distribution in all four species studied. In our case, differences were more marked at the higher dosage where most levels were higher but with the higher levels proportionately more so. Other rat studies are similar to ours but Edelfors (12) found high levels in the hypothalamus. The acute mouse study of Ebadi *et al.* (9) gave very similar results to our rat study. Results in monkey are of interest for the large number of brain regions measured. Where results can be compared they are close to our rat study. In monkey there are some significant differences even within regions, for example the thalamus. These regional differences are paralleled in the human brain study by the same author, though the marked difference within the human hypothalamus was not found in monkey.

It seems that we were justified in conducting our study on the species, and under the precise conditions, in which the later behavioural studies were to be performed.

References

1. Cade, J.F.J. (1949). *Med. J. Aust.,* **2,** 349
2. Schou, M. (1958). *Acta Pharmacol. Toxicol.,* **15,** 115
3. Birch, N.J. and Jenner, F.A. (1973). *Br. J. Pharmacol.,* **47,** 586
4. Birch, N.J. and Hullin, R.P. (1972). *Life Sci.,* **11,** 1095
5. Bond, P.A., Brooks, B.A. and Judd, A. (1975). *Br. J. Pharmacol.,* **53,** 235
6. Jackson, A.J., Michael, L.M. and Schumacher, H.J. (1972). *Anal. Chem.,* **44,** 1064
7. Chang, T.L., Gover, T.A. and Harrison, W.W. (1966). *Analyt. Chim. Acta,* **34,** 17
8. Glowinski, J. and Iversen, L.L. (1966). *J. Neurochem.,* **13,** 655
9. Ebadi, M.S., Simmons, V.J., Hendrickson, M.J. and Lacy, P.S. (1974). *Eur. J. Pharmacol.,* **27,** 324
10. Konig, J.F.R. and Klippel, R.A. (1963). *The Rat Brain* (Baltimore: Williams and Wilkins)
11. Morrison, J.M., Pritchard, H.D., Brau de, M.C. and D'Aguanno, W. (1971). *Proc. Soc. Exp. Biol. Med.,* **137,** 8898
12. Edelfors, S. (1975). *Acta Pharmacol. Toxicol.,* **37,** 387
13. Ho, A.K.S., Gershon, S. and Pinckney, L. (1970). *Arch. Int. Pharmacodyn.,* **186,** 54
14. Messiha, F.S. (1976). *Arch. Int. Pharmacodyn.,* **219,** 87
15. Spirtes, M.A. (1976). *Pharmacol. Biochem. Behav.,* **5,** 143
16. Francis, R.I. and Traill, M.A. (1970). *Lancet,* **ii,** 523

23

The Pharmacokinetics of Lithium in the Brain, Cerebrospinal Fluid and Serum of the Rat

O. WRAAE

In the treatment of patients for manic depressive disease it is normally assumed that the effectiveness of lithium salts is related to the concentration achieved in the brain. This cannot be monitored, and so it is usual to measure the concentration of the ions in the serum, which is the closest site in which repeated observations can be made safely. However, it has been shown in rats that when the lithium concentration in the serum changes rapidly, it does not correlate well with that found in the brain (1).

Recently, a high correlation was found at steady state between the lithium concentrations in the serum and in the cerebrospinal fluid in patients; the authors of this report assumed that the concentration in the cerebrospinal fluid would reflect the cerebral concentration better than that found in the serum (2).

Therefore, it was decided to compare directly in rats the concentration of lithium in the serum, the cerebrospinal fluid and the brain at steady state and also to examine the relationships between these concentrations during the uptake and elimination of lithium. These data could be compared with findings in patients and in previous experiments on cerebral slices of rats *in vitro* (3).

Male Wistar rats weighing 250-400 g were used. For the measurement of lithium at steady state they were given a powdered standard diet containing lithium carbonate. After 4 days they were anaesthetized with ether, and blood samples of approx 5 ml were taken by cardiac puncture. After exposing the atlanto-occipetal membrane approx. 100 micro.l of cerebrospinal fluid was drawn under slight suction. The rats were then killed by dislocation of the neck and the brain was rapidly removed. Measurement of lithium was made by atomic absorption spectrophotometry in duplicate, except for the samples of cerebrospinal fluid which are too small for double determination.

Whereas the concentration of lithium in the brain and in the serum were almost alike, that of the cerebrospinal fluid was much lower. The ratio of brain to CSF concentration was nearly 3 whilst the ratio of CSF to serum concentration was about 0.4. The variability of these ratios was relatively small because the results from each individual animal were compared. Almost identical ratios were found in a second experiment.

The ratios of the concentration of lithium between the cerebrospinal fluid and the serum compare reasonably well with values from a clinical material. Thus a mean ratio of 0.33 was found on patients in long term treatment with lithium (2). Most previous values given in the literature have been based on single administrations after which the ratios change continuously.

Results found *in vitro* are in partial agreement with the present findings. In rat cerebral slices, after incubation *in vitro,* the ratio of the tissue and the medium was found to be around 1.6 (3). The ratio was found to be dependent on metabolism. It is only about half that between the brain and the cerebrospinal fluid *in vivo.* However, the poorer ability of cerebral tissue *in vitro* to maintain a gradient is also apparent in the case of potassium.

The kinetics of lithium were examined in two series of experiments. In the first one a single injection of 5 mmol of LiCl/kg body wt was given i.p. and the rats were sacrificed 15 min to 48 h after the injection. Otherwise the procedure was as summarized before.

Several features of the findings are of interest. The concentration in the serum rose rapidly to more than 8 mmol/l, falling exponentially after 6-12 h. The results did not justify any compartmental analysis. In the brain the maximum concentrations (1.5 mmol/l) were seen between 12 and 24 h after the injection. The lithium in the cerebrospinal fluid was high enough to be measured after 15 min, reaching a maximum of 1.2 mmol/l in 2 h. For the first 2 h the concentration of lithium in the cerebrospinal fluid was greater than that of the brain. This is illustrated particularly clearly if one compares the ratios of the concentrations in the brain and in the cerebrospinal fluid, because the ratios vary less than the actual concentrations. The steady state level is reached after approx 20 h, illustrating the slow uptake in the brain. It is in striking contrast to the uptake of lithium in cerebral slices, in which the final distribution is reached within an hour.

Similar differences have been found in the uptake of potassium, and must be due to the blood-brain barrier. Looking at the temporal relationship between the ratios of concentration in the cerebrospinal fluid and in the serum, it becomes clear that one cannot make any inferences about the steady state situation by means of a single injection.

The elimination of lithium from the three different compartments took place at different rates even after 24 h, when the half life in the serum, the cerebrospinal fluid, and the brain was found to be 12 h, 10 h, and 7 h respectively, indicating that no equilibrium was reached during the period of observation. Therefore, the elimination was studied from a state of equilibrium in a second series of experiments. This time the rats were given subcutaneous injections of 0.9 mmol of LiCl/kg body wt. every 6 h for 2 days, corresponding to approx 8 half times. The elimination of lithium was followed from 6 h to 48 h after the last injection. The results from this experiment were plotted on semilogarithmic paper. At the starting point the same concentration ratios occurred as were found in the feeding experiment. The scatter of the points was considerable even for a semilog plot when the raw data were used, but again it is of some assistance to study a plot of the ratios. Assuming 1st order kinetics we would expect the ratios of the concentrations to be dependent on the elimination constants, as weel as the initial concentrations: $\mathbf{A}\ e^{-at}\ /\mathbf{B}\ e^{-bt}$. This expression becomes constant when the elimination constants a and b are equal, indicated by a horizontal plot of the ratios. The plots of the ratios of lithium in the brain and both in the serum and in the cerebrospinal fluid became horizontal after approx 24 h. Calculation of the elimination constants gave the following results expressed as half times:-6-24 h, serum 5.4 h (r = 0.89, n = 29), csf 7.2 h (r = 0.87, n = 27), brain 12.7 h (r = 0.80, n = 28), 24-48 h, serum 6.8 h (r = 0.28), n = 28), csf 7.6 h (r = 0.85, n = 22), brain 8.2 h (r = 0.9, n = 28).

The results from the kinetic experiments do not lend themselves to any compartmental analysis, but they are suggestive of a multi-compartmental system (4) in which there is a central and two peripheral compartments of which one is a so-called "deep" compartment with a slow equilibration. During the elimination of a drug from a steady state, achieved by repeated injections, the concentration in the deep compartment remains high, and the effects persist long after the concentration in the central compartment has fallen well below the minimum effective concentration, and may not even be measurable.

A similar system, with the brain as a deep compartment, could explain the common phenomenon in the initial phase after acute lithium intoxication when there are practically no symptoms despite high serum values of lithium. Also, the clinical signs of lithium intoxication often persist several days after successful haemodialysis leading to minimal concentrations of lithium in the serum.

According to the present animal experiments, measurements of lithium in the cerebrospinal fluid do not offer any advantages over measurements in the serum in predicting the concentration of lithium in the brain. This conclusion is supported by very recent findings during hemodialysis after lithium intoxication (5).

References

1. Frazer, A., Mendels, J., Secunda, S.K., Cochrane, C.M. and Bianchi, C.P. (1973). *J. Psychiat. Res.,* **10**, 1
2. Paul, H.-A. (1973). *Nervenarzt,* **44**, 210
3. Wraae, O. (1976). *J. Neurochem.,* **26**, 835
4. Kudsk, F.N. (1976). *Farmakokinetik,* (Copenhagen: F.a.d.L.'s Forlag)
5. Amdisen, A. (Personal communication)

24

EEG Changes During Lithium Treatment

F. ZERBI, L. FENOGLIO and P. TOSCA

INTRODUCTION

The EEGs of patients undergoing lithium therapy demonstrate a slowing of the background activity, an increase in amplitude and bilateral paroxysms of the syncronous slow waves. Mayfield and Brown (1) found EEG changes with serum lithium levels as low as 0.75 mmol whereas Platman and Fieve (2) found no correlation whatsoever between serum lithium levels and EEG changes. Andreani *et al.* (3) attribute the EEG changes to the CNS action of lithium, mainly on the reticular substance of the thalamus. Mayfield and Brown (1), however, find that a disturbance of the mechanism of central ionic exchange is difficult to demonstrate. Vacaflor (4), after an extensive review of the literature, concludes that the EEG characteristics most often associated with the neurotoxicity of lithium are: 1. the appearance of high voltage slow waves; 2. a decrease of alpha activity with an increase of theta and delta waves; 3. a correlation between the severity of EEG modifications and the clinical evidence of CNS damage; but a lower correlation with the serum levels of lithium; and 4. a high probability of EEG modifications (focal anomalies) in subjects who have shown anomalies prior to therapy.

Lithium salts have been shown to reduce psychomotor activity in manic patients and are presently used in manic depressive treatment (5). The observation that the administration of lithium increases the intracellular concentration of sodium (6) and the indirect data associating the depressive state with a high intracellular concentration of sodium ions, are of considerable interest in interpreting the electrophysiological modifications of depressed patients and patients undergoing lithium therapy.

Using the 'cortical recovery function' technique to study the action of lithium on cortical activity, Gartside *et al.* (7) observed that after administering lithium (1 g/day for 7 days) to normal subjects, the second response to paired stimuli with an interval of 10-25 mins became relatively much smaller, and this change in cortical recovery function resembles that seen in psychotic depressives. It is likely that the action of lithium on the cortical recovery function is related to the changes noted in the cuneate or thalamic relays or in the cortical grey substance.

Helmchen and Kanowski (8), over a 3-year period, reported EEG results, collected before and during lithium therapy, on 73 manic depressive psychotic patients who for the most part had had relapses and were treated, in part, on an out-patient basis. The changes seen most frequently were: 1. focal anomalies mainly on the left; 2. intermittent activity; 3. convulsive potentials; and 4. vigilance disturbances. The concept that the mechanism of action of lithium is one of membrane modification may be generalized to the peripheral nervous tissue (6). This concept is supported by the work of Pinelli *et al.* (9) who found, by tetanic stimulation of the median nerve, a different facilitative response in depressed patients treated with lithium carbonate in dose of 1200 mg/day. Such facilitation, while present in bipolar depressives, was lacking in unipolar depressives. This facilitation must be interpreted as a progressive reassumption of the normal maximal amplitude from an initial reversible block due to electrolytic inequilibria.

CLINICAL CASES

G.C. age 52 (case no. 42632)

Treated in this clinic in 1969-1971-1973 for depressive episodes with tricyclics and once with electroshock therapy, G.C. was readmitted on 16.4.74. The patient had been well for about 1 year after the last release but had now begun to be sad, to have microptic visual disturbances and not to sleep. No particulars were uncovered during the objective and neurological examination. As for psychological status, the patient was alert and orientated. The patient's mood was distinctly depressive — lifeless, lacking initiative, unable to sleep and without appetite.

Physical examinations revealed the following: electrolytes: K 4.219; Na 134; EEG: alpha rhythm 9.5 Hz, 60-80 mV in irregular sequence mixed with abnormal 6-7 Hz theta groups in all leads, sometimes with a syncronized appearance on the central regions, hyperpnea provoking a modest accentuation of the anomalies.

On 18.4.74, therapy was begun with 900 mg of lithium carbonate (three 300 mg tablets per day). The serum lithium level was determined every 7 days.

About a month later, since the patient had complained for a few days of cephalalgia and an accentuation of the preceding visual disturbances, and since there was an uncertain response to the plantar stimulus on the left, an EEG was performed on 13.5.74, with the following results; EEG: occipital-parietal activity at 6-8 Hz and disorganized background activity with voltage asymmetry higher on the right than on the left; partial bilateral reaction with eyes open, followed by the appearance of large polymorphic abnormalities with frequencies into the delta range and cuspid elements prevalently in the right hemisphere; hyperpnea accentuated the basal anomalies. Serum lithium level was 0.95 mmol/l; electrolytes: K 4.475; Na 126.5. Lithium therapy was suspended and periodic EEG control was begun (Figure 24.1).

On 21.5.74 the EEG was distinctly improved, the delta frequencies being no longer in evidence, and the background activity well organized with an alpha frequency of 8-9 Hz; the theta frequency was also reduced. Partial reactions occurred with eyes open.

The patient was released in good psychic condition on 25.5.74, but on 30.12.75 was readmitted due to complaints of depression, insomnia and

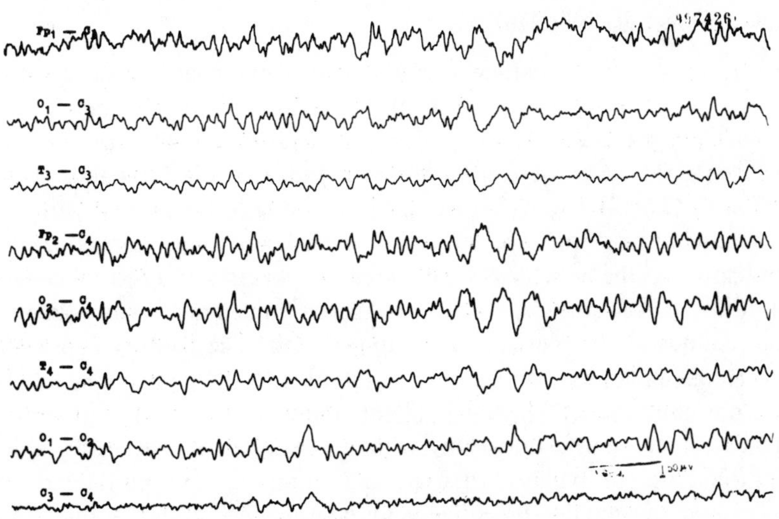

Figure 24.1 EEG of patient G.C.

inability to perform housework. Objective and neurologic examinations showed no change.

On 31.12.75 an EEG showed alpha rhythm 8.5-9.0 Hz, 30-70 mV, symmetric and stable. Normal reaction occurred with eyes open. There were few low voltage, diffuse, rapid rythms. Low voltage, 6-7 Hz rhythms, isolated or in short spurts were seen in the central-anterior regions. Hyperpnea produced no significant modifications.

Lithium carbonate therapy was again initiated on 2.1.76, 900 mg/day (three 300 mg tablets/day).

On 15.1.76 the patient complained of cephalalgia, but a neurological examination proved negative. An EEG was performed, showing occipito-parietal activity, 6-8 Hz, polymorphic medium voltage. No reaction occurred with eyes open. Slower sequences extending into the delta frequencies were noted, polymorphic mixed with background rhythm prevalently in the encephalic centre and bilateral. The lithium serum level was 0.95 mmol/l. The dose was reduced to 600 mg of lithium carbonate daily (300 mg tablets/day). The patient no longer complained of subjective disturbances.

The EEG on 2.2.76 showed an occipital alpha rhythm 10-10 5 Hz, which was fairly organized. Normal reaction occurred with eyes open. Persistent 6.5-7.5 Hz theta activity was recorded in the antero-central region, bilaterally, and was accentuated by hyperpnea. A lithium serum level of 0.38 mmol was recorded.

B.S. age 29 (Case No. 54070)

At the age of 20 this patient was admitted to the neurological ward with symptoms of vomiting, nausea, the sensation of an alimentary bolus, cephalalgia preceeded by clouded vision, and an overall depressed state. Two types of crises were intermittantly added to the foregoing symptomatology. The first was characterized by falling to the ground with a loss of consciousness for an imprecise period of time. Upon regaining consciousness the patient was pale, cold and sweaty. The second consisted of facial musculature spasms with speech impediment and cramp-like contractions of the muscles of the upper limb. The therapy consisted of antidepressant and antianxiety drugs. On 21.3.77 the patient was admitted into our clinic. For 15 days the patient complained of a sense of asthenia, malaise, precordial palpitation, with a sensation of not being able to swallow, loss of balance, nausea and vomiting. No particulars were uncovered during the objective and neurological examination. As for psychological status, the patient was alert and oriented. The patient's mood approached depression, with anxiety and marked psychosomatic disturbances. Physical examinations showed electrolytes: K 3.260; Na 143.5; EEG: alpha rythm 8.5-9.0 Hz, 30-50 mV, symmetric, stable, and with normal reaction with eyes open. Low voltage, diffuse, rapid activity was observed, which might have been pharmacological in origin, of frequency 7.5-8.0 Hz, posterio-central without hemispherical prevalence. hyperpnea caused no significant modifications.

On 2.4.77 therapy was initiated involving 1200 mg lithium carbonate daily (2 + 2 300 mg compresses daily). Three days later, on 5.4.77, intense tremors of the hands, irritability, and a bad mood appeared. At 20:30, the patient fell to the ground, lost consciousness, and exhibited generalized clonic tonic crisis, with a foamy mouth. Consciousness was regained after a few minutes. Lithium carbonate therapy was suspended.

On 6.4.77 the serum lithium level was 0.88 mmol/l. An EEG trace showed a further slowing of background activity with the appearance of isolated spikes of lower frequency and a voltage higher than the background rythm (Figure 24.2). Electrolyte examinations revealed K 3·516; Na 135. The tremors disappeared and convulsive crises no longer appeared in the succeeding days. On 5.4.77 the patient was released.

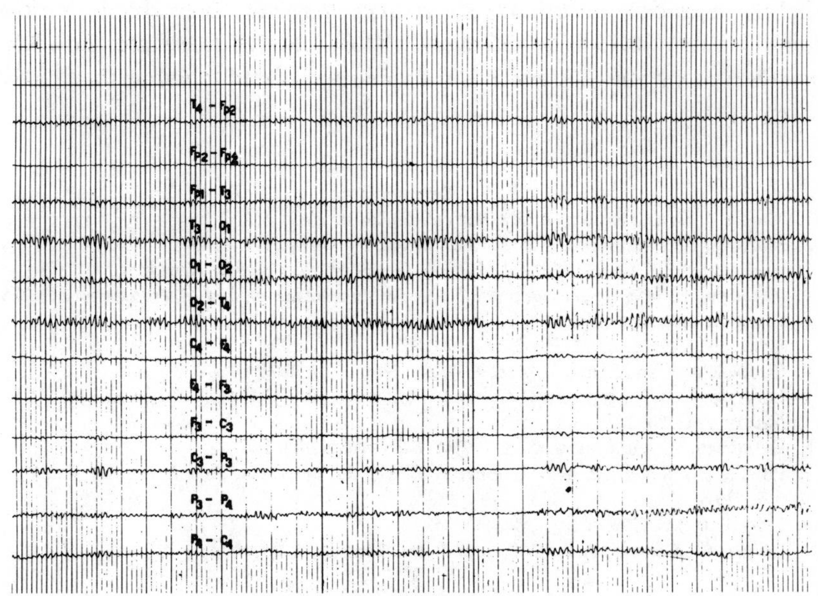

Figure 24.2. EEG of patient B.S.

DISCUSSION

As for the frequency and quality of EEG modifications, as well as their dependence on lithium or on psychopathological symptoms, different opinions exist. This may be due to the practical difficulty of a systematic, standardized and simultaneous EEG registration, observation of psychopathological symptoms, lithium determinations and acute or chronic intoxication. It has been known for some time that the action of lithium salts can reduce or block transmission at the level of certain synapses of the nervous system and that this action may be mediated by some cationic exchanges. In our two cases, it is interesting to note that the EEG alterations are always accompanied by a significant variation in the serum sodium level. We are not able to say, however, whether the EEG alterations observed are due to a non-specific action of lithium on the cerebral bioelectric activity or if instead it acts by unleashing a pre-existing neurophysiological situation or a latent epilepsy. With regard to the latter possibility, we recall the suggestive hypothesis held principally by Flor Henry (10) associating manic depressive psychosis with epilepsy of the non-dominant temporal lobe. Since it has already been demonstrated by Gartside (7), among others, it seems indisputable that lithium acts by modifying cerebral excitability. As for the relations between EEG modifications and neurotoxicity, we can say that EEG changes are only slightly dependent on lithium levels since they are observable at various levels between 0.15 and 1.25 mmol/l (1,8), though these are, however, always below 2 mmol/l, which is the value considered to define the limit of safety (11).

References

1. Mayfield, D. and Brown, R.G. (1966). *J. Psychiat. Res.,* 4, 207
2. Platman, J.R. and Fieve, R.R. (1969). *Br. J. Psychiat.,* 115, 1185
3. Andreani, G., Caselli, G.E. and Martelli, G. (1958). *G. Psychiat. Neuropat.,* 86, 273
4. Vacaflor, L. (1975). In: Johnson F.N., *Lithium research and Therapy* pp. 211-225, (London: Academic Press)
5. Schou, M. (1963). *Br. J. Psychiat.,* 109, 803
6. Coppen, A.J. and Shaw, D.M. (1963). *Br. Med. J.,* 2, 1439
7. Gartside, I.B., Lippold, O.C. and Meldrum, B.S. (1966). *Electroenceph. Clin. Neurophys.,* 20, 382
8. Helmchen, H. and Kanowski, S. (1971). *Nerventarzt,* 42, 144
9. Pinelli, P., Tonali, P. and Scoppetta, C. (1972). *Archivio. Psicol. Neurol. Psichiat.,* 5-6, 479
10. Flor-Henry, P. (1969). *Epilepsia,* 10, 363
11. Muniz, C., Forman, A.J., Wilder, B.J. and Ramsay, R.E. (1976). *Clin. EEG.,* 7, 31

25

Lithium and the Pineal-Adrenocortical Axis

S. PARVATHI DEVI, N. HARIHARASUBRAMANIAN and A. VENKOBA RAO

INTRODUCTION

It was the outcome of a 'hunch' during investigations relating to the endocrine sequelae of lithium administration that the possibility of lithium evoking changes in the pineal gland was thought of by one of us (SPD). This chapter will outline the involvement of the pineal gland and adrenal cortex during lithium administration.

The role of lithium in the treatment of affective disorders has been extensively studied. Its effects on ionic balance, on neurotransmitter dynamics and on endocrine mechanisms have also been documented (1-8). The influence of lithium on pineal gland activity as a possible mode of its therapeutic effect suggested itself to the present authors, who took note of the emergence of the pineal gland, in recent years, as a versatile neuroendocrine transducer. The actions of the pineal neurohumours (melatonin and serotonin) on behaviour are now being investigated by several workers (9). Reports have appeared which suggest that psychoactive drugs such as the phenothiazines (chlorpromazine), butyrophenones (haloperidol) and benzodiazepines (diazepam) may affect pineal function (10-14). Pineal parenchymal hyperplasia concomitant with adrenocortical hyperactivity has been observed (15). Many other aspects of the role of the pineal gland in reproduction and behaviour have been discussed (16).

The study reported here enquired into the manner in which lithium might activate the pineal adrenocortical axis to restore the electrolyte balance.

AIMS OF THE INVESTIGATIONS

The present set of investigations have been aimed at noting the effects of lithium in healthy laboratory-bred rats, suitably grouped and processed. Observations have been made in lithium treated rats on:

1. absolute eosinophil values as indices on adrenocortical oxycorticoid secretion;
2. adrenocortical cytology;
3. pineal cytological changes as possible indicators of fluctuations in aldosterone secretion;
4. pineäl gland RNA;
5. pineal gland histochemical fluorescence.

MATERIAL AND METHODS

Part A

Two sets each of 60 Wistar strain healthy adult male albino rats of 10-12 weeks age range, and 100-120 g weight range, housed under standardized conditions and on a regulated diet schedule, formed the material for the investigations. Two series of investigations were undertaken in succession, each involving 60 rats.

The first set of 60 rats were divided into four groups, viz. Groups I and II of 20 each for the investigations and Groups III and IV of 10 each to serve as controls for Groups I and II respectively. The dosage of lithium carbonate was set at 20 mg/kg body weight for parenteral administration at 09.00 h daily. Group I rats received lithium daily for 2 weeks while Group II had it daily for 4 weeks. Absolute eosinophil counts using Pilot's diluting fluid were done every morning at 08.30 h in all the animals of Groups I and II. Group I rats were subjected to unilateral adrenalectomy at the close of 2 weeks, while Group II rats had the same procedure at the end of 4 weeks. The adrenals were embedded, sectioned stained and cytological changes studied. The ten controls of Groups III and IV received no lithium. Their daily absolute eosiniphil counts were made at 08.30 h and they were subject to unilateral adrenalectomy at the end of 2 and 4 weeks respectively. Following these studies on the first set, a second series of 60 rats were subject to all the studies as for set I and in addition, at the end of 2 and 4 weeks, pinealectomy was done to study possible concomitant pineal cytological changes employing classic staining techniques. The respective controls had pinealectomy at the close of 2 and 4 weeks. Pineal glands were processed for staining the pinealocyte RNA using a modification of methyl green technique for nucleic acids (17). With this technique, the nucleolus and cytoplasm are purple while the rest of the nucleus is not stained.

Part B

36 adult Wistar strain male albino rats chosen and maintained in a normal day-night environment and divided into four groups of 9 rats each, formed the material for study. Group I served as controls;

Group II received parental injections of lithium carbonate at a daily dose of 20 mg/kg body wt for 1 week; Group III and Group IV rats were bilaterally adrenalectomized and maintained on adequate salt and fluid intake. Group III rats were administered lithium carbonate daily at the same daily dosage of 20 mg/kg body wt. for 1 week while Group IV rats were given a placebo-saline injection.

At the close of 1 week, the animals were sacrificed and their pineal glands removed for special histological and histochemical fluorescence study. Employing histochemical fluorescence techniques (18,19) changes in the noradrenaline and serotonin content within the pineal gland in rats administered lithium were observed (a qualitative study).

Part C

Five groups each of 10 healthy adult Wistar strain male albino rats (120-150 g) were selected and maintained under normal day-night environment and uniform ideal laboratory conditions for a week, following which they were divided for investigations.

Group I served as controls; Group II were subjected to continuous illumination for 2 weeks; Group III were subjected to continuous illumination for 14 weeks; Group IV received continuous illumination for 2 weeks during which lithium carbonate at a daily dosage for 20 mg/kg body wt. was administered. Group V received continuous illumination for 4 weeks during which lithium carbonate in the daily dosage of 20 mg/kg body wt. was administered.

At the end of the experimental schedules. the animals of groups II to V were sacrificed and their pineal glands removed for histochemical and histological study. Group I animals were similarly sacrificed, half the number at the end of 2 weeks and half at the end of 4 weeks.

OBSERVATIONS

1. A decrease occurred in absolute eosinophil count with the lowest values being observed between 10 and 14 days (2nd week) after lithium administration.

2. There was an hyperactive zona glomerulosa of the adrenal cortex during the 2nd week while on lithium.

3. Hyperactive zona glomerulosa and fasciculata of the adrenal cortex were noted during the 4th week of lithium administration.

4. In the second series of investigations where the rats were pinealectomized at the end of the 2nd and 4th weeks, pineal parenchymal cellular hyperplasia was manifest in both sets.

5. Pineal parenchymal hyperplasia followed lithium administration both in normal and in adrenalectomised rats.

6. The nucleoli of the pinealocytes in lithium treated rats were relatively larger and appeared darker. The cytoplasm appeared denser, diffuse and darker, indicating a deeper stain uptake and increased pinealocyte RNA.

7. Increased serotoninergic fluorescence occurred within the pineals of lithium treated rats.

8. The pineals of lithium treated rats housed under constant lighting schedules did not manifest pineal parenchymal regression characteristic of such changes in environmental illumination.

DISCUSSION

Lithium and adrenocortical changes

This study has been essentially experimental and our findings denote distinct adrenocortical responses to lithium. We recollect at this point Coppen's (20) findings relating to sodium accumulation within the body cells in depressive states being double that during normothymia, and that during manic episodes intracellular sodium may increase to 200%. Several recent studies have indicated that lithium rapidly alters cell membrane permeability, enters the intracellular compartment, and there becomes trapped, displacing mainly intracellular sodium. It may be that as lithium enters the cells, particularly those of the central nervous system, it replaces intracellular sodium. Once intracellular, lithium remains a non-functional substitute for the metabolically active ions such as sodium and potassium. In such a manner lithium could damp neural transmission. Under normal circumstances, such effects might result in no behavioural manifestations. However, under conditions of excessive intracellular sodium accumulation, such as occurs in affective disorders, the attenuating effects of lithium upon neural transmission may result in signs and symptoms of clinical improvement. It is relevant to point out that Goodwin and associates (21) have reported elevated urinary aldosterone values in patients with affective disorders receiving lithium therapy and this is suggestive of the response to ionic changes induced by lithium.

Hyperactivity of zona glomerulosa cells at the end of the second week with distinctly hyperplastic zona fasciculata of the adrenal cortex as observed in this study possibly denote:

1. A compensatory response to restore electrolyte balance through increased aldosterone output by the zona glomerulosa of the adrenal cortex;
2. As a consequence of the non-specific 'stressor' effect of disturbed electrolyte balance, stress-induced increased oxycorticoid secretion by zona fasciculata possibly evokes the eosinopenia noted in these rats. This observation fits in with the view that increased adrenal cortical activity in depression is perhaps non-specific in nature.

Lithium and pineal hyperplasia

Concomitant pineal parenchymal cell hyperplasia during the second and fourth week may indicate aldosterone secretion, possibly being regulated by the pineal body.

At this juncture, it may be mentioned that there have been references to the control of aldosterone secretion by neurohumours from around the diencephalon, particularly the pineal body which is said to respond to fluctuations in electrolyte homeostasis. This was pointed out by Farrell (22) who suggested an adrenoglomerulotrophin from the pineal for such control. The present observations on pineal cytological changes in rats on lithium tend to revive Farrell's views.

While lithium administration evokes an initial negative sodium balance, the effect is more pronounced in adrenalectomised rats. This electrolyte variation could step up pineal activity (22-24). In rats with intact adrenals, increased pineal activity causes aldosterone release and sodium retention thus diminishing brain excitability (25). In adrenalectomized rats, a direct effect of lithium on the pineal gland appears quite probable. This lithium-pineal-adrenal-electrolyte axis points to a possible mode of the anti-manic effects of lithium.

Lithium and increase in pineal RNA

The possibility is that lithium stimulates protein synthesis in the pinealocyte, through activation of ribosomal turnover in the nucleolus. The nucleoli of the pinealocytes in lithium-treated rats were relatively larger and appeared darker. The cytoplasm appeared denser, more diffuse and darker, indicating a deeper stain uptake and hence an increased pinealocyte RNA content. The size and stainability of the nucleolus is governed by its constituent nucleolonema which consists of ribosomal subunits.

It has been understood that the nucleolonemal ribosomal particles enter the cytoplasm through the nucleus, combining at some point with the mRNA already formed and constituting the cytoplasmic ribosomal RNA. The RNA content of ribosomes in the cytoplasm, the sites of protein synthesis imparts basophilia to the cytoplasm. Diffuse basophilia is indicative of the presence of a large number of free ribosomes and suggests that the protein synthesised by the cell is utilised for internal use by the cell or is stored in the cell (26).

The proteins thus synthesized could be pineal enzymes catalysing synthesis of melatonin or pineal proteins which might serve as carriers for pineal hormones or pineal polypeptides, like arginine vasotocin. Lithium could thus enhance the synthesis of melatonin and/or other pineal principles involved in pineal function.

It is of interest to note that lithium and melatonin have similar actions on both the central nervous system and endocrines. Both stimulate uptake of biogenic amines in the brain (27), inhibit stimulus-induced release of amines and induce EEG synchronization and sleep (9,28,29). They suppress L-Dopa-induced hypermotiltiy (30,31) and inhibit thyroid function (32,33). It seems quite possible to conclude that melatonin might mediate, at least in part, the therapeutic action of lithium and perhaps of other psychoactive drugs.

Lithium and increased pineal serotoninergic fluorescence

Increased serotoninergic fluorescence within the pineals of normal and adrenalectomised rats to which lithium has been administered, indicate that the pineal does respond to altered electrolyte balance. The pineals of the lithium-treated rats reveal increased serotonin content, with the histochemical fluorescence technique employed in this investigation. The presence of serotonin is indicated by the development of 5-HT fluorophores, yellowish-green in appearance. Pineal serotonin is converted into melatonin by the pineal enzyme hydroxyindole-O-methyl transferase (HIOMT). Melatonin has been shown to influence brain excitability. Its role in sleep-wakefulness rhythms and behavioural processes has already been reported (9). This observation of increased serotoninergic fluorescence in the pineals of rats on lithium is a pointer suggesting that the pineal gland does get involved in mediating the responses to lithium therapy.

Lithium and its prevention of pineal regression under conditions of constant lighting

The mammalian pineal is richly endowed with serotonin and norepinephrine. The organ also contains large amounts of the enzymes required for the synthesis and metabolism of these important biogenic amines. Within the pineal gland many of the constituents undergo daily fluctuations. One important factor determining these oscillations is the prevailing environmental photoperiod, acting by way of the sympathetic nervous system (34).

The concentration of norepinephrine in the pineal gland of the rat ranges from 3 to 12 micro.g/g. The catecholamine is almost exclusively confined to the postganglionic nerve terminals which abound in the pineal gland. The rhythm in pineal norepinephrine is abolished by depriving animals of light or by placing them under continuous illumination. When pineal norepinephrine is released, it causes a dramatic effect within the pinealocytes. Norepinephrine stimulates pineal adenyl cyclase while exposure of experimental animals to continuous light reduces the activity of the enzyme.

Within the pineal, norepinephrine stimulates formation of serotonin, the concentration of which is very high within the gland. Serotonin rhythm within the pineal gland also shows a circadian rhythm. This rhythm is abolished by constant light exposure, which inhibits the pineal enzyme hydroxyindole-O-methyl transferase (HIOMT) responsible for the conversion of serotonin into melatonin. Thus under constant lighting the pineal gland exhibits a hypoactive state. When lithium is administered to rats exposed to constant light, depression of pineal function is averted and pineal hyperplasia manifests itself. This serves as yet further evidence of pineal responses to lithium. These observations relating lithium to the pineal-adrenocortical axis could probably indicate the mechanisms underlying lithium action.

References

1. Cade, J.F.J. (1949). *Med. J. Aust.,* 36,349
2. Schou, M., Juel-Nilson, N., Stromgren, E. and Voldby, H. (1954). *J. Neurol. Neurosurg. Psychiat.,* 17, 250
3. Schou, M. (1957). *Pharmacol. Rev.,* 9, 17
4. Schou, M. (1958). *Acta Pharmacol.,* 15, 70
5. Schou, M. (1966). Proceedings of Excerpta Medica Foundation; Amsterdam

6. Maletzky, B. and Blachly, P.H. (1971). *Lithium in Psychiatry* (London: Butterworths)
7. Platman, S.R. and Fieve, R. R. (1968). *Arch. Gen. Psychiat.,* 18, 591
8. Schildkraut, J.J., Schanberg, S.M., Breese, G.R. and Kopin, I.J. (1967). *Am. J. Psychiat.,* 124, 600
9. Anton-Tay, F., Diaz, J.L. and Fernandez-Guardiola, A. (1971). *Life Sci.,* 10, 841
10. Hartley, R., Padwilk, D. and Smith, J.A., (1972). *J. Pharm. Pharmacol.,* 24, (*Suppl.*) 100
11. Hartley, R. and Smith, J.A. (1973). *J. Pharm. Pharmacol.,* 25, 751
12. Snyder, S.H. and Axelrod, J. (1965). *Science,* 49, 542
13. Wurtman, R.J., Axelrod, J. and Anton-Tay, F. (1968). *J. Pharmacol. Exp. Ther.,* 161, 361
14. Wurtman, R.J., Axelrod, J. and Kelly, D.E. (1968). *The Pineal* (New York: Academic Press)
15. Parvathi Devi, S., Venkoba Rao, A., Hariharasubramanian, N. and Srinivasan, V. (1973). *Ind. J. Psychiat.,* 15, 250
16. Parvathi Devi, S. and Venkoba Rao, A. (eds.) (1974). The Pineal in Reproduction and Behaviour: Commemoration volume. *International Pre Congress Satellite Symposium, Madurai,* 26th International Congress of Physiological Sciences, New Delhi
17. Roque, A.L., Jafarey, N.A. and Coulter, P. (1965). *Exp. Molec. Pathol.,* 4, 266
18. Falck, B., Hillarp, N.A., Thime, G. and Torp, A. (1962). *J. Histochem. Cytochem.,* 10, 348
19. Falck, B. and Owman, C. (1965). *Acta. Univ. Lund.,* 2, No. 7
20. Coppen, A. (1967). *Br. J. Psychiat.,* 113, 1237
21. Goodwin, F., Murphy, D.L. and Bunney, W.E. Jr. (1968). Presented at Annual Meeting of the American Psychiatric Association, Boston.
22. Farrell, G. (1959) *Recent Progr. Horm. Res.,* 15, 275
23. Machado, A.B.M. and DeSilva, C.R. (1963). *Experientia,* 19, 264
24. Panagiotis, N.M. and Hungerford, G.F. (1961). *Endocrinology,* 69, 217
25. Woodbury, D.M. (1958). *Pharmacol. Rev.* 10, 275
26. Toner, P.G., and Carr, K.E. (1968). *Cell Structure.* (Edinburgh: Livingstone)
27. Mendels, J. and Frazer, A. (1974). *Arch. Gen. Psychiat.,* 30, 447
28. Johnson, G., Maccario, M., Gershon, S. (1970). *J. Nerv. Ment. Dis.,* 151, 723
29. Small, J.G., Small, I.F. and Perez, M. (1971). *Biol. Psychiat.,* 3, 47
30. Segal, D.S., Callaghen, M. and Mandell, A.J. (1975). *Nature,* 254, 58
31. Minneman, K.P. and Wurtman, R.J. (1976). *Ann. Rev. Pharmacol. Toxicol.,* 16, 126
32. Baschieri, L., De Luca, F., Cramerosa, L., De Martino, C., Oliyerio, A. and Negri, M. (1963). *Experientia,* 19, 15
33. Schou, M., Amdisen, A., Eskjaer Jensen, S. and Olsen, T. (1968). *Br. Med. J.,* 3, 710
34. Reiter, R.J. (1973). In: L.W. Hedland, J.M. Franz, and A.D. Kenny (eds) *Biological Rhythms and Endocrine Functions* (New York: Plenum Press)

26

Lithium as a Regulator of Hormone-Stimulated Prostaglandin Synthesis

D. F. HORROBIN, J. P. MTABAJI, M. S. MANKU and M. KARMAZYN

INTRODUCTION

Our interest in lithium was triggered by the knowledge that it could increase urinary excretion of sodium, potassium and water. We used it to treat a woman with severe premenstrual syndrome who exhibited marked renal retention of all three substances (1). The initial response was favourable, but after several months of treatment lithium became ineffective. The woman subsequently responded completely to treatment with the inhibitor of prolactin secretion, bromocriptine (1). We therefore tested interactions between lithium, prolactin and vasopressin.

RENAL STUDIES

In sheep treated with cortisol we found that the kindneys became unresponsive to the water-retaining action of intravenous vasopressin (2). Normal responsiveness could be restored by pre-treating the animals with prolactin (2). We investigated the possibility that prolactin might also be able to restore renal responsiveness to vasopressin in lithium-treated rats (3). As with cortisol-treated sheep, prolactin could restore normal responses to vasopressin (4). The lithium-treated rats were resistant to aldosterone and in this case, too, prolactin could restore the normal action of the hormone.

Because in a vascular preparation we had demonstrated that prolactin acted by stimulating prostaglandin synthesis (5) we tested the possibility that a prostaglandin (PG) might be able to restore normal responses to vasopressin in lithium-treated animals. In acute experiments we demonstrated that infusion of very small amounts of PGA_2 (used because of its relative resistance to inactivation in the lungs) could restore the usual antidiuretic response to vasopressin in animals which, without the PG, were completely resistant (6).

VASCULAR STUDIES

In the isolated superior mesenteric vascular bed of the rat we have shown that low concentrations of prolactin up to 100 ng/ml potentiate responses to pressor agents while higher concentrations of above 200 ng/ml inhibit responses (5). Both effects seemed to be dependent on the stimulation of prostaglandin synthesis by prolactin. The prolactin dose/response curve could be exactly simulated by infusion of either PGE_1 or the precursor of PGE_1, dihomogammalinolenic acid. If lithium, in a concentration of 2 mM,was present in the perfusing buffer prolactin failed to change either vascular reactivity or prostaglandin synthesis. Lithium had no effect on basal vascular reactivity or basal levels of prostaglandin synthesis (7,8).

When vasopressin was added to the perfusing buffer it had little direct pressor activity until concentrations of over 1 ng/ml were used. However at concentrations of as little as 2 pg/ml it stimulated prostaglandin synthesis and potentiated responses to other pressor agents (8). Unlike the situation with prolactin, no concentration of vasopressin inhibited responses to other pressor agents. The effect of low concentrations of vasopressin on the preparation could be simulated by infusion of either PGE_2 or the precursor of PGE_2, arachidonic acid. Lithium at 2 mM had no effect on the direct pressor actions of vasopressin but did reduce the effect of vasopressin on prostaglandin synthesis and vascular reactivity. It was not as effective against vasopressin as against prolactin.

Lithium failed to affect prostaglandin synthesis or vascular reactivity in preparations perfused with maximal concentrations of arachidonic acid, dihomogammalinolenic acid, PGE_1 or PGE_2.

DISCUSSION

We believe that these results are consistent with the following concepts:-

1. Lithium at concentrations therapeutically effective in man is able to inhibit the effects of prolactin and vasopressin on prostaglandin biosynthesis;

2. Lithium probably acts at the level of the hormone stimulation of the phospholipase which splits the prostaglandin precursors, arachidonic acid

and dihomogammalinolenic acid from the membrane phopholipids. The evidence is: (a) prolactin, at least is known to stimulate PG synthesis by activating phospholipase; (b) lithium was ineffective in changing the responses of preparations in which an abundance of either arachidonic acid or dihomogammalinolenic acid was supplied exogenously; and (c) lithium had no effect on basal prostaglandin synthesis;

3. Lithium may be more effective in blocking the release of dihomogammalinolenic acid by prolactin than that of arachidonic acid by vasopressin.

How can these fundamental mechanisms help to explain the actions of lithium?

We suggest that most polypeptide hormones exert their effects by stimulating the intracellular generation of a second messenger (either a cyclic nucleotide or free calcium ions) and a prostaglandin. In the kidney, for example, vasopressin may act by generating cyclic AMP and an unknown prostaglandin while in blood vessels it may release calcium and prostaglandin E_2. Both the PG and the other second messenger are required for a fully normal response. In the absence of the PG stimulation the response may either not take place at all (as seems to happen with vasopressin and the kidney) or may be changed in amplitude or character (as seems to happen with vasopressin and blood vessels).

We have provided some evidence that this may be the mechanism of lithium action in the kidney. We have argued elsewhere that stimulation of prostaglandin synthesis by prolactin and other hormones may be an important factor in depression and mania. It is possible that depression may be associated with a concentration of a prostaglandin which produces an effect in one direction and mania with a higher concentration of the same prostaglandin which because of the nature of the dose/response curve produces exactly the opposite effect. The ability of lithium to reverse the potentiation of vascular reactivity produced by low prolactin levels, and the inhibition produced by high prolactin concentrations without having any effect on the normal reactivity has an interesting parallel in the ability of lithium to prevent both depression and mania without changing normal mood. There is recent good evidence that thyrotropin may exert part of its effect on the thyroid by stimulating PG synthesis. If lithium interfered with this it could explain some of its actions on thyroid function. A similar mechanism could account for some lithium actions in other tissues.

In conclusion we propose a completely new mechanism of lithium action, the blockade of hormone-induced prostaglandin synthesis without interference with basal levels of prostaglandin production. We believe that investigation of this idea will lead to fruitful new developments in lithium research.

References

1. Horrobin, D.F., Karmali, R.A., Mtabaji, J.P., Manku, M.S. and Nassar, B.A. (1976). *Postgrad. Med. J.*, **52**, (Suppl. 3), 79
2. Horrobin, D.F., Manku, M.S. and Robertshaw, D. (1973). *J. Endocrinol.*, 58, 135
3. Forrest, J.N., Cohen, A.D., Torretti, J., Himmelhoch, J.M. and Epstein, F.H. (1974). *J. Clin. Invest.*, 53, 1115
4. Mtabaji, J.P. Manku, M.S. and Horrobin, D.F. (1975). *J. Endocrinol.*, 67, 57P
5. Mtabaji, J.P., Manku, M.S. and Horrobin, D.F. (1976). *Canad. J. Physiol. Pharmacol.*, 54, 357
6. Mtabaji, J.P., Robinson, C.J., Manku, M.S., Cronin, D. and Horrobin, D.F. (1977). *J. Endocrinol.*, 73, 31
7. Horrobin, D.F., Manku, M.S., Mtabaji, J.P. and Nassar, B.A. (1975). *J. Physiol.*, 251, 24P
8. Karmazyn, M., Manku, M.S. and Horrobin, D.F. (1977). (Submitted for publication)

27

Renal Effects of Lithium

F. A. JENNER and P. R. EASTWOOD

INTRODUCTION

There have been a large number of important reviews of the pharmacology of lithium, some of which are listed in Bailey *et al.* (1). We have been associated with that review and with others (2,3). For little more than personal reasons this chapter continues the story in relation to renal physiology from where those articles leave it. We have found that we lack the erudition required to cope adequately with renal physiology, enzymology, physical chemistry, intermediary metabolism, etc. necessary for the production of an adequate review in this field. Nevertheless, we hope we can give signposts to the highlights of the literature, and we strongly recommend that castles should not be built on the shifting sands we offer but rather on the original mud and concrete we suspect we detected and that unfortunately we negligently overlooked.

Certain names and research units have made very outstanding contributions in this field, and we are bound to mention in this context Thomsen and (of course) Schou from Aarhus; and Forrest, Singer and Dousa from the States.

In very early studies, Schou (4) made careful attempts to identify the toxicological actions of lithium and he also studied its renal excretion. He had confirmed Cade's (5) great discovery of the antimanic effects of lithium ions and immediately appreciated the possible dangers and problems. In 1968 Schou (6) reported the polyuria and polydipsia which has been studied so intensively ever since.

STRUCTURAL DAMAGE TO THE NEPHRON

Now, however, the clinical relevance of the structural renal damage reported to be caused by lithium (7) is the subject of the most important current debate on the toxic effects of lithium. It is very important that the reported findings should be considered carefully. It is equally vital that this should be done dispassionately and with due regard to the fact that many patients have been helped for up to two decades by lithium treatment. Gross renal failure in them is not a common clinical finding. The state of their renal function needs assessing but it cannot be profoundly disturbed.

The results on which much of the new caution is based were produced by histological analysis of renal biopsy material from patients who were admitted for the treatment of acute lithium intoxication, or of lithium-induced nephrogenic diabetes insipidus. The initial study (8) involved 14 subjects with acute intoxication; none had any acute histological lesions but 13 showed focal nephron atrophy or interstitial fibrosis, or both. Blind histological analyses of the patients and age-related controls showed that sclerotic glomeruli were five times as common in patients as in controls, tubular atrophy was three times as common, and there was twice as much interstitial connective tissue. Post mortem studies in two patients also showed multiple small cysts mainly in the cortex. Evidence of glomerular- or chronic pyelo-nephritis and significant arteriosclerosis, as well as of obstructive urolithiasis, was excluded. Blood pressure was normal and proteinuria was only present during the period of the acute intoxication. The patients were said not to be taking analgesics regularly.

In that study there was doubt as to whether renal damage only arises in subjects who have from time to time toxic plasma levels. It is striking that five of the fourteen patients had had previous episodes of lithium intoxication with high plasma lithium levels. Patient compliance and/or monitoring may have been deficient in some of these persons.

In a second study, the same group (7) took the obvious next step of trying to correlate structural with functional defects. This involved studying 13 patients, eight of whom were also in the earlier series. Patients were selected who had polyuria or had had acute lithium intoxication. A further five patients, however, aged 31-69, were excluded because, although they had taken lithium for 1-15 years and had polyuria, renal function was normal, as was concentrating ability. Hence they were not submitted to a biopsy.

In these studies, osmolar clearance was calculated as well as free water clearance, creatinine, 125^{I}-iothalamate, and 131^{I}-hippuran clearance. All the 13 patients showed osmolar concentrating deficiencies. In five patients a slight increase of renal concentrating ability followed 6-12 months after stopping lithium treatment, whereas in two patients it decreased after resuming therapy. The authors conclude that lithium-induced reduction of renal concentrating ability cannot be considered as a harmless condition as it may well correlate with a chronic structural nephropathy.

The work reported above is consistent with the observations made by Lindop and Padfield (9) on a kidney from a patient who committed suicide. In that study the histological picture was described as predominantly a pleomorphism of the cells of the distal tubule, and it was postulated that this was the basis of the polyuria and vasopressin-resistant diabetes insipidus syndrome so frequently reported.

Further work by Rafaelsen, which is continuing, confirms to some extent the above findings. The problems presented by this work are considerable, and the need to view it in perspective is vital.

The central question of all medicine is to weigh the improved quality of life against the risks involved. If prophylactic lithium does reduce renal function over years of treatment, is this a reasonable price to pay for relief from manic-depressive psychosis? In some persons it is almost certainly so, but naturally we need to have more information to make the right informed judgements, especially if it is true that approximately 1/2000 of the population is taking lithium carbonate.

Perhaps the renal toxicity, if fully confirmed, may at least encourage more persons to check from time to time the need to continue lithium treatment for life.

EXCRETION OF LITHIUM

Saliva and sweat

Lithium is excreted in sweat and saliva as well as in urine. The urinary and salivary excretion are positively correlated if the subject is in a recumbent position. Urinary excretion, however, is posture-dependent (10) and in some ways analogous to sodium excretion dependent on glomerular filtration rate and proximal tubular function. The salivary excretion is more akin to active potassium excretion into saliva.

The renal excretion of lithium

Although administered lithium detectably appears in milk, sweat, tears and faeces, almost all that is administered can be recovered in urine, especially in normal or euthymic persons (11). The mode of excretion is essentially by glomerular filtration and proximal tubular reabsorption. It is possible that renal lithium excretion is reduced in mania (see Johnson (12) and Chapters 34 and 36 in this book). This might be due to differences in losses due to sweating, possibly to altered bone uptake, and of course could be a consequence of less reliable drug consumption and urine collections, extra sodium loss in sweat, dietary changes, and will be influenced by steroid changes due to altered posture. The area remains one of controversy and will not be discussed further here.

Thomsen *et al.* (13), Thomsen and Schou (14), as well as Steele *et al.* (15), have all shown that lithium is mainly reabsorbed in the proximal renal tubules. Further, as would be expected, Baer *et al.* (16) have also shown that mineral corticoids have differential effects on sodium and lithium excretion. They essentially affect distal tubular function. Some reservations have, nevertheless, been expressed by Steele *et al.* (15) on the suggestion that lithium is only reabsorbed proximally and that therefore proximal reabsorption can be measured using lithium (13). However, if the major reabsorption is proximal, the general outlook so carefully worked out by Thomsen is not seriously threatened.

Clinically this leads to the important fact that reduced glomerular filtration or an increased proximal tubule reabsorption will lead to an increased plasma lithium, which may at times be dangerous. Altered proximal tubular reabsorption may, of course, be primary or secondary but is almost always secondary. The special exception arises in cases of structural damage to the proximal tubule due to lithium itself, as for example reported by Lavender, Brown and Berrill (17). That report is a rare example of structural change based on biopsy evidence taken from a patient before recovery.

Lithium clearance almost certainly decreases with increasing age, probably due to reduced glomerular filtration. Lehmann and Merten (18) reported a reduced lithium clearance to 60% in a group of patients of mean age of 58, compared to one of mean age of 25. Hewick *et al.* (19) have studied the problem and give some rule of thumb guides to the relation between age and weight-related daily doses required to give approximately 1 mmol/l plasma values. They feel a 50% dosage reduction is commonly required for age-related decreases in lithium excretion. They point out that age as such explains a small part of the variance. Clearly, the age relation itself is a factor influenced by the likelihood of increased specific pathology with age. Lithium excretion is clearly reduced with most renal deficiencies.

Because of the essentially proximal tubular reabsorption of lithium, clearance is not greatly affected by simple changes of urine volume. Unfortunately, we (20) are among those in print who have previously failed to appreciate this so clearly demonstrated by Thomsen and Schou (21). The therapeutic level is affected by sodium in the diet but toxic levels are negligibly reduced by acute sodium administration in man.

RENAL EFFECTS OF LITHIUM

Secondary effects on proximal tubular reabsorption of lithium

The key to much which is relevant in the renal handling of lithium seems to depend on grasping the relation between proximal tubular reabsorption of sodium and lithium by essentially sodium transport pathways. When whole body sodium is depleted, proximal tubular reabsorption of sodium and lithium is increased. The mechanism worked out by Thomsen (22) for the vicious circle in lithium intoxication illustrates what may be involved.

Essentially he postulates that lithium inhibits distal tubular reabsorption of sodium. In the rat at least with lithium serum levels much above 1 mmol/l (man is less sensitive) the sodium loss by the distal tubule induces compensatory sodium reabsorption by the proximal tubules. The simultaneous consequent proximal lithium reabsorption leads to an increase in serum lithium levels. The equally inevitable water reabsorption reduces the urine volume. The high lithium levels make things worse. The processes are clearly part of a very dangerous vicious circle. This is made even more harmful by reduced renal glomerular filtration rate, as demonstrated by the decrease of creatinine clearance (23).

The decrease of distal sodium reabsorption induced by lithium is very strongly suggested by Thomsen, Jensen and Olesen's (24) demonstration that lithium inhibits the renal action of aldosterone. That this would lead to 'attempted' compensatory activity by the proximal tubules is in line with general views of renal responses to reduced body sodium (25).

Further, sodium alone will increase the urine volume and decrease the lithium clearance in the intoxicated animal (23). It is daring but not unreasonable therefore for Thomsen to imply that the changes in kidney function during lithium intoxication can be completely accounted for 'by lithium-induced inhibition of reabsorption of sodium in the distal parts of the nephron. No further mechanisms seem to be involved' (26).

Later we will discuss some reasons for also suspecting a primary proximal tubular effect on sodium transport and/or inhibition of chloride transport in the ascending limb of the loop of Henle, as reasonable explanations of the inhibition by lithium of the antidiuretic action of vasopressin.

Urine volume, however, depends on the action of vasopressin which also depends on the concentrating activity of the loop of Henle, which also requires the delivery of suitable volumes of saline, the concentration of which is itself of relevance. Lithium probably acts at every level of this complicated reverberating renal system. Our task is to elucidate the relative significance of each action. As far as lithium intoxication is concerned, the views of Thomsen seem to be unrivalled. Part of the reduced urine volume may also be due to the reduced delivery of fluid to the loop of Henle, because of the increased proximal tubular reabsorption of water. This would then make the action of excess lithium analogous to that of distal tubular diuretics in nephrogenic diabetes insipidus.

Renin and lithium intoxication

In 1974 Kierkegaard-Hansen (27) showed that non-toxic doses of lithium administered to the rat caused no change in plasma renin and plasma renin substrate. Toxic doses, however, cause a fall of substrate and a rise in renin. Nephrectomized animals (28) showed the same rise of substrate whether lithium-intoxicated or not, hence the changes in renal renin production explain the initial findings. A high sodium diet in intact animals counteracts the effects in the renin system but it also increases lithium clearance. If the increased lithium clearance is also counteracted by yet higher doses of lithium, renin plasma levels are higher than those of rats lithium treated with low sodium intake. Plasma renin substrate, however, is the same in the two groups. Sodium, it is postulated, may therefore also act on the lithium-induced renin release by kidney tissue, as well as on lithium excretion (cf. Gutman *et al.* (29)). In considering renin angiotensin systems and lithium, it should be remembered that Altamura and Morganti (30) showed that plasma renin activity is significantly reduced in depression and lithium compensated for this reduced activity.

Phosphates, calcium, magnesium, parathyroid, and lithium

Steele and Dudgeon (31) showed that lithium excretion is not dependent on or affected by phosphate excretion or parathormone.

Arruda *et al,* (32) are among those showing that lithium does inhibit the parathormone-sensitive adenyl cyclase in the renal cortex. These studies were in dogs and the results seem in conflict with those of Olesen and Thomsen (33) studying rats. Arruda *et al.* (32) also show that lithium does inhibit the direct phosphate excretion effects induced by cAMP.

Plasma phosphate is reduced after acute or chronic administration of lithium in man and animals (34,35). *In vitro* studies have suggested that intracellular phosphate uptake is increased secondarily to an effect of lithium analogous to insulin on carbohydrate metabolism. Hence the reduced phosphate levels in plasma.

The plasma magnesium levels are increased during lithium therapy (36,37). Further decrease of calcium following a phosphate load can be prevented by lithium chloride ingestion (38). Mellerup and Rafaelsen (39) therefore suggest that the magnesium and calcium changes are secondary to altered phosphate metabolism.

There may, however, be a more direct competition between renal handling of calcium and lithium. Crammer (40) showed a very quick response of calcium excretion to lithium administration, and Mellerup *et al.* (36) themselves drew attention to a correlation between serum lithium levels throughout the 'daynite' and calcium and magnesium excretion in the absence of any induced changes of phosphate excretion. One finds it difficult to doubt the probability that in view of the chemical relation between lithium, magnesium and calcium (41,42) at least some of the changes induced in excretion result from direct renal interactions.

Diuretics and lithium

The Thomsen model of the consequences of excess lithium causing a reduction in its own excretion, which becomes particularly dangerous when it develops an unstable positive feed-back loop, helps considerably in understanding the toxic effects of diuretics or other substances inhibiting sodium reabsorption in the distal tubule.

Petersen *et al.* (43) showed that lithium clearance is reduced to 24% by simultaneous administration of thiazides in man and rats. This leads to increased plasma lithium. As lithium itself causes oedema in some subjects (44), and as in some populations 11% over 50 take diuretics, it is important to know about the dangers of the combination of lithium and diuretics, especially those inhibiting distal tubule sodium reabsorption. In this situation the reduction in urine volume is probably largely due to the reduced delivery from the proximal tubule.

Levy, Forrest and Heninger (45) reported on a patient who developed lithium induced diabetes insipidus and who was enabled to continue in therapy by the judicious simultaneous administration of chlorothiazide. The lithium dosage though had to be reduced.

Several further studies of thiazide-type diuretics effects have been subsequently published. Earlier work showed that mercurial diuretics had little effect on lithium excretion, nor did furosemide, bendroflumethiazide, nor ethacrynic acid, these latter being thought to act on the ascending limb of the loop of Henle. On the other hand, aminophylline and urea profoundly increase lithium excretion. This would be consistent with their presumed proximal tubular function (46).

Lithium-induced polyuria and polydipsia

Knowledge about the excretion of lithium itself is of central importance in the understanding of the pharmacokinetics and proper therapeutic use of the ion. The side effect of induced polyuria has, however, attracted at least as large a literature. Lithium tends to produce a defect in urine-concentrating mechanisms and leads to a hypotonic increased urine volume, not infrequently amounting to a frank but reversible nephrogenic diabetes insipidus which is resistant to vasopressin.

Lindop and Padfield (9) emphasize a structural alteration of the distal tubules due to lithium. In a patient they studied after suicide they demonstrated a pleomorphism also reported earlier in dogs by Radomski *et al.* (47) and in the rat by Evan and Ollerich (48). Such faulty tubules they argue would develop slowly and be vasopressin resistant. However, their report is based on very limited case material and it is difficult to be confident about what a person who kills himself has done. Further, the rapid reversibility of the syndrome when one stops taking lithium might argue against their view. Indeed, even the paradoxical effect of thiazides, still able partially to reverse the polyuria, suggests the damaged tubules are still very significantly reabsorbing sodium. Naturally, further evidence is required to assess this hypothesis.

Some renal effects related to catecholamines

Beck and Kim (49) showed that lithium inhibits the antidiuretic activity of isoproterenol, an adrenergic beta-blocking agent. They also showed that animals showing the inhibition had a reduced rise of renal medullary cyclic AMP. Hence they postulated that part of the inhibitory effect of lithium on the renal concentrating mechanisms depends on inhibition of catecholamine-dependent systems.

Smith and de Jong (50) showed that rats exposed to a cold environment (4 °C for 3 h) showed increased excretion of water, lithium and sodium, but not of potassium. Renin changes correlated with volume but not electrolyte changes. The workers suggest that renal lithium clearance could be raised in human beings during exposure to the cold. They suggest the simplest explanation of the mechanisms involved would be to postulate increased catecholamine responses to the cold; these are then the mediators of renal effects. They also report work showing that adrenaline administered to the adrenalectomized rat does elevate lithium and sodium excretion.

Thirst

There seems little doubt that lithium produces some degree of polydipsia by extra-renal actions, presumably on the hypothalamus. The direct effects are of less significance than the renal-mediated action on thirst (51). Nevertheless, thirst precedes the increased urine flow (52) and occurs in animals with ligated ureters (53). See also Galla *et al.* (54).

Hochman and Gutman (55) also showed that lithium causes increased fluid intake in Brattleboro rats without any vasopressin, and in normal rats without any change in plasma osmolality. Singer and Rotenberg (56) suggested that lithium might inhibit hypophyseal vasopressin release but Torp-Pedersen and Thorn (57) showed that lithium does not inhibit sodium stimulated vasopressin release *in vitro*. Hochman and Gutman (55) showed that *in vivo* lithium tends to deplete hypophyseal vasopressin and does not prevent increased release following hypertonic injections. Histological studies (58) are in essential agreement with these statements.

Perumal and Rao (59) showed that the thirst in rats induced by lithium is partially blocked by haloperidol and propranolol but not by atropine. They conclude that the mechanism depends on beta adrenergic and dopaminergic pathways. This interesting observation does not, however, add greatly to the debate of whether thirst is secondary to a renal effect. This has been clearly resolved, if too frequently discussed.

Kerry, Liebling and Owen (60), Schou *et al.* (61) and O'Connell (62) have all drawn attention to the weight gain induced by lithium treatment. Kerry, Liebling and Owen (60) postulated that lithium might allow the patients to achieve their non-morbid normal weight. However, it seems that the weight gains are too large and the persons certainly consider themselves excessively overwheight. Vendsborg, Bech and Rafaelsen (63) showed a marked correlation between thirst and weight gain. They very reasonably suggest that the patients showing the increased obesity do so because they quench their thirst with high calorie containing fluids.

Lithium and the antidiuretic hormone

Lithium can produce the well-known gross polyuria but in that state and with lower doses, or before any increase in urine volume has occurred, the kidney can become insensitive to the antidiuretic action of vasopressin. Indeed, in rats Dousa and Barnes (64) have shown that the antidiuretic hormone can even have a diuretic effect, presumably due to inhibition of electrolyte and iso-osmotic water reabsorption in various nephron segments proximal to the collecting ducts. This diuresis occurs without significant effect on free water clearance but with a reduced urine osmolality, and an increase of renal medullary lithium. The adenyl cyclase from the renal medulla of animals treated with vasopressin and lithium was less responsive to vasopressin *in vitro* than the enzyme from animals treated with lithium alone.

MacNeil *et al.* (20) showed that renal excretion of vasopressin increased when rats or men were given lithium. They postulated that the degree of polyuria was the result of a comparative compensation by increased hypothalamic production for the renal inhibition of ADH. They also presented data suggesting that the enormous polyuria which can occur might do so when the hypothalamic response begins to drop off. Padfield *et al.* (65) in concordance, reported raised arginine vasopressin levels and angiotensin II in the plasma of a patient dying with high serum lithium.

Padfield *et al.* (66) then went on to show high plasma vasopressin levels in several patients treated with lithium. As has been stated, they felt this was a response to cellular damage which they feel explains the diabetes insipidus. While occasionally this may be true, some doubts have already been expressed on that group's views. On the other hand, Padfield *et al.* (65) did show that high levels of plasma vasopressin can be increased in states of marked polyuria by fluid deprivation. In those circumstances, the hypothalamus cannot be completely exhausted as work from our unit has certainly implied might be the 'cause' of the large urine volumes becoming the enormous diuresis of diabetes insipidus.

While there is something more than a semantic issue involved in distinguishing the structural from the functional explanation of lithium's production of renal insensitivity to vasopressin, the structural theorist still requires an explanation for the damaged cells' loss of function. It is equally important to draw attention to the conflicting reports of proximal and distal tubular damage (9,17).

Lithium and renal adenyl cyclase

Physiologically a number of renal effects have been demonstrated but their relevance to which problems remains in doubt. The dominant view was that the vasopressin-sensitive adenyl cyclase was inhibited by lithium ions. This reduced the cAMP response to ADH and hence the mechanisms for increasing permeability of capillary pathways for osmotic water movements.

Christensen *et al.* (67) studied the effects of lithium chloride on plasma cyclic AMP in rats. They found that it caused a slight but significant increase associated with a small but also significant drop in cAMP/creatinine ratio in the urine, and an equally significant increase in urine creatinine/24 h. Twenty-four hour cyclic AMP excretion in the urine dropped but not statistically significantly, and the authors conclude that the results obtained are certainly not consistent with a generalised effect of lithium on the production of cAMP.

Beck and Davis (68) showed that, while lithium inhibited the vasopressin augmented medullary cyclic AMP in the rat renal medulla, it had no such effect on parathormone-dependent cAMP level in the kidney cortex. Further, there was no effect of lithium on the renal medullary vasopressin-dependent adenylate cyclase level. Nevertheless, lithium did augment the AMP-phosphodiesterase activity. Hence they propose that lithium increases cAMP catabolism rather than decreasing anabolism. Jenner and MacNeil (69), however, failed to show any effect of lithium on the antidiuretic response to theophylline (a phosphodiesterase inhibitor); they also showed that, although the antidiuresis due to infused ATP could be inhibited by lithium, increasing the dose of ATP did not reduce the inhibition. Dousa (70) also failed to show any influence of lithium ions on cyclic AMP-dependent adenyl cyclase. Several workers have also shown that lithium inhibits the antidiuresis due to cyclic AMP (69).

Hormone-sensitive adenyl cyclase is reported to be inhibited by lithium ions in therapeutic concentrations. The studies have, however, largely been performed by measuring cyclic AMP production in incubated tissues in the presence of lithium ions (71,72). Further, after prolonged treatment of the intact animal with lithium, the renal adenyl cyclase activity is decreased in the rat (73), as well as in man (74).

Olesen, Jensen and Thomsen (75) showed, however, that lithium enhanced the increased cyclic AMP excretion produced by glucagon administration. Geisler *et al.* (76) showed that lithium increased the unstimulated and the glucagon stimulated excretion of cyclic AMP. In man lithium produced no effect on cyclic AMP excretion, nor on glucagon degeneration. The authors see these results as also offering no support to the view that lithium has *in vivo* a general effect on hormone-sensitive adenyl cyclases. They are cautious because, as they put it, there are complex regulatory mechanisms which could alter glucagon-sensitive adenyl cyclase *in vivo*.

Christensen and Geisler (77) studied the urinary cyclic AMP responses to ADH in lithium-treated polyuric rats and normal animals. They obtained varied results from the normal rats, less than 50% showing a rise; none of the animals with lithium-induced polyuria, however, showed any cyclic AMP response to vasopressin and all had 85% inhibition of the action of vasopressin. They take this to be compatible with the view that ADH acts by altering intracellular cAMP, and that in some way alteration to this system causes the vasopressin-resistant diuresis. They remark on the greater resistance of their rats to vasopressin-induced (85% inhibition) antidiuresis, compared to the 50% reported by Harris and Jenner (78). However, their animals are not receiving alcohol and are possibly already under the influence of much higher circulating levels of vasopressin (17). Perhaps under these conditions extra vasopressin is supramaximal. It does seem that the results they obtained could be used to question their adenyl cyclase hypothesis, as well as support it.

THE ROLE OF PROSTAGLANDINS

Mtabaji *et al.* (79) make the very interesting suggestion that prostaglandins are necessary for the action of cAMP release following ADH administration. The relevant prostaglandin is controlled by prolactin or the other lactogenic hormones. Lithium, it is postulated, exerts its influence on the effect of the hormones on prostaglandin release. In support of this view, it is demonstrated that prostaglandin A_2 at low rates of infusion restores the antidiuretic effect of vasopressin in lithium-treated rats. If confirmed, this novel approach might considerably alter our views, although if correct it is probably not the site of action of lithium which has been discovered, but just yet another site. The hypothesis does, however, explain why lithium inhibits the effects of cAMP as well as of vasopressin.

ELECTROLYTE EFFECTS OF LITHIUM AND THEIR IMPORTANCE FOR THE ACTION OF ADH

The fact that free water clearance in rats (80) and in man (81) is unaltered by lithium excludes a gross change of chloride reabsorption in the ascending loop of Henle. However, the increased diuresis of Brattleboro rats with the associated increase of free water clearance to glomerular filtration rate (82) indicates an important ADH-independent factor in lithium polyuria due to reduced sodium and water reabsorption in the proximal tubule, a mechanism equally independent of the vasopressin-sensitive adenyl cyclase.

Carney, Rayson and Morgan (83), studying isolated papillae of rats taken from normal and lithium-treated animals, failed to show any difference in permeabiltiy between normal and lithium-treated animals, nor any significant effect on permeability following addition of lithium to the test media. They did, however, show that the cyclic AMP response to ADH in renal tissue from lithium-treated animals was defective. They argue, however, that this is not very relevant as it had no effect on the change in permeability. They further quote Jenner and MacNeil (69) that there is anyway a high ADH level in rats (and men) treated with lithium, and so the permeability of the collecting ducts is probably already high. ADH cannot, therefore, further profoundly influence it. Hence lithium seems to be affecting sodium transport proximally in the nephron. Precisely that view is also postulated by Martinez-Maldonado *et al.* (84) and by Harris and Dirks (80). The authors also point out that a failure to show any change in renal medullary sodium is equally damaging to a hypothesis primarily explaining the diuresis as secondary to insufficient cAMP in the distal and collecting tubules as to one explaining the results by more primary sodium changes more proximally.

Harris and Jenner (78) showed that the inhibition of the renal effect of vasopressin in the rat infused intravenously commences within 10 minutes. Species differences and the delay in onset of clinical problems, as well as multiple effects of lithium on the kidney, have raised the question of the relevance of such studies to the clinical problems. The work of Webb *et al.* (85) on acute effects of lithium on renal concentrating mechanisms in the primate (*Galago crassicavdatus pagamiensis*), however, suggests a similar response occurs in primates (and hence probably in man). They showed that lithium very quickly reduces solute-free water reabsorption without affecting free water clearance. Amiloride reverses almost completely this effect and the results are reported as highly consistent with an effect of lithium depending on its entry into cells of the distal tubules and collecting ducts, where it antagonises the effect of vasopressin.

Although Torp-Pedersen and Thorne (57) reported difficulties in demonstrating rapid recovery of the renal responsiveness of the rat to vasopressin in the presence of high serum lithium values, when the infusion contained no more lithium, Jenner and MacNeil (69) confirmed Harris and Jenner's (78) finding that acute inhibition of the action of vasopressin was dependent on a rising plasma lithium level and not on the absolute concentration.

Explanation of this phenomenon would be simpler in terms of physical chemical rather than enzymic effects. It is most easily explained if lithium disturbs a compensated equilibrium which has a lag in its response. Clearly, it is optimistic speculation to suggest this depends on sodium disturbances proximal to the distal tubule but that remains our hunch. It would certainly explain the very acute animal studies. However, there is no adequate support for this, the author's view and the situation itself is not necessarily very relevant to the clinical problems, even if correct.

Lithium and pH

Angielski *et al.* (86) performed interesting studies comparing the effects on renal function of maleate and lithium. Maleate has a marked affinity for renal tissue whereas lithium has a more general effect. Acute injections of either in rats produced a bicarbonaturia and a rise of urine pH and PCO_2. In addition, lithium caused a rise in plasma chloride and a fall of plasma bicarbonate and phosphate. Maleate produced a small increase in pyruvate, lactate and alpha-ketoglutarate but had no effect on plasma citrate. Lithium had a much more marked effect, increasing plasma lactate, pyruvate, citrate and alpha-ketoglutarate. The renal clearances of the dicarboxylic acids, alpha-ketoglutarate and citrate were increased to many times the control values, and there was a much smaller increased excretion of lactate and pyruvate. Renal ATP levels dropped after maleate or lithium though cAMP levels rose, and the ATP/ADP ratio was greatly reduced. The decreased total production of energy in the kidney is not, however, adequate to explain the specific effects as other metabolic inhibitors produce different results.

Further studies showed that in rats with ligated ureters the loss of lithium from the extracellular spaces was equimorlarly associated with increased hydrogen ion concentration. These results suggest that the intracellular alkalosis induced by lithium administration may be fundamental in explaining the renal effects of lithium ions.

The results also suggest that we (87,88) have over-emphasized the purely renal role in causing changes in the handling of $C_{4\text{-}6}$ dicarboxylic acids following lithium, by the body. Perhaps an intracellular alkalosis in the brain and the consequent metabolic effects are of more significance, even of therapeutic significance.

Roscoe *et al.* (89) showed that even in severe acute acidosis in rats lithium still increases bicarbonaturia and also reduces the urine minus blood carbon dioxide pressure. The latter they interpret as evidence that the impaired urinary acidification is almost entirely due to a severe distal tubule defect in hydrogen ion secretion. However, they clearly indicate that the bicarbonaturia can be due to a mild defect of hydrogen ion secretory effect in the proximal tubule.

Studies in our own unit (mainly by Askew, MacNeil and Thompson) have shown that one cannot detect any intracellular pH changes in red cells in men and rats with therapeutic lithium levels. This work was, however, done using 5,5-dimethyl 2,4-oxazolidinedione; it leaves much to be desired and would miss small changes. Further work with intracellular electrodes in *Helix pomatia* showed no change in intracellular pH with quite large alterations in intra and extracellular lithium levels. However, lithium seems to affect transport of many drugs and probably many other weak acids and weak bases. Mandelic acid and ammonium chloride both reverse the inhibition of ADH and pH seems possibly, though complicatedly, relevant to the effects on the tricarboxylic acid cycle metabolite excretion. These results of our own studies led us to postulate interference with inter-cellular pH. Hence, applying Jackson's hypothesis (90) for the transport of weak acids and bases, this might explain some of the findings. This degree of theoretical sophistication would be unnecessary, however, if a pH change could be demonstrated intracellularly, then the theory need not depend on the unmeasurable postulated pH change in inter-cellular canaliculi.

Olesen, Jensen and Thomsen (91) showed that high potassium intake in the rat can partially compensate for the lithium-induced retardation of growth and the polyuria. This occurred without influencing the serum lithium levels, high sodium intake produced less striking but similar effects, but these were associated with reduced serum lithium concentrations which would be adequate to account for the results obtained. Lithium induced a shift of urine pH towards alkalinity and this was counteracted by the high potassium intake. Lowering pH also affects the changed water permeability of the toad bladder (96).

Lithium and inappropriate ADH secretion

White and Fetner (93) used lithium successfully to reverse the effect of inappropriate antidiuretic hormone secretion following head injury. They reported no change in urine cyclic AMP during reversal of the water retention. However, Hendler *et al.* (94) draw attention to objections to this treatment preferring demeclocycline. Long-term in contrast to short-term lithium treatment no longer leads to increased aldosterone and hence sodium retention.

References

1. Bailey, E. *et al.* (1975). *Progr. Medicinal Chem.,* **11**, 193
2. MacNeil, S. and Jenner, F.A. (1975). In: F.N. Johnson (ed.) *Lithium Research and Therapy,* pp. 473-484 (London: Academic Press)
3. Jenner, F.A. (1973). *Biochem. Soc. Trans.,* **1**, 88
4. Schou, M. (1958). *Acta Pharmacol. Toxicol.,* **15**, 85
5. Cade, J.F.J. (1949). *Med. J. Aust.,* **36**, 349
6. Schou, M. (1968). *J. Psychiat. Res.,* **6**, 67
7. Hansen, H.E. *et al.* (1977). *Proc. Eur. Dialysis Transpl. Assoc.,* **14**, (in press)
8. Hestbech, J. *et al.* (1977). *Kidney Int.,* (in press)
9. Lindop, G.B.M. and Padfield, P.L. (1975). *J. Clin. Pathol.,* **28**, 472
10. Shimizu, M. and Smith, D.F. (1976). *Clin. Pharmacol. Ther.,* **21**, 212
11. Saran, B.M. and Russell, G.F. (1976). *Psychol. Med.,* **6**, 381
12. Johnson, F.N. (ed.) (1975). *Lithium Research and Therapy.* (London: Academic Press)
13. Thomsen, K. *et al.* (1969). *Pflügers Arch. Ges. Physiol.,* **308**, 180
14. Thomsen, K. and Schou, M. (1973). *Am. J. Physiol.,* **215**, 823
15. Steele, T.H. *et al.* (1975). *Am. J. Med. Sci.,* **269**, 349
16. Baer *et al.* (1971). *J. Psychiat. Res.,* **8**, 91
17. Lavender, S., Brown, J.N. and Berrill, W.T. (1973). *Postgrad. Med. J.,* **49**, 277
18. Lehmann, K. and Merten, K. (1974). *Int. J. Clin. Pharmacol.,* **10**, 292
19. Hewick *et al.* (1977). *Br. J. Clin. Pharmacol.,* **4**, 201
20. MacNeil, S. *et al.* (1976). *Br. J. Clin. Pharmacol.,* **3**, 305
21. Thomsen, K. and Schou, M. (1975). In: F.N. Johnson (ed.) *Lithium Research and Therapy,* pp. 227-236. (London: Academic Press).
22. Thomsen, K. (1976). *J. Pharmacol. Exp. Ther.,* **199**, 483
23. Thomsen, K. (1973). *Acta Pharmacol. Toxicol.,* **33**, 92
24. Thomsen, K., Jensen, J. and Olesen, O.V. (1976). *J. Pharmacol. Exp. Ther.,* **196**, 463
25. Dirks, J.H., Cirksena, W.J. and Berliner, R.W. (1966). *J. Clin. Invest.,* **45**, 1875
26. Thomsen, K., Jensen, J. and Olesen, O.V. (1974). *Acta Pharmacol. Toxicol.,* **35**, 337
27. Kierkegaard-Hansen, A. (1974). *Acta Pharmacol. Toxicol.,* **35**, 370
28. Kierkegaard-Hansen, A. (1976). *Acta Pharmacol. Toxicol.,* **39**, 97
29. Gutman, Y., Tamir, N. and Benzakein, F. (1973). *Eur. J. Pharmacol.,* **24**, 347
30. Altamura, A.C. and Morganti, A. (1975). *Psychopharmacologia,* **45**, 171
31. Steele, T.H. and Dudgeon, K.L. (1974). *Kidney Int.,* **5**, 196
32. Arruda, J.A.L. *et al.* (1976). *Am. J. Physiol.,* **231**, 1140
33. Olesen, O.V. and Thomsen, K., (1974). *Acta Pharmacol. Toxicol.,* **34**, 225
34. Mellerup, E.T. and Plenge, (1976). *Int. Pharmacopsychiat* (in press)
35. Vendsborg, P.B., Mellerup, E.T. and Rafaelsen, O.J. (1973). *Acta Psychiat. Scand.,* **49**, 97
36. Mellerup, E.T. *et al.* (1976). *Acta Psychiat. Scand.,* **53**, 360
37. Birch, N.J. and Jenner, F.A. (1973). *Br. J. Pharmacol.,* **47**, 586
38. Karniol, I.G. and Rafaelsen, O.J. (1976). (to be published)
39. Mellerup, E.T. and Rafaelsen, O.J. (1975). In: F.N. Johnson (ed.) *Lithium Research and Therapy* pp. 381-389. (London: Academic Press)
40. Crammer, J. (1975). *Lancet,* i, 215
41. Williams, RJ.P. (1973). In: S. Gershon (ed.) *Lithium, Its Role in Psychiatric Research and Treatment.,* (New York: Plenum Press)
42. Birch, N.J. (1970). *Br. J. Psychiat.,* **116**, 461
43. Petersen, V. *et al.* (1974). *Br. Med. J.,* **3**, 143
44. Demers, R. and Heninger, C. (1970). *J. Am. Med. Assoc.,* **214**, 1845
45. Levy, S.T., Forrest, J.N. and Heninger, G.R. (1973). *Am. J. Psychiat.,* **130**, 1014
46. Fyrö, B. and Sedvall, G. (1975). In: F.N. Johnson (ed.) *Lithium Research and Therapy,* pp. 287-312 (London: Academic Press)

47. Radomski, J.L. *et al.* (1950). *J. Pharmacol.*, **100**, 429
48. Evan, A.P. and Ollerich, D.A. (1972). *Am. J. Anat.*, **134**, 97
49. Beck, N. and Kim, S. K. (1975). *Endocrinology*, **96**, 744
50. Smith, D.F. and de Jong, W. (1975). *Pharmacopsychiat.*, **8**, 132
51. Christensen, S. (1974). *Acta Pharmacol. Toxicol.*, **35**, 201
52. Smith, D.F. and Balagura, S. (1972). *Life Sci.*, **11**, 1021
53. Gutman, Y., Benzakein, F. and Livneh, P. (1971). *Eur. J. Pharmacol.*, **16**, 380
54. Galla, J. N. *et al.* (1975). *Yale J. Biol. Med.*, **48**, 305
55. Hockman, S. and Gutman, Y. (1974). *Eur. J. Pharmacol.*, **28**, 100
56. Singer, I. and Rotenberg, D. (1973). *N. Engl. J. Med.*, **289**, 254
57. Torp-Pedersen, C. and Thorn, N.A. (1973). *Acta Endocrinol.*, **73**, 665
58. Ellman, G.L. and Gan, G.L. (1973). *Toxicol. Appl. Pharmacol.*, **25**, 617
59. Perumal, T.A. and Rao, P.J. (1974). *Br. J. Pharmacol.*, **51**, 107
60. Kerry, R.J., Liebling, L.I. and Owens, G. (1970). *Acta Psychiat. Scand.*, **46**, 238
61. Schou, M. *et al.* (1970). *Br. J. Psychiat.*, **116**, 615
61. O'Connell, H. (1971). *Comprehens. Psychiat.*, **12**, 224
63. Vendsborg, P.B., Bech, P. and Rafaelsen, O.J. (1976). *Acta Psychiat. Scand.*, **53**, 139
64. Dousa, T.P. and Barnes, L.D. (1976). *Am. J. Physiol.*, **231**, 1754
65. Padfield, P.L. *et al.* (1975). *Clin. Nephrol.*, **3**, 220
66. Padfield, P.L. *et al.* (1977). *Br. J. Psychiat.*, **130**, 144
67. Christensen, S. *et al.* (1977). *Acta Pharmacol. Toxicol.*, **40**, 455
68. Beck, N. and Davis, B.B. (1975). *Endocrinology*, **97**, 202
69. Jenner, F.A. and MacNeil, S. (1975). *Br. J. Pharmacol.*, **55**, 527
70. Dousa, T.P. (1974). *Endocrinology*, **95**, 1359
71. Wolff, J., Berens, S.C. and Jones, A.B. (1970). *Biochem. Biophys. Res. Commun.*, **39**, 77
72. Forn, J. and Valdecasas, F.G. (1971). *Biochem. Pharmacol*, **20**, 2773
73. Geisler, A.O., Wraae, O. and Olesen, O.V. (1972). *Acta Pharmacol. Toxicol.*, **31**, 203
74. Murphy, D.L., Donnelly, C. and Moskowitz, J. (1973). *Clin. Pharmacol. Ther.*, **14**, 810
75. Olesen, O.V., Jensen, J. and Thomsen, K. (1974). *Acta Pharmacol. Toxicol.*, **35**, 403
76. Geisler, A. *et al.* (1976). *Acta Pharmacol.*, **38**, 433
77. Christensen, S. and Geisler, A. (1977). *Acta Pharmacol. Toxicol.*, **40**, 447
78. Harris, C.A. and Jenner, F.A. (1972). *Br. J. Pharmacol.*, **44**, 223
79. Mtabaji, J.P. *et al.* (1977). *J. Endocrinol.*, **73**, 31
80. Harris, C.A. and Dirks, J.H. (1973). *Fed. Proc.*, **32**, 381
81. Singer, I., Rotenberg, D. and Puschett, J.B. (1972). *J. Clin. Invest.*, **51**, 1081
82. Rahn, D.W. and Forrest, J.N. (1975). *Clin. Res.*, **23**, *602A*
83. Carney, S., Rayson, B. and Morgan, T. (1976). *Pflügers Arch.*, **366**, 19
84. Martinez-Maldonado, M. *et al.* (1975). *J. Lab. Clin. Med.*, **86**, 445
85. Webb, R. K. *et al.* (1975). *Am. J. Physiol.*, **228**, 909
86. Angielski, S. *et al.* (1976). In: U. Schmidt and U.C. Dubach (Eds.) *Renal Metabolism in Relation to Renal Function* (Bern: Huber)
87. Bond, P.A. and Jenner, F.A. (1974). *Br. J. Pharmacol.*, **50**, 283
88. Bond, P.A. *et al.* (1972). *Br. J. Pharmacol.*, **46**, 116
89. Roscoe, J.M. *et al.* (1976). *Kidney Int.*, **9**, 344
90. Jackson, M.J. (1974). In: D.H. Smyth (ed.) *Biomembranes*, pp. 673-709 (New York: Plenum Press)
91. Olesen, O.V., Jensen, J. and Thomsen, K. (1975). *Acta Pharmacol. Toxicol.* **36**, 161
92. Singer, I. and Franko, E.A. (1973). *Kidney Int.*, **3**, 151
93. White, M.G. and Fetner, C.D. (1975). *New Engl. J. Med.*, **292**, 390
94. Hendler, N. *et al.* (1976). *N. Engl. J. Med.*, **294**, 446

ADDENDA TO CHAPTER 27

1. A Note on Reports of Nephrotoxic Effects of Lithium

M. SCHOU

With regard to the possibility of kidney damage produced by lithium, the observations of morphological changes have obviously put us on the alert, but like Professor Jenner I recommend that the matter is viewed in perspective. Progressive development of kidney insufficiency does not seem to be at all frequent among lithium treated patients, not even those treated for many years. The question is, of course, what functional alterations the morphological changes are associated with, for it is presumably too much to hope that this is a purely cosmetic phenomenon. The functional damage may be at different levels. It may, for example, involve merely the renal capacity to concentrate urine, and if this remains the only defect, it may be unpleasant and troublesome for the patients but does not endanger their lives. If , on the other side, the glomerular filtration rate is affected, this may, if the affection is progressive, lead to renal insufficiency and the patient's death. The patient sample examined in Aarhus is a highly selected one, most of them having had previous intoxications. We therefore do not know whether the findings are representative. In order to find that out, and also to examine the functional and prognostic significance of the morphological changes, extensive international studies are at present under way to investigate a large unselected sample of lithium treated patients with various kidney function tests.

2
A Note on Animal and Human Studies of Possible Kidney Damage Caused by Lithium

N. J. BIRCH

Professor Jenner has referred to studies in which lithium-induced renal damage has been reported. Some comment on our own experience on this matter may be appropriate. We have been unable to demonstrate any evidence of progressively decreasing renal efficiency in 90 patients receiving lithium prophylactically.

Recently, I sent to Dr Jytte Hestbech some post-mortem kidney specimens from male and female rats who had received from weaning either tap-water or lithium chloride (1 mmol/kg body weight/day) as drinking fluid for about 18 months. Lesions, similar in character to those seen in the human lithium-treated kidneys, have now been reported in some of these rat specimens though they occurred in both control and lithium animals. Of the five rats who had severe lesions, four were male, two lithium treated and two control. The female rat with lesions was of low body weight for her age and might have been suffering from lithium toxicity. Two control female rats were reported to have very slight lesions and the remaining animals, all female, were normal. There were three lithium and two control rats in this group.

These results are on a small number of animals. There has not been sufficient time to receive a reply from Dr Hestbech and it may be that her interpretation will be different from mine. However, it seems that we have observed differential effects of ageing in the rat kidney. The normal rat lifespan is from 2½ to 3 years and females have a longer life expectancy than males. I understand that rats are particularly susceptible to glomerulonephritis and that this and arteriosclerosis are the most common cause of death in old age. The lesions which Dr Hestbech has reported might be the early signs of the onset of ageing in the male rat.

Two points should be considered with regard to the human renal lesions which have been reported to be associated with lithium treatment. The lesions are not specific to lithium and perhaps one might question whether those patients affected were already suffering from sub-clinical renal disease which was exacerbated by lithium. The controls used in the human study were from donors for renal transplant who had been specifically screened to exclude kidney disease and hence might give a false reference point when compared with a psychiatric population who may have been treated with a variety of potentially nephrotoxic drugs over many years. Secondly, I would raise again the question of whether polyuria is actually a harmless side effect of lithium or whether it is really a warning of marginal toxicity. Perhaps we should reconsider the question of otimal plasma lithium concentrations for prophylaxis since the present recommendations were derived empirically from the doses used in the acute treatment of mania. Continuous treatment at high plasma levels greater than 1 mmol/l) may prove not only to be unnecessary but may lead periodically to unrecognized marginal toxicity. In addition the cardinal rule must be frequent (less than 10 weeks) monitoring of plasma lithium with systematic recording of data so that any gradual tendency for a rise in concentration may be seen quickly and the dose adjusted.

28

Lithium Effect on Various Diurnal Rhythms in Manic Melancholic Patients

E. T. MELLERUP, H. DAM, G. WILDSCHIØDTZ and O. J. RAFAELSEN

INTRODUCTION

Several rhythmic phenomena are characteristic for manic melancholic disorders. Firstly, the occurrence of attacks during a lifetime is periodic and may be rhythmic in many patients. Secondly, the single affective episode may show a phasic course with gradual divergence from the normal level of mood towards the mania or depression, and then, in a more or less symmetrical way, return to the base line of mood. Thirdly, during the depressive period many patients may experience diurnal variaton in symptoms, and furthermore show changes in various circadian rhythms (1). It has been suggested that the desynchronization, which can take place when one or more of the biological rhythms follows its own endogenous or free running circadian period, may be of aetiological importance for manic depressive psychosis (2,3). Lithium treatment may influence all of these rhythmic phenomena. The relapse preventive effect of lithium *by definition* changes the overall pattern of attacks, and the course of the single attack may likewise be changed by lithium both with respect to length and amplitude. With respect to circadian rhythms lithium has been found to change the length of some circadian periods in plants, animals (4), and man (5).

The aim of the present work was to study the effects of lithium on the diurnal variation in manic melancholic patients.

MATERIALS AND METHODS

Patients and control persons were divided into three groups. Group I consisted of 91 normal control persons. Group II consisted of 88 psychiatric controls, most of them were manic melancholic patients; they were treated with antidepressants, neuroleptics, or no medical treatment was given at the time of investigation. Group III comprised 78 lithium treated manic melancholic patients. These patients normally took their whole dose of lithium at bedtime. During the investigation the time of administration was fixed at 22.00 h except for a small group (20), who had their intake postponed 12 h to 10 h.

Blood samples were obtained through an indwelling catheter. The catheter was connected to a drip with physiological saline (without heparin) in order to keep the catheter open. The blood sampling started at 21 h and 17 samples were collected during the next 24 h. The subjects were allowed to walk around in the research ward (6), with the drips hanging in a moveable rack. During the night when the subjects were in bed, the catheters were led through tubes in the wall, allowing blood samples to be obtained from the adjoining room.

All urine samples were collected and analyzed separately. Oral temperature was recorded seven times during the investigation. Self-rating on a mood-scale and reaction time determination were performed in the evening, in the morning, and in the afternoon.

Analysis of sodium, potassium, calcium, magnesium, lithium, and phosphate was performed on plasma, erythrocytes, and urine samples. Protein and glucose determination was performed on plasma. Urine pH was measured. Student's t test was used to compare the mean values.

RESULTS AND DISCUSSION

Serum

It has previously been found that a single injection of lithium to rats was followed by changes in electrolyte metabolism. Serum phosphate decreased, serum calcium, and serum magnesium increased (7). A similar picture was seen in patients who had been on lithium treatment for several years (8). About 1 hour after the intake of the daily dose of lithium at 22.00 h serum phosphate decreased compared with both normal and psychiatric controls and returned to control levels in the morning. Serum calcium rose slightly some hours after the lithium intake and returned to control levels during the day. Serum magnesium was elevated all the time.

The increase in serum calcium and serum magnesium may be due to a lithium induced increase in parathyroid hormone secretion (9,10), but other mechanisms may also be working because the increase in serum calcium and serum magnesium was observed in thyro-parathyroidectomized rats (11). We have previously suggested (7,8) that the changes in calcium and magnesium metabolism were secondary to the changes in phosphate metabolism, which in turn were secondary to lithium induced changes in carbohydrate metabolism.

Urine

After the intake of the lithium dose, urine calcium decreased, and the excretion for the next 12 h was reduced to about half the excretion of control groups. The excretion during the rest of the day was not significantly lower in urine from the lithium patients, but the total excretion remained lower. With respect to magnesium, urine excretion during the night was similar in the three groups, but increased significantly in the lithium-treated patients during the day. These results are in agreement with the results from long-term balance studies of lithium-treated patients (12).

Determination of pH in the urine showed that pH rose shortly after the intake of the lithium and remained higher for the next 16 h. This result is in agreement with earlier reports, and it may be due to lithium-produced inhibition of the hydrogen ion secretion in the nephron (13).

Temperature

The lithium-treated patients had higher oral temperatures than the normal controls at all times; this difference was statistically significant except at 16.00 h where the control group had its maximum temperature. The lithium group had its maximum at 12.00 h.

The lithium-treated patients, who during the day of investigation had their lithium-intake postponed for 12 h, showed a much steeper decrease in temperature during the night than the patients, who took their lithium at the usual time (22.00 h). At 8.00 h the former group had decreased their temperature to the level of the normal controls, however, after the delayed lithium intake (10.00 h) the oral temperature rose again and reached the value of the other lithium group in the evening.

The lithium-induced increase in temperature, which is in agreement with previous reports (14,15), may be secondary to changes in electrolyte metabolism, or it may be due to a direct lithium effect on the temperature regulation centre in the hypothalamus. The latter possibility may be of importance due to the probable involvement of the hypothalamic area in affective disturbances.

References

1. Mellerup, E.T. and Rafaelsen, O.J. (1977). (In press)
2. Halberg, F. (1968). In: J. de Ajuriaguerre (ed.) *Cycles Biologiques et Psychiatrie,* pp. 73-126 (Paris: Masson & Cie)
3. Pflüg, B. (1976). *Acta Psychiat. Scand.,* 53, 148
4. Engelmann, W. (1973). *Z. Naturforsch.,* 28, 733
5. Atkinson, Martha, Kripke, D.F. and Wolf, S.R. (1975). *Chronobiol.,* 2, 325
6. Rafaelsen, O.J., Lauritsen, B., Plenge, P. and Mellerup, E.T. (1976). In: E. Usdin and I.S. Forrest (eds.) *Psychotherapeutic Drugs,* Part 1. Psychopharmacology Series Vol. 2, pp. 581-604. (New York: Marcel Dekker)
7. Mellerup, E.T., Plenge, P., Ziegler, R. and Rafaelsen, O.J. (1973). *Int. Pharmacopsychiat.,* 8, 360
8. Mellerup, E.T., Lauritsen, B., Dam, H. and Rafaelsen, O.J. (1976). *Acta Psychiat. Scand.,* 53, 360.
9. Christiansen, C., Baastrup, P.C. and Transbøl, I. (1976). *Lancet,* ii, 969
10. Christensson, T.A.T. (1976). *Lancet,* ii, 144
11. Plenge, P. and Mellerup, E.T. (1976). *Psychopharmacology,* 49, 187
12. Bjørum, N., Hornum, I., Mellerup, E.T., Plenge, P.K. and Rafaelsen, O.J. (1975). *Lancet,* i, 1243
13. Roscoe, J.M., Goldstein, M.B., Halperin, M.L., Wilson, D.R. and Stinebaugh, B.J. (1976). *Kidney Int.,* 9, 344
14. Tupin, J.P. (1970). *Int. Pharmacopsychiat.,* 5, 227
15. Williams, R.J.P. (1973). In: S. Gerhson and B. Shopsin (eds.) *Lithium: Its Role in Psychiatric Research and Treatment.* (New York: Plenum Press).

29

Lithium Effects on Leukocytosis and Lymphopenia

J. PEREZ-CRUET, J. T. DANCEY and J. WAITE

INTRODUCTION

Except for two studies (1,2), numerous investigators have reported a consistent leukocytosis during treatment with lithium salts (3-8). The increase in white blood cells (WBC) is associated with a neutrophilia and no shift to immature myeloid cells. This indicates that the leukocytosis is not due to infection. The increase in WBC can be relative or intermittent (2); it is not associated with blood lithium levels (6,9) or cytogenic effects of the cation on marrow chromosomes (8); and it is not permanent, returning to normal after discontinuation of lithium (4-6).

Two mechanisms by which lithium can produce a leukocytosis have been postulated:

1. Some studies have shown that lithium stimulates adrenocortical activity and increases cortisol output (10,11) whereas others have shown no effect (12). Also lithium stimulates transitorily aldosterone output (13) by a direct action on the adrenal cortex (14). Although steroids can produce a leukocytosis (15) there is no consistent evidence that lithium stimulates adrenocortical activity in man.

2. The initial report that lithium produces hyperplasia of the bone marrow (3) has not been duplicated by others (7,8,16). Others have reported that lithium can induce marrow cell proliferation *in vivo* and can increase the granulocyte pool *in vivo* (17). The neutrophilia observed during lithium treatment is quite small and modest (5,6,8). Some

investigators have reported that lithium is effective in increasing the number of granulocytes in patients with granulocytopoenias (18,7); others, however, have been unable to duplicate these effects (8). It is doubtful that either granulocyte proliferation or adrenocortical activation are sufficient to explain the leukocytosis during lithium therapy and more research is needed.

Although much attention has been placed on the neutrophilia as the main cause of the leukocytosis less attention has been placed on the contribution of lymphocytes to this effect. All reports, with the exception of one (7), report a consistent leukopenia which accompanies the leukocytosis. In the dog, lithium induces a significant lymphopenia (19). No study is yet available on the effects of lithium on T and B lymphocytes. The T lymphocytes are thymus dependent and the B lymphocytes participate in the production of humoral antibodies. A recent report has already shown a significant involution of the thymus gland in mice during treatment with lithium (20). Evidence that lithium may have a cytogenic effect on human lymphocytes has been reported (21), but others have not been able to duplicate these findings (22).

It is the main purpose of this chapter to present further evidence that lithium exerts a definite effect on WBC, neutrophils and lymphocytes, and to advance a hypothesis that lymphocytes may be involved.

METHODS AND MATERIALS

Human studies

The retrospective human studies consisted of examining the records of over 250 inpatients admitted to a general hospital, the Montreal General Hospital (MGH) and a mental state hospital, St. Louis State Hospital (SLSH), who had been treated with lithium. About 96% of the inpatients met the research diagnostic criteria for manic, hypomanic, or depressive disorder, and 4% met the criteria for schizo-affective disorders as described elsewhere (23). The patients were selected at random and all routine haemograms, including differential counts, were examined before, during and after treatment with lithium. The MGH inpatient population consisted of 62% females and 38% males with an age range of 17-65 years, and a mean age of 39 years. The SLSH inpatient population consisted of 61% females and 39% males with an age range of 24 to 63 years and a mean age of 42 years.

In our study, due to the severity of the illness requiring hospitalization, the majority of inpatients were treated with other psychotropic drugs (phenothiazines, butyrophenones or tricyclics). For this reason, another scrutiny of haemograms in 50 severely ill manic depressive inpatients not treated with lithium, but receiving other drugs, was done.

None of the above inpatients have any history of infectious disease during the period studied.

In addition to retrospective studies, an additional group of inpatients admitted to the MGH in the manic phase of a manic depressive disorder were followed with routine haemograms before and during lithium therapy. Whenever possible the doses of lithium were maintained between 1800 g and 2100 g/day. Reliability of haemograms and differential counts was reassessed by selecting patients with known haematological disorders and infections.

Animal studies

Swiss and CBA male mice weighing 30 g were used. Lithium chloride (LiCl) was given orally or intraperitoneally in doses of 1 and 3 mmol/kg twice a day for at least 4 days. An additional series of experiments were done with doses of 1 and 3 mmol/kg twice a day i.p. for periods up to 32 days. Determinations of WBC were done with a Coulter apparatus on days 4, 10, 18, 24, and 32 after obtaining blood by orbital puncture. The addition of lithium chloride to control blood samples did not alter WBC counts in the Coulter instrument. In addition, differential counts were done by a haematology technician on peripheral blood and marrow aspirates. Lithium levels were determined with a flame spectrophotometer. In addition, thymus glands were examined as described elsewhere (20).

Mean, standard deviation and two tailed Student's t tests for statistical significance were done as described elsewhere (24).

RESULTS

As illustrated in Table 29.1, a significant ($p < 0.05$) leukocytosis, neutrophilia and lymphopenia was observed in both inpatient populations treated with lithium. The SLSH inpatients showed a more significant leukocytosis ($p < 0.01$) and higher levels of lithium than the MGH inpatients.

Both groups showed a slight neutrophilia (MGH: + 6.5%; SLSH: + 2.6%) and lymphopenia (MGH: - 4.9%; SLSH: – 3.0%). The increase in leukocytes was almost identical in both groups (MGH: + 1641; SLSH: + 1623), as shown in Table 29.1.

Table 29.2 shows nine selected patients showing an increase in WBC

Table 29.1. WBC, neutrophils, lymphocytes and lithium levels in an inpatient population in a general and state mental hospital: means ± standard deviations

Hospital	Tx	No.	WBC	% Neutrophils	% Lymphocytes	Serum Lithium
A. MGH	None	30	7118.0 (68) ±2466.0	64.1 (54) ±14.1	24.7 (54) ±11.41	0
MGH	Lithium	23	8759.5 (37)* ±2216.0	70.6 (23)* ±9.9	19.8 (23)* ±7.3	0.64 (30) ±0.13
MGH	Other psychotropics	78	7069.23 ±2491.14	66.89 ±12.64	23.03 ±9.77	
B. SLSH	None	40	8465.0 (73) ±2801.0	66.3 (65) ±8.1	30.1 (65) ±8.7	0
SLSH	Lithium	57	10088.0 (104)*** ±4348.0	68.8 (98)* ±7.9	27.1 (98)*** ±8.6	0.89 (65) ±0.32**

Number in parenthesis represent the number of determinations
Tx = Treatment. *$p < 0.05$; **$0.05 > p > 0.02$; ***$0.01 > p > 0.001$.

Table 29.2. WBC, neutrophils and lymphocytes in selected bipolar manic depressive inpatients before and during lithium treatment

No.	Sex	White blood cells Pretreatment	White blood cells Li	Neutrophils Pretreatment	Neutrophils Li	Lymphocytes Pretreatment	Lymphocytes Li	Serum lithium
1.	Female	5600	7600	62	76	36	26	1.0
2.	Female	4300	7700	56	73	38	20	0.9
3.	Male	5600	8500	53	74	39	16	0.6
4.	Female	7700	9200	48	77	37	15	0 6
5.	Female	8900	10600	68	73	30	23	0.2
6.	Male	8600	11000	61	68	36	29	0.4
7.	Male	6400	13500	69	75	27	23	0.6
8.	Male	9600	14500	57	74	43	26	0.8
9.	Female	9700	23000	54	81	41	10	1.9

during lithium therapy. A relative leukocytosis (i.e. counts less than 10 800) was observed in patients 1, 2, 3, 4, 5, and a true leukocytosis in patients 6, 7, 8, and 9. The increase in WBC was not correlated with increments in neutrophils, serum lithium levels, the decrease in lymphocytes, age or sex. A significant ($p < 0.05$) negative correlation between the increments in neutrophils and the decrease in lymphocytes was observed. These results suggest a possible interaction between lymphocytes and neutrophils.

The effects of lithium on WBC in mice are summarized in Table 19.3 LiCl produces a significant leukopenia and lymphopenia during acute and chronic lithium treatment. The leukopenia is dose related because 2 mmol/kg/day did not produce any significant change in WBC. These results show a different leukocyte response in the mouse.

Table 29.3. Changes in WBC in Swiss mice during chronic lithium treatment

Group	Dose	Day 4	Day 10	Day 18	Day 24
A. Control A	None	3376 ± 180	4048 ± 310	5440 ± 260	4982 ± 295
LiCl	1 mmol/kg	3484 ± 230*	4061 ± 260*	4940 ± 140*	4897 ± 330*
B. Control B	None	4895 ± 367	5264 ± 332	4772 ± 187	4325 ± 350
LiCl	3 mmol/kg	3682 ± 160**	3623 ± 257**	3559 ± 210*	5026 ± 588*

Each WBC value is the mean ± standard deviation of 8 mice. * changes not statistically significant; ** $p < 0{\cdot}05$

Table 29.4. Changes in neutrophils (N) and lymphocytes (L) in Swiss mice during chronic lithium treatment

Group	Dose	Day 4		Day 10		Day 18		Day 24	
		N	L	N	L	N	L	N	L
Control	None	760 ±100	3820 ±242	980 ±198	4460 ±310	1650 ±200	3980 ±177	2100 ±235	3440 ±177
LiCl	3 mEq/kg	970 ±200	2840 ±185	800 ±168	2300 ±122	770 ±107	1900 ±140	870 ±200	2900 ±98
% Change		+22*	-26**	-23*	-48**	-53*	-52**	-59**	-16*

N and L represents the number of neutrophils and lymphocytes per cu.mm. ± standard deviation. *$p < 0{\cdot}05$, **$p < 0{\cdot}01$

The changes in neutrophils and lymphocytes during lithium treatment and accompanying the WBC changes reported in Table 29.3(B) are shown in Table 29.4. LiCl produced a significant depression of neutrophils and lymphocytes. The depression of neutrophils intensifies with the duration of lithium treatment whereas the lymphocyte and WBC depression begin to recover by Day 24. These results suggest a definite effect of lithium on lymphocytes and neutrophils and a possible influence of lymphocytes on WBC recovery.

DISCUSSION

About 65% of our patients developed an increase in WBC during lithium treatment of which only 44% developed a true leukocytosis (WBC greater-than 10 800). A decrease in WBC during lithium treatment was observed in 22% of the patients. It was usually associated with initial high counts probably secondary to the various emotional states as reported elsewhere (25).

The modest neutrophilia and the mild lymphopenia during lithium therapy in our patient population is in agreement with the findings of others (2,5,6). The negative correlation (Pearson correlation coefficient: -0.93) between neutrophils and lymphocytes has not been reported previously although a mild lymphopenia was observed in several studies (2,4-6). Lymphocytes must be involved in the response to neutrophil proliferation. Animal experiments support this view showing that the marked leukopenia observed in our mice was accompanied by a significant neutropenia and lymphocytopenia.

Experiments in the mouse showing that lithium produces a significant involution of the thymus gland in normal and adrenalectomized mice (20) suggest that lithium may also have some effect on T lymphocytes. It is possible to hypothesize on the basis of our findings that in the mouse, lithium may interfere with the thymus and produce a suppression of lymphocytes. The suppression of lymphocytes stimulates the proliferation of neutrophils. A study of the effects of lithium on T and B lymphocytes may provide more information on the effects of lithium on lymphocytes.

Our retrospective studies are open to criticism because of the many uncontrolled variables encountered. Other reports have shown that major tranquilizers (6) or tricyclics (2) do not produce leukocytosis. Likewise our drug control with major tranquilizers and tricyclics did not show evidence of leukocytosis. The retrospective study has advantages in that it represents observations encountered under normal hospitalization and theoretical prejudices are not imposed on the data collection. Furthermore, the agreement of the data between the MGH and SLSH suggest that the leukocytosis is a real phenomenon observed in general and state mental hospitals. These WBC differences must be associated with lithium treatment, and not to hospitalization variables and they agree with other investigations which have utilized controlled research wards (5,6).

SUMMARY

Studies of haemograms in a general and state mental hospitals showed significant increases in WBC, a neutrophilia, and a lymphopenia. The lymphopenia was negatively correlated with the neutrophilia. Experiments in mice showed that lithium suppressed WBC, neutrophils and lymphocytes. It is hypothesized that lithium produces a lymphocytic suppression which may be associated with direct effects of lithium on the lymphocytes.

References

1. Johnson, G., Gerson, S. and Hekimian, L.J. (1968). *Compr. Psychiat.,* 9, 563
2. O'Connell, R.A. (1970) *Int. Pharmacopsychiat.,* 4, 30
3. Bille, A.M. and Plum, C.M. (1955). *Ugeskr. Laeg.,* 117, 293
4. Mayfield, D. and Brown, R.G. (1966). *J. Psychiat. Res.,* 4, 209
5. Murphy, D.L., Goodwin, F.K. and Bunney, W.E. (1971). *Am.J. Psychiat.,* 127, 135
6. Shopsin, B., Friedmann, R. and Gershon, S. (1971). *Clin. Pharmacol. Ther.* 12, 923
7. Gupta, R.C., Robinson, W.A. and Smyth, C.J. (1975). *Rheum.,* 18, 179
8. Bille, P.E., Jensen, K.K., Jensen, J.P.K. and Poulsen, J.C. (1975). *Acta Med. Scand.,* 198, 281
9. Watanabe, S., Taguchi, K., Nakashina, Y., Ebara, T. and Iguchi, K. (1974) *Folic Psychiat. Neurol. Jap.,* 28, 161
10. Platman, S.R. and Fieve, R.R. (1968). *Arch. Gen. Psychiat.,* 18, 591
11. Shopsin, B. and Gershon, S. (1972). *Arch. Gen. Psychiat.,* 24, 230
12. Sachar, E.J., Hellmann, L., Kream, J., Fukushima, D.K. and Gallagher, T. (1970). *Arch. Gen. Psychiat.,* 22, 304
13. Murphy, D.L., Goodwin, F.K. and Bunney, W.E. (1969). *Lancet,* ii, 458
14. Fleischer, K., Binick, E., Klaus, D. and Tolle, R. (1971) *Arzneim. Forsch.,* 21, 1363
15. Bishop, C.R., Athens, J.W., Boggs, D.R., Warner, H.R., Cartwright, G.E., and Wintrobe, M.M. (1968). *J. Clin. Invest.,* 47, 249
16. Schou, M. and Kissmeyer-Nielsen, F. (1955). *Ugeskr. Laeg.,* 117, 234
17. Tisman, G., Herbert, V. and Rosenblatt, S. (1973). *Br. J. Haemat.,* 24, 767
18. Jacob, E. and Herbert, V. (1974). *J. Clin. Invest.,* 53, 35a
19. Radomski, Jack, Fuyat, H.N., Nelson, A.A. and Smith, P.K. (1950). *J. Pharmacol.,* 100, 429
20. Perez-Cruet, J. and Dancey, J.T. (1977). *Experientia,* 33, 646
21. Friedrich, U. and Nielsen, J. (1969). *Lancet,* ii, 435
22. Genest, P. and Villeneuve, A. (1971) *Lancet* ii, 1132
23. Spitzer, R.L., Endicott, J., Robins, Eli, Kuriansky, J. and Gurland, B. (1975). In: Sudilovsky, A., Gershon, S. and Beer, B. *Predictability in Psychopharmacology: Pre-clinical and Clinical Correlations.* pp 1-48 New York: Raven Press
24. Snedecor, G.W. (1956). *Statistical Methods.* (Ames: Iowa State College Press)
25. Milorat, A.T., Small, S.M. and Diethelm, O. (1942). *Arch. Neurol. Psychiat.,* 47, 779

30

Effect of Maternal Lithium Ingestion on Biochemical and Behavioural Characteristics of Rat Pups

J. M. HSU and A. A. RIDER

INTRODUCTION

In 1948 a calming action of lithium (Li) salts was demonstrated in guinea pigs (1). A follow-up of these original findings led to the use of Li in the treatment of manic-depressive illness and today it is an important drug in the therapy of this disorder. Since a patient may become pregnant, whilst on Li medication it is important to ascertain the possible effects of the therapy on the future well-being of the offspring. Early work (2) has revealed no anatomical anomalies in rat progeny after the ingestion of pharmacological doses of Li by the dam during pregnancy. We now report an extension of these studies in which we have determined the effect of maternal drinking of Li on certain aspects of behavioral and biochemical characteristics of rat offspring.

MATERIALS AND METHODS

Preparation of animals

4-month-old female rats of McCollum strain were mated with males of similar age and strain. On the day when sperm were seen in the vagina, the females were housed individually and divided into two groups, all of which consumed Purina rat chow *ad libitum.* During pregnancy Group 1 of 13 rats received Li in tap water (20 mmol Li as Li citrate per litre) *ad libitum* whereas Group 2 of 10 rats drank tap water only and were used as control mothers. In the experiment for behavioural studies, all female rats receiving Li, and their respective controls, were maintained on a nutritionally adequate formulated diet.

At birth the dams and their offspring were weighed. One pup from each litter of the control and the Li groups were sacrificed. Haematocrit and serum protein (3) were determined. The weights of the spleen, kidney and liver were recorded. Four pups from each litter of the control and the Li groups were nursed by control mothers and four were nursed by lithium drinking mothers. Thus, four groups of progeny were formed as follows:

CC: dam received no Li during pregnancy and lactation
CL: dam received Li during lactation only
LC: dam received Li during pregnancy only
LL: dam received Li during pregnancy and lactation

All rats were weaned at 3 weeks of age, weighed and the male offspring of all groups were used in subsequent experiments.

Behavioural measurements

Maze performance

When the male offspring were 4½ months old, 18 males representing six litters from each of three groups were deprived of water overnight and then tested in a platform T maze containing four choice points. Water was used as the reward. Immediately following each trial the rats were returned to their home cages and water was provided. Two trials per week were run on each rat until a total of five trials had been completed. Starting time, running time and total errors were recorded.

Avoidance response

10 days after completion of the maze experiment the same animals, after being deprived of water overnight, were placed in the 'start' area of a box divided into two sections. After 2 min a gate was opened to allow access to the drinking chamber. Time elapsing before crossing the gate and time in the drinking chamber before the first lick of water were measured. Seven trials were run on each rat, 24 h elapsing between each set of trials (1-3), and (4-7). 72 h elapsed between trials 3 and 4. On the fourth trial, a single shock of approximately 0.75 ma was delivered via the water. This was the only shock given to the animals. Following this, the above parameters were again measured. This test is similar to the one recently described by Hughes and Annau (4).

DNA, RNA and protein contents in tissues

After overnight fasting the 3-week-old pups were sacrificed and the brain, liver and kidney were immediately removed, weighed and stored at -75°C. The contents of DNA, RNA and protein were measured as described previously (5).

Incorporation of [^{3}H] tyrosine into tissue protein

Each weaning pup was fasted for 16 h and injected intramuscularly with L-tyrosine-3,5-^{3}H (20 micro Ci/100 g body weight, Sp. A. 60.3 Ci/mmole. 3 h later the pups were sacrificed and the radioactive protein in the brain, liver and kidney were measured according to the method of Wannamacher *et al.* (6).

Incorporation of [^{3}H] uridine into tissue RNA

After overnight fasting and two hours prior to decapitation each three-week-old pup was injected intramuscularly with uridine-5,6-^{3}H (50 micro Ci/100 g body weight, Sp. A. 41 Ci/mole). RNA in the brain, liver and kidney was isolated and assayed for radioactivity (7).

Statistical analysis

Data were analysed using Student's t test except for the values obtained on the 'shock' experiment. In this case the median test, a variation of Fisher's exact test, was used (8).

RESULTS

Physical measurements

The data in Table 30.1 indicate that survival to weaning was adversely affected by Li intake during pregnancy, whereas weaning weight and the age of eye opening were significantly delayed in the progeny of Li drinking mothers during lactation irrespective of Li intake during pregnancy. The weight gain by the Li ingesting dams during lactation was about 12% less of that of the dams who were not consuming Li, a fact which correlated with the lower weaning weight of pups nursed by Li treated females.

From Table 30.2 we see that, except for a lower weight of liver, the organ weights measured in the newborn were unaffected by Li in the dams' drinking water. Neither serum protein nor hematocrit levels differed between the two groups.

Table 30.1. Characteristics of pups in postnatal period

Group	No. of pups	Survival to weaning (%)	Weaning weight (g)	Eye opening day of age
CC	9	100 ± 0[a]	42.4 ± 1.7	14.3 ± 0.3
CL	9	100 ± 0	31.3 ± 2.3[c]	15.2 ± 0.2[c]
LC	11	84 ± 7[b]	38.0 ± 1.7	14.5 ± 0.3
LL	11	82 ± 8[b]	30.4 ± 5.8[c]	15.5 ± 0.2[c]

a. Mean ± SEM
b. Significantly different from CC and CL groups $p < 0{\cdot}05$
c. Significantly different from CC and LC groups $p < 0{\cdot}01$

Table 30.2. Mean organ weights, serum protein and hematocrit level of newborn

Group	CC	LC
No. of pups	8	11
Birth weight (g)	6.31 ± 0.33[a]	6.06 ± 0.32
Organ weight (mg/g body weight)		
Spleen	3.53 ± 0.34	3.51 ± 0.30
Kidney	7.58 ± 0.33	7.99 ± 0.34
Liver	46.8 ± 1.2	40.6 ± 2.2[b]
Haemotocrit (%)	37.6 ± 2.7	38.5 ± 1.5
Serum protein (g/100 ml)	6.21 ± 0.71	5.90 ± 0.47

a. Mean ± SEM
b. Significantly different from CC group $p < 0.05$

Behavioral measurements

Maze performance

By the fifth trial on the maze, the running time of 38.0 ± 3.1 (SEM) seconds for the CC group was significantly ($p < 0.05$) shorter than for any of the other groups (LL: 87.0 ± 11.4, LC: 111.7 ± 32.3). There was no significant difference in starting time or total errors between any of the groups on any of these trials.

Avoidance behavior

The results of the time spent in the chamber before the first lick show that all groups quickly learned to run the straight path to the water. On the trial immediately following the one in which the shock was administered, the pups who had been exposed to Li during both prenatal and neonatal life returned more quickly to drinking water in this situation than did their counterparts who had been subjected to Li prenatally only or not at all. When these results were analysed according to the median test, a significant difference was seen between the rats exposed to Li during both prenatal and early neonatal life and those never exposed to Li. A similar reaction was seen in the time elapsing before crossing the gate into the drinking chamber.

Brain analysis

Mean brain weight of the CL progeny was lower than that of the control CC progeny. When brain weight was calculated on the basis of 100 g body weight, control progeny had a lower mean value than the progeny of the other three groups. There was a significant increase of both RNA and protein contents in the CL and LC progeny when compared to CC and LL progeny. DNA content was unaffected by Li ingestion.

Table 30.3. Effect of maternal Li ingestion on brain of the 3-week-old male progeny

Group	Brain weight (g/100 g body wt)	Brain DNA	Brain RNA	Brain protein
		(mg/g)		
CC	3.062 ± 0.313[a]	0.68 ± 0.34	2.31 ± 0.24	98 ± 13
CL	3.598 ± 0.721	0.69 ± 0.09	2.68 ± 0.20[c]	117 ± 13[c]
LC	3.441 ± 0.482	0.64 ± 0.06	2.75 ± 0.19[c]	112 ± 11[c]
LL	4.236 ± 0.386[b]	0.60 ± 0.06	2.32 ± 0.18	97 ± 7

a. Mean of six pups ± SD
b. Significantly different from CC group $p < 0.05$
c. Significantly different from CC and LL groups $p < 0.03$

Liver analysis

The progeny from the CL, LC and LL groups all displayed a marked decrease in their mean liver weights as compared to the progeny from the CC group. However, the ratio of liver weight to body weight was similar in all groups. Livers of the CL and LC progeny had a higher DNA content than either the CC or LL progeny. No difference was observed in RNA and protein contents among the four groups.

Kidney analysis

There was no difference between control group and Li treated groups in terms of DNA, RNA and protein contents with the exception of the LL progeny which had a lower mean value of DNA than the CC and LC progeny.

Incorporation of [^{3}H] uridine into tissue RNA

The uptake of ^{3}H by brain of the CL progeny was significantly higher than that of the CC progeny. On the other hand, the radioactivities in the livers of the LL progeny and in the kidney of the LC progeny were substantially reduced. Table 30.4 demonstrates the specific activity of RNA in three selected tissues. At the end of two hours, significantly more (^{3}H) uridine was incorporated into brain RNA of the LC and LL progeny that that of the CC progeny. However, among the four groups, no detectable difference was observed in the incorporation of uridine into liver or kidney RNA

Table 30.4. Effect of maternal Li ingestion on incorporation of uridine-5,6-^{3}H into tissue RNA of the 3-old week male progeny

Group	Brain	Liver	Kidney
	(DPM/mg RNA)		
CC	744 ± 105[a]	2082 ± 195	11125 ± 3028
CL	784 ± 152	1958 ± 519	9333 ± 2760
LC	957 ± 142[b]	1888 ± 655	9222 ± 1043
LL	958 ± 132[b]	1787 ± 690	9671 ± 3506

a. Mean of six pups ± SD
b. Significantly different from CC group $p < 0{\cdot}05$

Incorporation of [^{3}H] tyrosine into tissue protein

The amounts of radioactivity, three hours after tyrosine-3,5-^{3}H injection in the brain, liver and kidney of Li reared pups were approximately the same as those of pups receiving no Li. Results of the incorporation of tyrosine-3,5-^{3}H into protein as shown in Table 30.5 reveal that the pups in the CL and LC groups had significantly more radioactive protein in their brain and kidney than those in the CC group.

DISCUSSION

The suckling pups from Li ingested mothers showed reduced growth. The degree of growth reduction increased with age of the nursing pups and thus with exposure to the Li ion. The growth depression reduced the weight of organs examined when compared with those from pups of non-Li ingested mothers. The organ weights expressed as percentages of

Table 30.5. Effect of maternal Li ingestion on incorporation of tyrosine-3,5-^3H into tissue protein of the 3-week-old male progeny

Group	Brain	Liver	Kidney
		(DPM/mg protein)	
CC	390 ± 80[a]	592 ± 66	689 ± 62
CL	473 ± 72[b]	557 ± 71	1096 ± 300[b]
LC	510 ± 86[c]	538 ± 62	1025 ± 74[c]
LL	404 ± 83	535 ± 97	653 ± 125

a. Mean of six pups ± SD
b. Significantly different from CC group $p < 0.02$
c. Significantly different from CC and LL groups $p < 0.001$

body weight did not vary significantly among the four groups.

The behaviour of 4½-5½-month-old male rat pups is affected by the ingestion of pharmacological doses of Li by the dam during pregnancy and lactation. This is shown by a significant decrease in performance when tested on a T maze. A difference in avoidance behaviour as exhibited by a significantly faster return to a drinking tube after shock was also seen in the offspring of dams receiving Li during pregnancy and lactation.

Recently other workers (4) have also reported that a potentially toxic substance administered to the dam during pregnancy can affect the subsequent behaviour of the offspring. When they were 56 days old, progeny of mice who had been injected with methylmercury on day 8 of gestation showed behavioural differences including a diminished response to an electric shock in a situation comparable to the one reported here.

The maternal Li ingestion showed various influences on the composition of three organs of the progeny, namely, the brain, liver and kidney. In brain, RNA and protein concentrations were elevated in CL and LC groups and RNA/DNA ratios were increased in LC group suggesting a stimulation in RNA and protein synthesis. The protein/DNA ratio, representing the cell size, was not changed by Li supplement. The pups from mothers receiving Li during pregnancy and lactation also did not show significant changes in the concentrations of RNA, DNA or protein when compared to the pups born and nursed by normal females. Thus, it appears the time and dose of Li administration are important in regulating RNA and protein metabolism.

In liver, the concentrations of RNA and protein were unaffected by Li supplementation. DNA concentrations were elevated in the CL and LC groups suggesting a reduced cell size and RNA/DNA ratios were also reduced perhaps implying a depression in RNA and protein synthesis. The hepatic cell sizes were smaller in LC group than in CC group as reflected in a reduced ratio of protein/DNA.

Li ingestion during pregnancy and lactation had no effect on RNA and protein concentrations but had a reduced DNA concentration in the kidney. This later change, however, did not alter the ratios of RNA/DNA and protein /DNA. The apparent ambiguity in response to Li ingestion in the brain, liver and kidney is not clear.

Li given the pregnant females (LC) or to the mothers during pregnancy and lactation (LL) stimulated the incorporation of [^{3}H] uridine into brain RNA (DPM/mg RNA) of the offspring. The specific activity (DPM/mg RNA) in LC group was about the same as in LL group and the values between CC and CL groups were not significantly different; therefore; the effects of Li on RNA metabolism would appear to be more pronounced in fetus development than in suckling pups. Li ingestion had no influence on RNA synthesis of the liver and kidney. Thus, organ specificity would indicate a basis for the relationship of Li and brain function. The increased incorporation which we observed could be due to increased RNA synthesis or to increased RNA turnover. Our results agree with the findings of Dewar and Reading (9) indicating that Li treated rats showed an elevated RNA synthesis at two hours following intraventricular injection of 6- ^{14}C-orotic acid. Since the labelling in cerebral RNA fractions observed at 8 and 24 h after orotic acid injection was progressively decreased in the Li treated rats, these authors suggested that Li induced an enhancement in RNA turnover. If this were the case, one would expect to observe a normal or a possible decrease of brain RNA concentration in Li treated rats. The present results showing that a high concentration of RNA and an increased incorporation of uridine into brain RNA in Li treated suckling pups (CL and LC groups) do not support their view. Our findings, however, indicate that Li has a stimulating effect on RNA synthesis. More detailed studies to clarify this issue should be done.

Protein synthesis in brain and kidney was also enhanced by Li administration. This was demonstrated in CL and LC rats showing an increase in protein concentration of brain and an increased tyrosine incorporation into brain and kidney protein (DPM/mg protein). Whether the effect of Li on the metabolism of brain protein is the result of the changes of RNA metabolism remains to be studied. The increased incorporation, which we observed, could also be due to increased synthesis or to decreased degradation of the amino acid. Variation in pool size may be another important factor. Nevertheless, it is evident that Li ingestion of the dams during pregnancy and lactation caused alterations in the response to brain RNA and protein metabolism of the growing progeny.

CONCLUSION

There is clearly a great need for further studies in the area of the effects of Li ingestion on the translation process which in turn affects protein synthesis. The findings which have been produced to date are undoubtedly intriguing, but they are not sufficiently detailed to draw any conclusions. As more knowledge becomes available, additional theories will be formulated so that a new understanding of how lithium acts on biological systems can be modulated for the benefit of the patient.

Although it is not possible to apply the results of studies on rats directly to the human situation, Li ingestion by dam or pup during the early development of the organism carries with it the threat of physical, behavioural and biochemical abnormalities in the progeny. Others (10) have also expressed concern over maternal Li ingestion especially during lactation and we concur with them in the belief that breast feeding by women on Li medication should be discouraged.

ACKNOWLEDGEMENTS

The authors wish to acknowledge the assistance of Dr. Maria Simonson, Miss Lurline Walker and Mr Y. S. Weng of the Johns Hopkins University in the performance of the behaviour experiments and Mr William Anthony of the Veterans Administration Center, Bay Pines, Florida, in the performance of isotopic experiments.

This work was supported by the Medical Research Service of the Veterans Administration and aided, in part, by a grant from the National Foundation March of Dimes.

References

1. Johnson, F.N. and Cade, J.F.J. (1975). In: F.N. Johnson (ed.). *Lithium Research and Therapy,* pp. 9-22 (London: Academic Press)
2. Rider, A.A. and Hsu, J.M. (1976). *Nutr. Rep. Int.,* **13**, 567
3. Henry, R.J., Sobel, C. and Berkman, S. (1957). *Anal. Chem.,* **29**, 1491
4. Hughes, J.A. and Annau, Z. (1976). *Pharmoc. Boichem. Behav.,* **4**, 385
5. Hsu, J.M., Kim, K.M. and Anthony, W.L. (1974). *Adv. Exp. Med. Biol.,* **48**, 347
6. Wannemacher, R.W. Jr., Banks, W.L. Jr. and Wunner, W.H. (1965). *Anal. Biochem.,* **11**, 320
7. Hsu, J.M. and Anthony, W.L. (1974). *Trace Subst. Environ. Hlth,* **8**, 387
8. Siegel, S. (1956). *Non-parametric Statistics,* pp. 111-115 (New York: McGraw-Hill Press)
9. Dewar, A.J. and Reading, H.W. (1971). *Psychol. Med.,* **1**, 254
10. Weinstein, R.M. and Goldfield, M.D. (1975). In: F.N. Johnson (ed). *Lithium Research and Therapy* pp. 237-264 (London: Academic Press)

31

Models of Lithium Action Based on Behavioural Studies Using Animals

P. E. HARRISON-READ

INTRODUCTION

In attempting to devise an animal model of the mood stabilizing property of lithium, two aspects of the action of lithium merit particular attention, especially if it is assumed that a single biological mechanism is involved. Firstly, lithium can prevent and treat apparently opposite behavioural and emotional disorders which characterize mania and depression, without producing marked effects in normal people (1). Secondly, it is well known that there is a delay of days or weeks before lithium has any beneficial effect in these conditions.

In a recent theory, Mandell and Knapp (2) attempt to explain these points, basing their arguments on the different neurochemical effects of short-term and long-term lithium administration in rats (3). After prolonged pre-treatment with a high daily dose of lithium (5 mmol/kg), extremes of activity in 5-hydroxytryptamine (5-HT) pathways are thought to be precluded by the maximal operation of two mechanisms with opposing effects on 5-HT synthesis. The first of these mechanisms is a facilitation of tryptophan uptake into the brain, which appears shortly after beginning lithium treatment. Initially 5-HT synthesis is increased, but with more prolonged lithium treatment, the activity of the 5-HT synthesizing enzyme tryptophan hydroxylase decreases and brings 5-HT synthesis back to normal. The reduction in tryptophan hydroxylase activity is thought to be a negative feedback mechanism resulting from increased 5-HT receptor stimulation.

Results from the present behavioural experiments, using a lower dose of lithium (2 mmol/kg), also suggest that prolonged lithium treatment stabilizes activity in 5-HT pathways, but the mechanisms appear quite different. After short-term lithium, behavioural effects are compatible with reduced availability of 5-HT at synapses in the brain. As treatment continues, an increase in 5-HT receptor sensitivity appears to develop, and probably restores transmission in 5-HT pathways back to normal levels. However the new equilibrium may be reached at the expense of accommodating large increases and decreases in neural transmission. Since abnormal acitivity in 5-HT pathways may underly the affective psychoses (4), these results suggest an explanation for the therapeutic effects of lithium.

PRETREATMENT OF RATS WITH LITHIUM

Hooded male rats were allocated at random to groups of four per cage. They were housed in a temperature-controlled room (21 °C), which was partially soundproof and lit by artificial light on a 12 h on, 12 h off cycle. An air conditioning unit produced a constant background noise. The rats were left undisturbed, except for weekly weighing and cage cleaning, for a minimum of 2 weeks before starting injections. Food and water was available *ad libitum* throughout. When they had reached a body weight of about 200 g, the four rats in each cage were injected daily with either saline or lithium chloride, 2 mmol/kg i.p. (13 ml/kg of 0.154 M solutions). Rats injected with lithium gained weight normally and showed no overt toxic symptoms, although after a week they were drinking 2-3 times more water than controls. On day 11, half of the saline pretreated rats were switched to lithium injections. This produced three chronic pretreatment groups: saline (S), short-term lithium (SL), and long-term lithium (LL), all rats having received the same number of injections. Lithium plasma concentrations measured after 8 and 18 days of pretreatment, and 3-4 h after the last injection, were 0.91 ± 0.22 and 0.88 ± 0.15 (mean ± SD) respectively.

EXPLORATORY BEHAVIOUR IN THE Y MAZE

On day 15, the rats were tested in a Y maze, in random order, 3-5 h after the morning injection. 1 hour before the trial, approximately half the rats from each group were injected i.p. with 100 mg/kg L-tryptophan, suspended in saline containing 0.5% Tween, whereas the remainder received the vehicle solution alone. The Y maze was open-topped, and illuminated by a 150 W ceiling light directly overhead. The arms of the maze were 38 cm long, 13 cm wide and 33 cm high, and were painted grey with a matching floor. At the end of each arm was a conical earthernware pot, which was painted either black or white. At trial 1, all three pots were the same colour. Rats were placed individually in the maze and allowed to explore freely for 3 min. Their behaviour was scored by an observer sitting above the maze as previously described (5). In addition to arm entries and rears onto the hind legs, head-dips into the pots were recorded, as was the time spent investigating individual pots. At the end of the trial, rats were removed from the maze and placed in an empty cage whilst one of the pots, selected at random, was changed for one of the opposite colour. After an interval of about 1 min, the rats were replaced in the maze and observed for another 3 min.

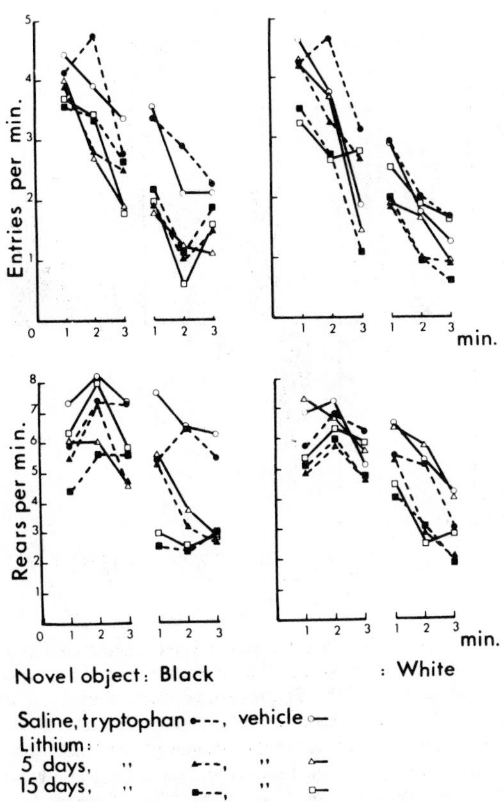

Figure 31 1. Entries and rears in the Y maze. Both activity measures were reduced by lithium pretreatment, (entries, $F(2,95) = 6.94$, $p < 0\ 01$; rears, $F(2,95) = 8.12$, $p < 0\ 01$).

The numbers of entries and rears made per minute by the rats are shown in Figure 31.1. Lithium pretreated rats were generally less active than controls. Reaction to the introduction of the novel pot at trial 2 was assessed by calculating the time spent investigating this pot as a percentage of the time spent investigating all three pots. Figure 31.2 illustrates the mean scores expressed as differences from the scores at Trial 1, when the pot considered was the same colour as the other two. Despite their tendency to be relatively inactive, rats injected with lithium for 5 days spent more time investigating the novel pot than either of the two more familiar pots. This effect was greatest with the white novel pot, which control rats tended to avoid, and the effect was completely abolished by additional pretreatment with tryptophan. These results suggest that lithium reduces the availability of 5-HT at synapses within the brain. This conclusion is supported by reports that lithium reduces release of 5-HT from neural tissue (6-8), and by increases in reactivity to novel stimulus

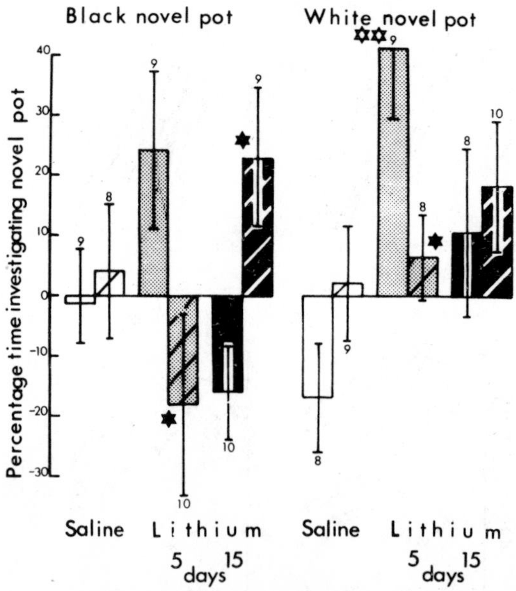

Figure 31.1. Time spent investigating the novel pot at Trial 2, calculated as a percentage of the total time for all three pots, and expressed as the difference from the score at Trial 1 when all the pots were the same, (means ± SEM). Figures above each column give the number of rats per group. Analysis of variance on arcsine transformed percentages showed an interaction between the chronic pretreatments and acute tryptophan pretreatment (hatched columns), F (2,95) = 8.78, $p < 0.001$. When percentage scores at Trial 2 were analysed without subtracting the Trial 1 scores, there was also a significant main effect of the chronic pretreatments, F (2,95) = 3.19, $p < 0.05$. t tests, 2 tailed: difference from saline-vehicle group, **$p < 0.01$; difference from SL or LL vehicle group *$p < 0.05$.

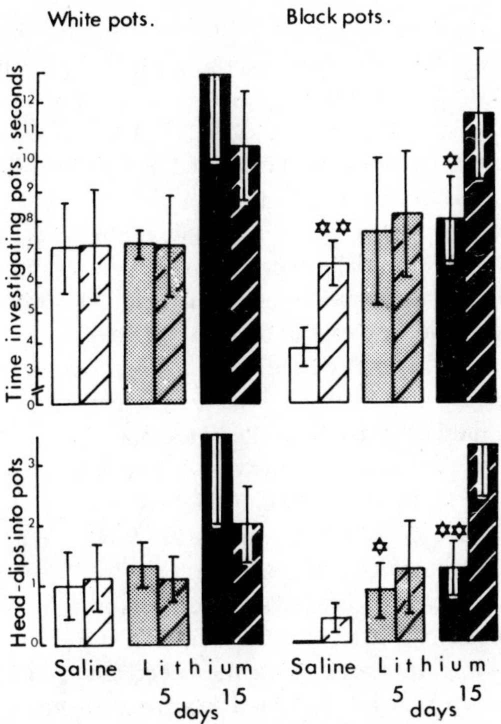

Figure 31.3. Exploration of the three similar pots at Trial 1 was increased by 15 days pretreatment with lithium. Analysis of variance revealed significant main effects of the chronic pretreatments: for time investigating the pots (log transformed data), $F(2,95) = 6.60$, $p < 0.01$; for head-dips into the pots (square root transformed data), $F(2,95) = 8.15$ $p < 0.01$. Tryptophan injections 1 h before the trial (hatched columns) tended to increase the time spent investigating the black pot, as shown by a significant interaction between acute pretreatment and the colour of the pots, $F(2,95) = 4.10$, $p < 0.05$. t tests, 2 tailed: difference from saline-vehicle group: *$p < 0.05$, **$p < 0.01$.

change which have been observed following depletion of brain 5-HT (9,10). Also previous work (11) has demonstrated that, in common with treatments which deplete brain 5-HT, lithium increases rats' sensitivity to footshock, an effect which is abolished by 5-hydroxytryptophan (5-HTP). Presumably tryptophan and 5-HTP counteract the effects of lithium by increasing the amount of 5-HT available for release from nerve endings.

Rats pretreated with lithium for 15 days did not show any preference for the novel pot unless they were administered tryptophan before the trial. These results after long-term lithium suggest that a chronic reduction in receptor stimulation may have increased the sensitivity of 5-HT receptors

(12). Increased receptor sensitivity could compensate for reduced 5-HT release, and restore neural transmission to normal. This might explain the failure of long-term lithium to enhance rats' response to novelty. Tryptophan increases the synthesis of 5-HT and its release from nerve endings, and causes feedback inhibition of 5-HT nerve cells as a result of increased receptor activation (13).

After long-term lithium, tryptophan might cause exaggerated feed-back inhibition, and despite initially increased receptor stimulation, transmission across 5-HT synapses may subsequently fall. This would be expected to produce the observed increase in response to novelty.

Both tryptophan and long-term lithium treatment increased the time rats spent exploring all three pots at Trial 1, (Figure 31.3). The effect of tryptophan was only apparent with the black pots, to which controls paid little attention. As has been seen, increased time spent exploring the pots at Trial 1 did not lead to an increase in selective investigation of the novel pot by these rats. Interestingly, increased 5-HT receptor sensitivity following withdrawal of chronic methysergide treatment has also been found to produce increased investigation of pots in a Y maze, (results to be published). Behaviour after long-term lithium therefore seems compatible with, if anything, increased rather than decreased 5-HT activity.

The results which indicate increased reactivity to novelty after short-term lithium are of particular interest since it has been argued previously (14) that lithium reduces rats' awareness of their environment. This interpretation is based on observations of reduced exploratory activity, particularly rearing, after acute injections of lithium. These observations, if not their interpretation, are compatible with the present findings of reduced activity in lithium pretreated rats. The results imply that the amount of exploratory activity does not always reflect the extent to which rats attend to their environment.

EXPLORATORY ACTIVITY IN THE HOLE-FIELD

On day 16 all rats were tested in another novel environment, the hole field. As on the day before, rats were run 3-4 h after saline or lithium injections, and those rats which had previously received tryptophan were given a second injection 1 h before the trial. The hole field consisted of a circular arena 58 cm in diameter, with a 33 cm high wall. A central circle 29 cm in diameter was marked out on the floor, and radial lines divided the inner circle into 4 segments, and the outer into 8 segments. The field was painted grey, and was illuminated by an overhead 150 W ceiling light. In the centre of each segment was a hole 3.2 cm in diameter, and 18 cm deep. The field stood on a box with a translucent plastic top, which was 4.5 cm below the surface of the arena floor. The box contained two electric lamps located one above the other beneath the centre of the field. A thyristor-controlled circuit enabled the lamps to be switched on and off at a variable rate. In the usual condition, a 25 W lamp was on continuously. In one of the two stimulus conditions, the 25 W lamp was flashed on and off at a rate of twice a second, with an approximately equal light-dark cycle. In the other stimulus condition, a 40 W lamp flashed on when the 25 W lamp went out. The stimulus conditions were thus equivalent to an intermittent decrease and increase in the brightness of the light visible through the holes in the floor of the field. Rats were placed individually in the centre of the field, and observed for 4 min. The following types of behaviour were scored: the number of floor segments entered (walking), the number of rears onto the hind legs, the number of head-dips into the holes, and finally the number of seconds rats spent with the whole of their heads in the inner circle. At the end of 4 min one of the flashing light stimuli was switched on for 2 min, followed by another 2 min with the holes continuously illuminated.

Figure 31.4 summarizes the activity measures obtained. Analysis of variance revealed a significant reduction in activity due to lithium, either in the stimulated period only, (rears, $F(2,93) = 5.66$; $p < 0.01$), or in both stimulated and unstimulated periods, (walking, $F(2,93) = 3.64$, $p < 0.05$; and $F(2,93) = 15.80$, $p < 0.001$ respectively). During stimulation with novel light flashes of increasing brightness, the saline pretreated rats (S) tended to increase the time they spent in the centre of the field, and to increase the number of head-dips in the centre of the field. In this situation head-dips probably reflect exploratory behaviour (15). With flashes of decreasing brightness, the control rats did not increase their exploration of the centre of the field. In contrast, the short-term lithium rats (SL) showed a marked increase in exploration of the field centre during decreasing-intensity flashes, but failed to respond to flashes of increasing intensity. Rats in the long-term lithium group (LL) showed no apparent response to either kind of stimulus. In the analysis of variance these results were reflected by significant interactions between chronic pretreatments and the two types of stimuli, (for head-dips in the centre, $F(2,93) = 3.38$, $p < 0.05$; for time spent in the centre, $F(2,93) = 3.69$, $p < 0.05$). Response to novel stimulation was best illustrated by the difference between the score during the period of stimulation and the average score for the unstimulated periods, expressed as a percentage of the average score for the trial as a whole (Figure 31.5). It can be seen that additional pretreatment with tryptophan completely abolished the effect of short-

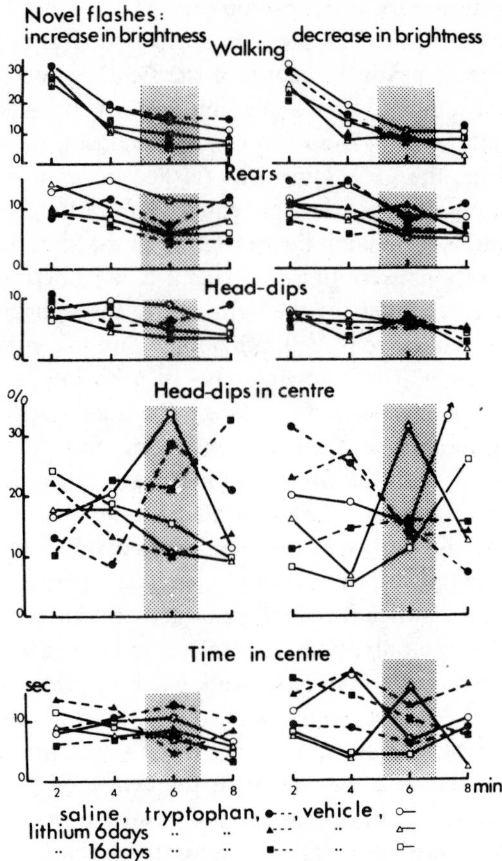

Figure 31.4. Summary of behavioural measures in the hole field. Each trial lasted 8 min. During the 5th and 6th min, rats were exposed to novel light flashes visible through the holes in the floor of the field.

term lithium, whilst having no effect in the S and LL groups. In the analysis of variance of arcsine transformed percentages, this was reflected by significant interactions between the chronic pretreatments and tryptophan pretreatment (see Figure 31.5). These results support the Y maze data in that short-term lithium appears to increase rats' sensitivity to relatively subtle novel stimuli which leave control rats unaffected, probably by reducing the availability of 5-HT within the brain. The tendency for more intense stimulation to suppress the exploratory behaviour of SL and LL rats in an open field type environment is supported by previous findings (16).

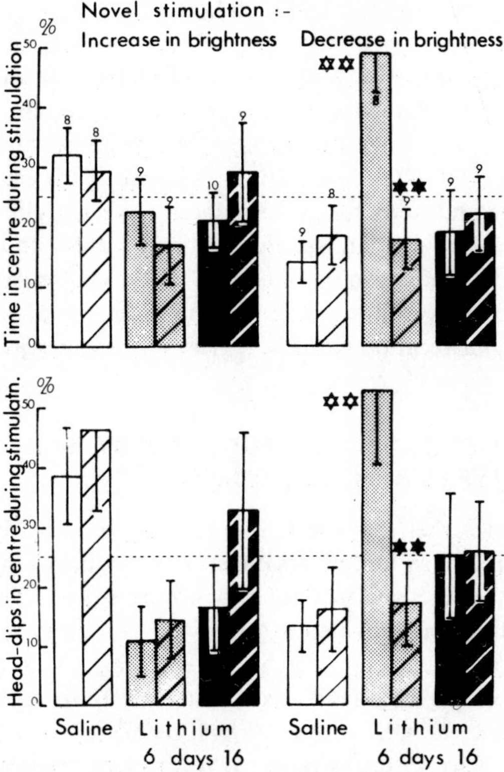

Figure 31.5. Measures reflecting exploration of the centre of the hole field during novel stimulation lasting 2 min (5th and 6th min of the trial), compared with that during the whole trial which lasted 8 min. Differences between scores obtained during the period of stimulation, and the average scores for the unstimulated periods were expressed as a percentage of the average score for the trial as a whole. The columns and vertical bars represent means ± SEM, the figures indicating the number of rats per group. Arcsine transformation of percentages was carried out before analysis of results. Values below 25% indicate a lack of response to stimulation, and reflect the decline in exploration over the course of the trial. Values above 25% indicate a clear increase in exploratory response during stimulation. There were significant interactions between the chronic pretreatments and the type of stimulation used: % time in centre, $F(2,93) = 5.20, p < 0.01$; % head-dips in centre, $F(2,93) = 6.61, p < 0.01$; and interactions between chronic pretreatments and acute tryptophan pretreatment (hatched columns): % time in centre, $F(2,93) = 4.19, p < 0.02$; % head-dips in centre, $F(2,93) = 3.56, p < 0.05$
t tests, 2 tailed: differences from saline vehicle group, **p < 0 01;
differences from SL vehicle group, **p < 0 01

Time spent in the centre of the field during unstimulated periods was reduced in both lithium pretreated groups, but only in trials when flashes of decreasing brightness were used during the stimulus period. The dependence of this effect on the stimulus condition is puzzling, because it was apparent *before* the onset of stimulation, when test conditions were identical for the two types of trial. The effect of lithium in reducing time spent in the centre of the field was abolished by tryptophan. These results were reflected in an interaction between stimulus condition and acute and chronic pretreatments which just failed to reach statistical significance, $F(2,93) = 3.07, p = 0.051$). The relative avoidance of the centre of field by lithium pretreated rats may be due to reduced availability of 5-HT. This is supported by the finding that depletion of brain 5-HT with the neurotoxin 5,6-dihydroxytryptamine causes rats to avoid the centre of an open-field (10). The effect may indicate that lithium pretreated rats were more fearful, although defecation in the hole field was not increased.

HEAD-SHAKE BEHAVIOUR PRODUCED BY 5-METHOXY-N, N-DIMETHYLTRYPTAMINE, (5MeODMT)

It was suggested earlier that the failure to observe enhanced reactivity to novelty after prolonged lithium treatment may be due to the development of a compensatory increase in 5-HT receptor sensitivity. Further evidence for this suggestion was provided by observing rats' head shake behaviour following a small dose of the direct acting 5-HT agonist 5-MeODMT (17). On the day after the hole-field trial, some rats from each pretreatment group were injected with 0.75 mg/kg 5-MeODMT dissolved in saline (2 ml/kg, i.p.). This dose was expected to produce little effect in control rats. After 1 h, the rats were placed in the Y maze used previously, but with the pots removed, and head shake responses were counted for 5 min. Head shakes were defined as stereotyped rotatory movements of the head, as distinct from the jerking movements often associated with sneezing. Some of the rats, (5 to 7 from each group selected at random) were also observed 2 h after injection. Differences between pretreatment groups were more marked at 2 h, so only these results will be considered here. Figure 31.6 shows that lithium pretreatment clearly increased the frequency of head shakes, and that the increase was related to the duration of lithium pretreatment. This result suggests that 5-HT receptors become supersensitive during prolonged lithium treatment. There was also an indication that previous treatment with tryptophan increased the frequency of head shakes in control rats. It is possible that the feed-back inhibition of 5-HT cells that occurs after tryptophan (13) leads to an increase in 5-HT receptor sensitivity. However, it must be assumed that the feed-back inhibition of 5-HT far outlasts the direct stimulation of postsynaptic receptors by 5-HT, and that receptor supersensitivity develops rapidly.

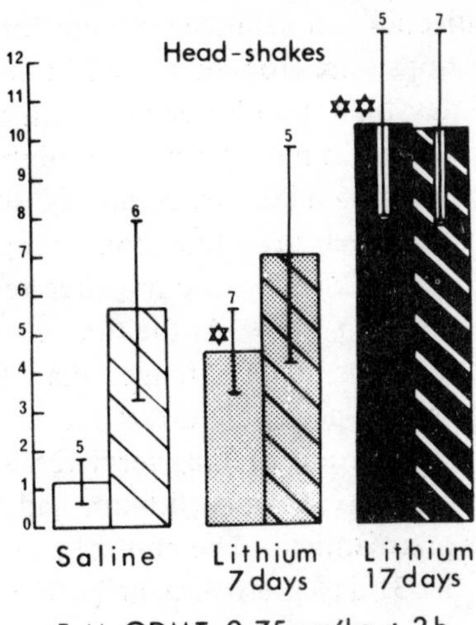

Figure 31.6. Mean number of head shakes (± SEM) counted over 5 min. Lithium pretreatment increased the number of head shakes after a small dose of 5-methoxy-N, N-dimethyltryptamine: analysis of variance on square root transformed data, $F(2,29) = 5.82$, $p < 0.01$. The increase was greater in rats pretreated for 17 days than in those pretreated for 7 days, t test, 2 tailed, $p < 0.05$. Tryptophan administered on the 2 previous days (hatched columns) had no significant effect overall, although head shakes were increased in the saline group, t test, t tailed, $p < 0.02$.
t tests, 2 tailed, differences from saline-vehicle group, $*p < 0.05$; $*p < 0.05$; $**p < 0.01$

HEAD-SHAKE AND BODY-SHAKE RESPONSES INDUCED BY 5-HTP

High doses of 5-HTP induce head shaking in mice (18), and in rats shaking of the whole body including the head occurs (19). Body shakes, which are also called 'wet-dog' shakes, appear at doses lower than those required to produce the characteristic behavioural syndrome including limb rigidity, tremor and stereotyped movements (20). At still lower doses, 5-HTP produces head shakes which only occasionally develop into 'wet-dog' shakes. The essential difference therefore between body shakes and head shakes appears to be quantitative rather than qualitative. Both responses presumably result from stimulation of 5-HT receptors by 5-HT synthesized from 5-HTP within nerve endings containing aromatic acid decarboxylase.

In order to observe the effect of long-term lithium treatment on 5-HTP-induced behaviour, the rats which had received 5-MeODMT on day 17 continued to receive injections of saline or lithium for another 14 days. In some rats lithium injections were stopped after 11 days, and were replaced by saline for the last 3 days. On the 14th day of extra pretreatment, all rats were injected with carbidopa (25 mg/kg i.p.), an inhibitor of extracerebral decarboxylase (21), followed ½ h later by 50 mg/kg dl-5-HTP. Both drugs were dissolved and suspended in saline containing 0.5% Tween, and injected in a volume of 5 ml/kg. Two hours after receiving 5-HTP, rats were observed for 5 min in the Y maze. At the time of testing some rats had received lithium injections for 10 days longer than the rest. This extra period of pretreatment had a negligible effect on the results, so the data were combined to give one group of long-term (21 and 31 days) lithium pretreated rats, and one group in which lithium had been withdrawn for 3 days after long-term pretreatment. The control rats had received saline injections throughout the 31 day pretreatment period. Figure 31.7 shows

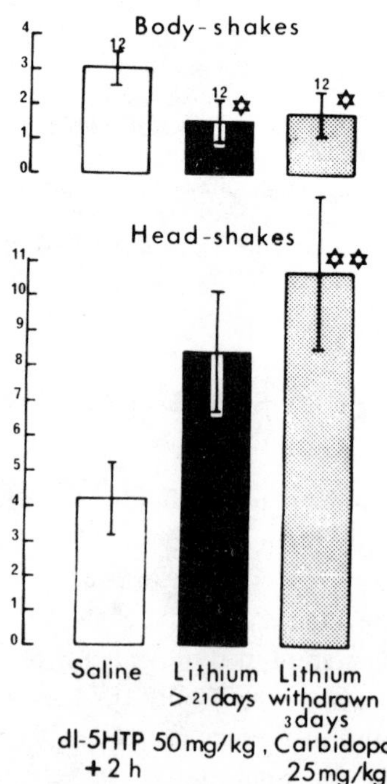

Figure 31.7. Body shakes and head shakes induced by 50 mg/kg 5-HTP, (means ± SEM). Body shakes in both lithium groups were significantly reduced compared to the control group, but overall analysis of variance on square root transformed data was not significant, F (2,33) = 3.04. Analysis of variance of head shakes showed a significant overall effect, F (2,33) = 4.07, p< 0.05
t tests, t tailed, differences from control, *p< 0.05, **p< 0.01

that whereas head shakes were increased by long-term lithium, particularly if injections were withdrawn 3 days before testing, body shakes were reduced. The increase in head shakes was not simply a result of an increased number of potential body shakes failing to develop fully, since the total number of head and body shakes also tended to be increased in the lithium pretreated rats. The increase in head shakes after 5-HTP confirms the hypothesis of increased 5-HT receptor sensitivity after prolonged lithium treatment. The reduction in body shakes suggests that under conditions when 5-HT release is potentially high, lithium-induced reduction of 5-HT release predominates over increased receptor sensitivity. This prediction was tested in another experiment using a higher dose of 5-HTP.

On the day after testing in the hole field, some rats were injected with carbidopa (25 mg/kg) followed ½ h later by 100 mg/kg dl-5-HTP. One hour after receiving 5-HTP, the rats were observed in the Y maze for 5 min. As is shown in Figure 31.8, in control rats the number of head shakes and body shakes was more than double the number recorded 2 h after 50 mg/kg 5-HTP. As expected, body shakes were reduced by long-term lithium pretreatment, but head shakes were unaffected. In the SL rats a reduction in body shakes only occurred when tryptophan had been given on the two preceding days. Since an increase in the rate of intraneuronal synthesis of 5-HT occurs after short-term lithium (2,8), the increased conversion of 5-HTP into 5-HT may compensate for reduced 5-HT release. After tryptophan pretreatment, 5-HT synthesis may be reduced as a result of feed-back inhibition of 5-HT neurones (13), so that inhibition of 5-HT release predominates.

CONCLUSIONS

The results of these experiments are compatible with the following hypothesis. At low to moderate levels of activity in 5-HT neurones, receptor supersensitivity produced by prolonged lithium administration predominates over, or just compensates for, the lithium-induced reduction in 5-HT release. At potentially high levels of 5-HT activity, inhibition of 5-HT release and exaggerated feedback inhibition of 5-HT neurones effectively reduces transmission at 5-HT synapses. As a consequence of these changes following prolonged lithium administration, large transient increases or decreases in activity in 5-HT pathways are buffered, whereas normal activity is little affected.

The behavioural experiments on which these conclusions are based admittedly give only indirect information about interactions between lithium and activity in brain 5-HT pathways. However, this is also true of

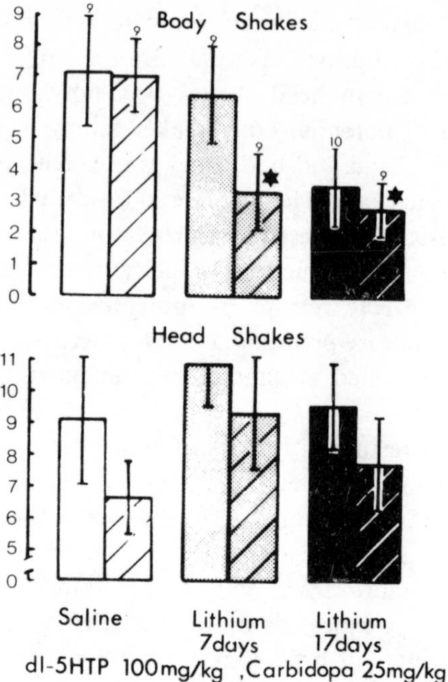

Figure 31.8. Body shakes and head shakes induced by 100 mg/kg 5-HTP, (means ± SEM). There were no significant differences between groups for head shakes. For body shakes analysis of variance on square root transformed data showed a significant main effect of the chronic pretreatments, $F(2,49) = 4.46$, $p < 0.02$. Hatched columns represent groups treated with tryptophan on the two preceding days. t tests, 2 tailed, differences from saline-tryptophan group, $^*p < 0.05$

many neurochemical studies, since it is not clear what aspects of 5-HT metabolism are relevant to the function of 5-HT as a possible neurotransmitter (22). One possibility arising from the interpretation of the results is that behaviour dependent on 5-HT pathways in the brain, although overtly normal after long-term lithium, may be resistant to disruption, for example, by environmental disturbance. This prediction suggests one approach to testing a model of the mood-stabilizing effects of lithium.

ACKNOWLEDGEMENTS

I thank Professors Hannah Steinberg and J.W. Black for the use of laboratory facilities in the Pharmacology Department at University College London. Mr A. Davies gave statistical advice, and Mr R. Croxton and Mr M. Warren helped make some of the apparatus. This work was aided by a grant from the Central Research Fund of the University of London.

References

1. Schou, M. (1968). *J. Psychiat. Res.,* 6, 67
2. Mandell, A.J. and Knapp, S. (1977). *Pharmakopsych.,* 9, 116
3. Knapp, S. and Mandell, A.J. (1976). *J. Pharmacol. Exp. Ther.,* 193, 812
4. Lapin, I.P. and OxenKrug, G.F. (1969). *Lancet,* i, 132
5. Cox, C., Harrison-Read, P.E., Steinberg, H. and Tomkiewicz, M. (1971). *Nature,* 232, 336
6. Katz, R.I., Chase, T.N. and Kopin, I.J. (1968). *Science,* 162, 466
7. Corrodi, H., Fuxe, K and Schou, M. (1969). *Life Sci.,* 8, 643
8. Schubert, J. (1973). *Psychopharmacologia,* 32, 301
9. Brody, J.F. Jr (1970). *Psychopharmacologia* 17, 14
10. Diaz, J., Ellinson, G. and Masuoka, D. (1974). *Psychopharmacologia* 37, 67
11. Harrison-Read, P.E. and Steinberg, H. (1971). *Nature New Biol.,* 232, 120
12. Trulson, M.E., Eubanks, E.E. and Jacobs, B.L. (1976). *J. Pharmacol. Exp. Ther.,* 198, 23
13. Gallagher, D.W. and Aghajanian, G.K. (1976). *Neuropharmacology,* 15, 149
14. Johnson, F.N. (1975). In F.N. Johnson (ed.) *Lithium Research and Therapy* pp. 315-350 (London: Academic Press)
15. File, S.E. and Wardill, A.G. (1975). *Psychopharmacologia,* 44, 53
16. Gray, P., Solomon, J., Dunphy, M., Carr, F. and Hession, M. (1976). *Psychopharmacologia,* 48, 277
17. Fuxe, K., Holmstedt, B. and Jonsson, G. (1972). *Eur. J. Pharmacol.,* 19, 25
18. Corne, S.J., Pickering, R.W. and Warner, B.T. (1963). *Br. J. Pharmacol.,* 20, 106
19. Bedard, P. and Pycock, C. (1977). *Br. J. Pharmacol.,* 59, 450P
20. Jacobs, B.L., Eubank, E.E. and Wise, W.D. (1974). *Neuropharmacologia,* 13, 575
21. Bartholini, T. and Pletscher, A. (1969). *J. Pharm. Pharmac.,* 21, 323
22. Grahame-Smith, D.G. (1974). *Adv. Bioch. Psychopharmacol.,* 10, 83

32

The Variety of Models Proposed for the Therapeutic Actions of Lithium

F. N. JOHNSON

INTRODUCTION

In the chapters of this book there are three important questions being asked:

1. What does lithium do?
2. How does it do it?
3. What light does such information throw on the nature of the conditions which lithium is used to treat?

Meetings such as the First British Lithium Congress, and books like the present volume, are necessary because the answers to such questions are, at the moment, either inadequate or incomplete: moreover, such answers as *are* available are many, varied, and couched in such widely different terms that it is not always easy to see how they interrelate.

Why should there be so many different models of lithium action? Because, in general, research workers approaching the topic have quite different views about what is, or should be, the primary focus of investigation. The nature of the problem is illustrated diagrammatically in Figures 32.1, and 32.2 and 32.3. In Figure 32.1 the rectangular boxes represent the outer boundaries of organisms; every organism is subjected to stimulation from the surrounding environment (represented in the figure by **S**) and, in reacting to that stimulation, organisms make responses (represented by **R**). Within each organism there is some mechanism which links the response (**R**) to the stimulation (**S**) (Figure 32.1a). We may conceive of this mech-

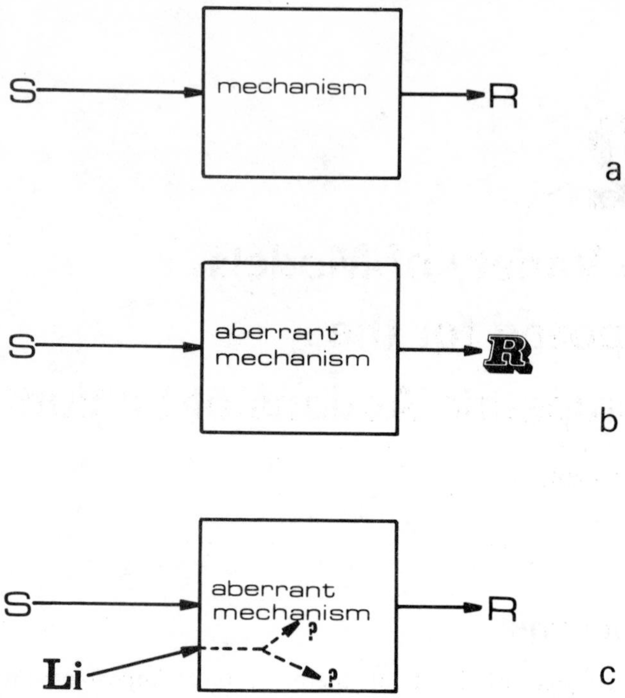

Figure 32.1. Input stimulation leads to a response, the response selection being determined by an intraorganismic mechanism (a); when the mechanism becomes aberrant, stimulation leads to an abnormal response (b); lithium, acting either directly upon the aberrant mechanism, or indirectly via an effect upon some other intra-organismic process, restores the normal response to stimulation (c).

anism as being in part genetically determined and in part subject to modification as a result of experience, the balance depending on what exactly **S** and **R** represent.

In psychopathological conditions it may be reasonable to assume that the mechanism linking **S** and **R** becomes (or is genetically) aberrant (Figure 32.1b) in which case environmental stimulation leads not to the expected (normal adaptive) response, but to one which is unexpected (abnormal, maladaptive). Successful treatment with a drug, e.g. lithium, restores the connection between the input stimulus and the output response (Figure 32.1c). How exactly this comes about — whether by a direct action of the drug upon the aberrant mechanism itself, or indirectly as a result of some other mechanism being stimulated or suppressed by the drug (Figure 32.1c) — is not always clear.

The terms in which statements about the **S-R** linking mechanism are couched may be of several different kinds. Thus a biochemist will see the mechanism as consisting of a chain of chemical changes and energy transduction processes, whereas a psychologist may use a description employing notions which have no physiological counterparts. Whilst both biochemist and psychologist will be talking about the same thing, the statements of the one may nevertheless be virtually incomprehensible to the other.

The matter is complicated further if we consider what sources of information may be used to derive details of the **S-R** linking mechanism and the actions of drugs within the organism. Whilst much of the information — where therapeutic agents are concerned — comes directly from studies involving patients, other studies may make use of normal (i.e. non-patient) volunteers. When lithium is given to someone who is not showing aberrant (abnormal, maladaptive) responses, lithium cannot be acting upon an aberrant mechanism, but instead upon the *normal* mechanism linking stimulation and response (or indirectly via some other mechanism which then affects the normal **S-R** linking mechanism). The result is that, in such studies, input stimulation leads to a response being elicited which differs from the normal response and from responses elicited in the psychopathological condition (Figure 32.2b).

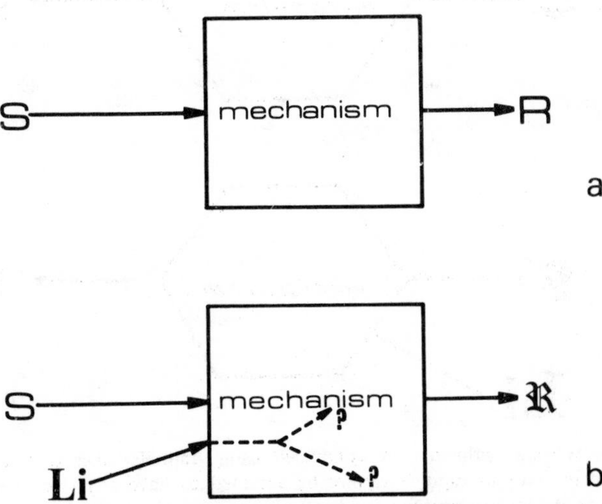

Figure 32.2. When lithium is given to a normal volunteer in whom stimulus input is related to response output by a normally functioning intra-organismic mechanism (a), the lithium acts either directly upon that mechanism, or indirectly via some other process (b), to produce a response to stimulation which is unlike either the abnormal response (Figure 32.1) or the normal response to stimulation.

Nor is that the end of the matter, for many of those who undertake investigations into lithium either do not have access to patients or wish to carry out studies which, for technical or ethical reasons, cannot be performed either on patients or on human volunteers. In such circumstances the investigator has to have recourse to some other experimental medium—either using a different species of animal or resorting to *in vitro* tests of one kind or another. If animals of a different species (rats, mice, guinea pigs, etc.) are used, not only are the environmental stimuli and the animals' response repertoire (**s** and **r** in Figure 32.3) different from those in the human situation, but it cannot be assumed that the mechanism linking stimulus and response in the two conditions have close identity. Even less can it be assumed that the response which an infra-human animal makes to stimulation whilst under the influence of lithium (Figure 32.3b) has any direct relationship to either the normal or aberrant human response to stimulation, with or without lithium. The best that can be hoped for from animal experiments is that the effects observed are to some extent *analogous to* the human situation.

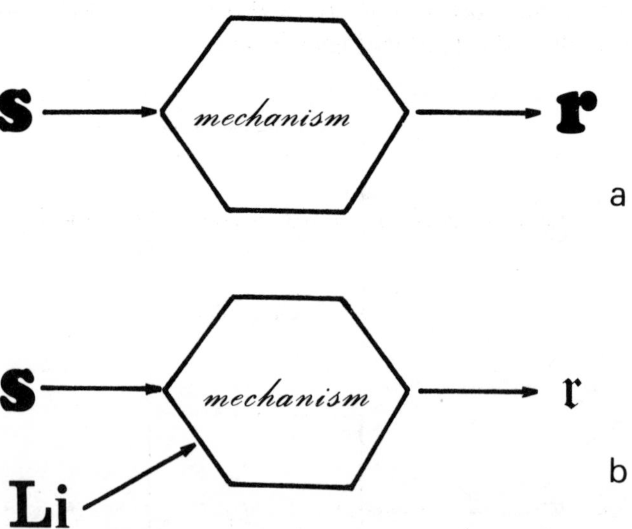

Figure 32.3. When experiments are conducted using animals other than man, the input stimulus and the output response cannot be assumed to have any close relation to those encountered in the human situation, and the mechanism linking stimulus and response must therefore also be assumed to differ from human mechanisms in at least some particulars (a); when lithium is administered to animals, it either directly affects the *S-R* linking mechanism or has an effect upon some other intra-organismic process, producing a response to stimulation which does not have any necessary relationship to responses produced in normal or abnormal human situations, either with or without lithium being administered.

When the position is stated baldly in this way, it is easy to see why so little agreement exists between lithium research workers on what exactly is going on within the lithium-treated manic depressive patient.

MODELS AT DIFFERENT CONCEPTUAL LEVELS

The terms in which lithium researchers have conceptualized the mechanisms (and the aberrant forms of such mechanisms) underlying normal and abnormal behaviour and the effects of lithium on such mechanisms, may be seen as lying along a conceptual continuum.

Models at the molecular level

It is well-known that DNA and RNA are structurally very cation sensitive, and that therefore lithium could affect the molecular conformation of these substances (with, presumably, consequences for such processes as cell division and protein synthesis). A model of lithium action which concentrated on this type of property of lithium, would be one at the molecular level.

Models at the biochemical system level

Figure 32.4 indicates some of the ways in which lithium might affect carbohydrate metabolism (1). Here we are dealing not simply with a molecular conformation change, but with a modification in the conformation of a complex of molecular interactions. Another example is given in Figure 32 5 which illustrates a model of lithium action proposed by Mandell and Knapp (2): this model suggests that lithium may affect cellular tryptophan uptake, with consequent repercussions upon the enzyme activity responsible for converting tryptophan into 5-hydroxytryptamine. Here the effect of lithium is not localized at the level of a molecular change, but on a *system* of biochemical changes, feed-back links, and other forms of molecular interaction.

Models at the organ level

Whatever lithium may be doing molecularly or on biochemical systems, certain organs are more likely than others to be subject to the influence of lithium. The nature of the changes thus produced by lithium in whole organs provides the object of study for some investigators.

It is not unreasonable, for example, to look for lithium effects on overall brain functioning, and for this purpose electroencephalographic techniques may be used. Lithium does indeed modify EEG patterns but (to

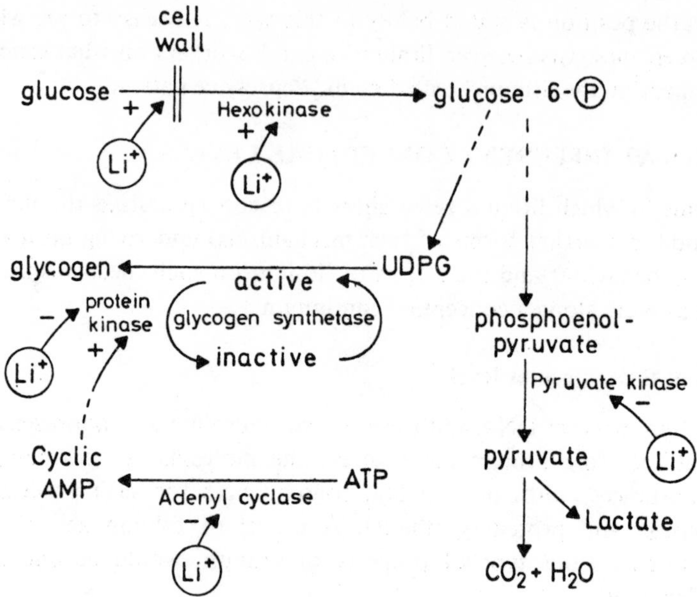

Figure 32.4. A model of lithium action on carbohydrate metabolism, put forward by Mellerup and Rafaelsen (1): lithium has multiple actions at a variety of sites in the pathways outlined in this figure

date, at least) studies of the changes so produced have been relatively disappointing in leading to a model of lithium action, though more modern recording and analysing techniques may change the picture in the near future.

More encouraging, perhaps, have been studies on *parts* of the brain, particularly on synaptic processes (transmitter release and re-uptake, receptor sensitivity, and so on). From such work may be derived models expressed in terms of what lithium does on organ functioning, rather than on the molecular or biochemical system changes which underlie such functioning.

Models at the level of organ systems

The operation of any body organ is linked directly to ongoing levels of activity in other organs, Recognition of this fact leads investigators to seek for changes in *patterns* of organ interaction when lithium treatment is administered. A splendid example of this is provided by the recent work of Dr S. Parvathi Devi (see Chapter 25) on changes induced by lithium in the pineal-adrenocortical axis. In models derived from work such as this, the

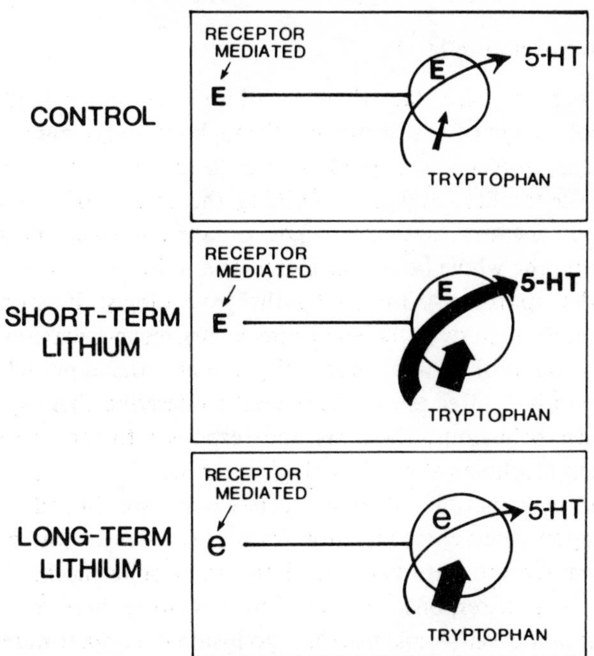

Figure 32.5. A model of lithium action on tryptophan metabolism, put forward by Mandell and Knapp (2) who describe the model as follows: In the control neuron, tryptophan hydroxylase (E) is optimal in both cell body and nerve ending. Tryptophan is taken up through the neuronal membrane and converted by E to 5-HT, which is released from the nerve ending. After short-term lithium treatment tryptophan uptake is augmented and consequently synthesis and release of 5-HT are increased, since intraneuronal enzyme is not saturated with regard to substrate. After long-term lithium treatment, "amount" of enzyme has been reduced (E ⟶ e) to compensate for the enhanced bombardment of the receptor. Tryptophan uptake is still augmented, but 5-HT synthesis and release at the nerve ending have returned to control levels because of the enzyme deficit (e instead of E)

reference is not to molecular, biochemical, or single organ functioning, but to the effects of lithium on the *interaction* between several organs.

In the ultimate analysis, of course, all organs are functionally related more or less directly to each other: changes in one lead *necessarily* to changes in others. This being so, it is difficult (and in practical terms may be impossible) to distinguish between a primary effect of lithium on one organ and an effect produced secondarily upon a second organ because of changes in the first. Tertiary, quaternary and higher order effects (including feedback effects on the primarily affected target organ) are even more difficult to disentangle. Models at the organ system do not attempt the disentanglement: they simply look at a system of organs as a whole and, irrespective of what changes are primary, secondary, or whatever, describe lithium action in terms of modifications produced in the whole complex network of organ interactions.

Models at the organism level

Once one has recognized that whatever lithium does in the body there will result a whole range of readjustments throughout a vast number of interacting systems, it becomes a simple matter to take the step of recognizing the body as a totality, and of describing the effects of lithium not on molecules, biochemical systems, single organs, or even on systems of organs, but on the whole body considered as a unit.

This is the approach adopted by the psychologist in studying drug action. The unit of study is the environment-organism-behaviour complex, and from the point of view of practical psychiatry the approach has much to recommend it — after all, patients tend to describe their symptoms in terms of their behaviour, thoughts and responses to their surroundings, rather than in biochemical or physiological terms.

From an examination of what behaviours are linked to, or are dependent upon, what environmental features or changes, the psychologist attempts to infer the nature of the intra-organismic mechanism linking stimulus input and response output. The key word here is 'infer'. The psychologist *qua* psychologist does not go inside the organism in his search for information about the **S-R** linking mechanism, nor does he say, when proposing a model for such mechanisms, 'this is what *is* going on inside the organism': what he says, in effect, is 'given the observed relationships between the organism's environment (including such inputs as lithium administration) and the organism's behaviour, the organism may be conceived of *as though* it had a particular kind of internal mechanism'.

The stimulus significance model of lithium action

An example of model construction at this level is provided by work carried out by myself and various colleagues in which we looked at lithium effects on the behaviour of rats (3). We concluded from that work that the behaviour of animals might be divided into two major categories: 1) actions which were essentially responses or reactions to environmental circumstances, and 2) actions which were spontaneous and hence independent of stimulus input. Lithium, we suggested, affected certain behaviours within the former category but was less effective on behaviours in the latter category. From this we went on to propose a model of lithium action (Figure 32.6). We inferred from our behavioural studies that lithium behaved as though it affected some internal stimulus analyser mechanism (we argued on other grounds that neither receptor nor effector mechanisms were involved): it was as though lithium reduced the

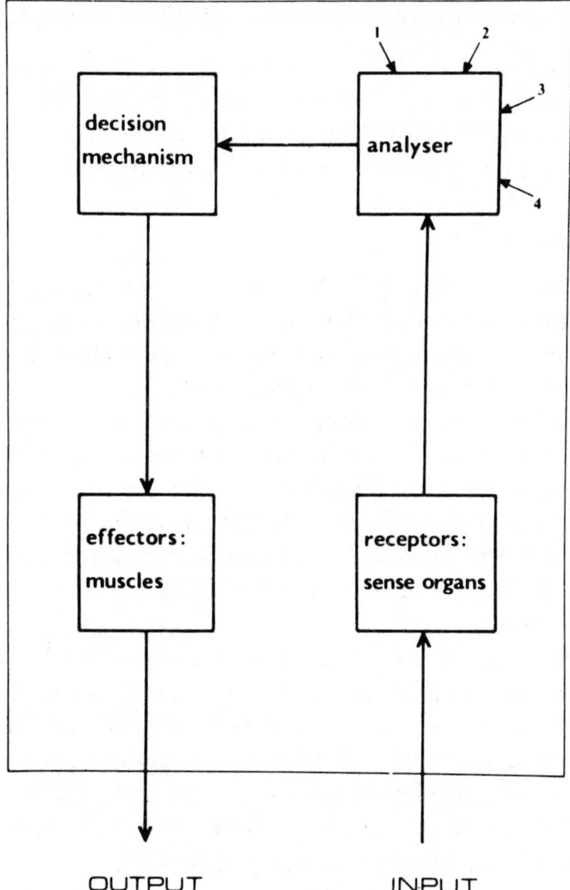

Figure 32 6. A stimulus-significance model of lithium action: see text for discussion

significance (meaning, importance) which our animals attached to stimulus input from their environment.

A stimulus significance model of affective disorders

On the basis of our model of lithium action I proposed a related model of manic depression (4). Mania, it was suggested, might be conceived of as a condition of hyper-active stimulus processing, leading to a flight of ideas, over-reaction to input, and so on: depression, on the other hand, was to be seen as a state of hypo-active stimulus processing, leading to a lack of responsiveness, lethargy, and all the other behavioural characteristics of melancholia.

A catastrophe model of manic depression and lithium prophylaxis

On the basis of the stimulus significance model of lithium action and manic depression, an even more ambitious model was subsequently developed. This model, its derivation and the empirically testable predictions to which it leads, will be expounded in some detail.

The catastrophe surface

Within the last few years there has become available a versatile and intriguing mathematical model which, when applied to a wide range of physical, biological, sociological and psychological phenomena, permits some insight into the way in which sudden changes or discontinuities may occur in the observed function even when the underlying causative forces are essentially continuous. This mathematical model has been given the name 'catastrophe theory' and whilst the detailed arguments upon which it is founded are mathematically sophisticated and difficult (5-7) the model may nevertheless be expressed diagrammatically in a form which can be readily appreciated even though it lacks the status of a formal proof of the underlying theorem.

Briefly, catastrophe theory states that phenomena which demonstrate sudden quantitative jumps from one state to another (such as the sudden switch from the resting potential to the action potential in the neurone, the eruption of heated water into the boiling state, an outburst of aggression or anger, and so on) may be thought of as being under the control of two more or less independent mechanisms neither of which themselves show temporal discontinuities (sudden jumps) in magnitude.

The graphical representation of this relationship between three variables takes the form of a partially folded surface as illustrated in Figure 32.7 and it is this surface (referred to as a 'cusp catastrophe' surface) which provides the basis for a new description of manic-depressive psychosis. If the phenomenon in which discontinuities exist is indicated quantitatively by **z**, represented by the vertical axis of a three-dimensional graph, and the underlying continuous processes (the two horizontal axes of the graph) are represented quantitatively by **x** and **y** respectively, the relationship between the three measures has the general form:

$$\mathbf{z}^3 = \mathbf{x} + \mathbf{y}\mathbf{z}$$

and the existence of such a relationship is a fundamental property of all forms of physical (animate and inanimate) system.

Some fundamental properties of the cusp-catastrophe surface are shown in Figure 32.7. Consider point 1 on the cusp catastrophe surface: a change

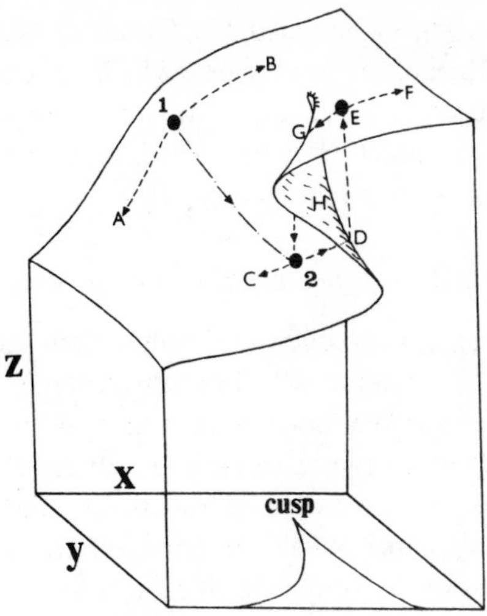

Figure 32.7. A cusp catastrophe surface: see text for a full discussion

in the value of **x** causes the point to move smoothly along the line AB. If however, a change occurs in the value of **y** such that point 1 moves to point 2 on the surface, subsequent variations in **x** have quite different effects upon the point's movements than was the case for point1. Thus if **x** decreases in value, point 2 moves smoothly over the surface towards C: an *increase* in **x**, however, causes point 2 to move to the edge of the fold in the catastrophe surface (D) and any further increase leads to point 2 making a sudden jump from D to the upper surface of the fold (represented in the figure by E). This jump is the 'catastrophe' or switch process, a discontinuity in the value of **z** (intermediate values of **z** between points D and E do not exist: the surface H will be mentioned briefly later) which results from a smooth, continuous change in the value of **x**. When point 2 has moved to position E further increase in **x** leads it back to the upper edge of the fold (at G) and eventually results in a second catastrophe, or discontinuity, in the value of **z** as the point drops back again to the lower surface of the fold. The point does not pass from either upper or lower surfaces to the reflected fold surface, H, which, whilst representing possible **z** values between the upper and lower surfaces, is a low probability surface. The point oscillates between the two extreme fold surfaces as **x** increases and decreases in value.

One point of nomenclature may be made before proceeding to the application of the cusp catastrophe surface model to manic depression. The factor arranged along the **x** axis is referred to as the 'normal' factor, whilst that along the **y** axis is called the 'splitting factor'. It is usual to choose as the splitting factor that process which changes the more slowly under normal circumstances, and to put the more labile variable along the normal factor axis, though this is not, of course, the only criterion for deciding which factor is which.

Application of the catastrophe model to manic depression

In Figure 32.8 the cusp catastrophe surface has been adapted to provide a descriptive model of the changes which occur in manic depression. For the purposes of this exercise the normal (**x** axis) factor has been labelled anxiety (**a**) and the splitting factor (**y** axis) as self esteem (**e**). It should be noted that whilst, for the purposes of the theory being presented here, these dimensions are quantitatively inverted on the axes, passing from high at the origin to low at points distal from the origin, this in no way affects the application of the model. The **z** axis, or the behaviour space as it is sometimes called, is taken to be the efficiency of stimulus analysis (**s**), i.e. the readiness with which the individual attaches importance, meaning, or significance to observed external events. The catastrophe model of manic depression makes the basic assumption that, as a fundamental biological property,

$$\mathbf{s}^3 = \mathbf{a} + \mathbf{es}$$

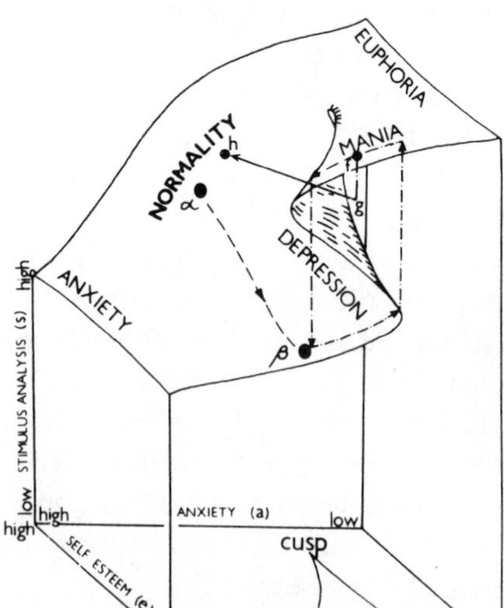

Figure 32.8. A catastrophe model of manic depression and prophylactic action of lithium (see text for a full discussion)

so that the three variables are related by a cusp catastrophe surface.

In the 'normal' individual (i.e. the individual whose mood states fall within the limits of personal and social acceptability) it is assumed that moderately high anxiety levels can be coped with provided that self-esteem levels remain also high. This will place the individual at point A on the cusp catastrophe surface, where the efficiency of stimulus analysis is also moderate and perceived events are neither passed over nor imbued with undue importance. Provided that no change occurs in the individual's level of self esteem (which may be regarded as a relatively stable characteristic supported by various psychological defence mechanisms) variations in anxiety level will cause the individual to swing between mild euphoria (low anxiety) and high anxiety: depression will not be involved.

If, however, a change occurs in the splitting factor such that, for one reason or another, self esteem drops (as a result of repeated experience of failure, for example) the individual may move to a point B on the cusp catastrophe surface where subsequent variations in anxiety level do have implications for depressive and manic mood states. At B, stimulus analysing efficiency is fairly low, which means that the individual tends to under-process information which he receives about the environment: this prevents his attaching excess importance to such information and he therefore ceases to worry unnecessarily about it. There thus occurs a steady fall in anxiety level and point B moves to the right until it reaches the lip of the fold in the cusp catastrophe surface. Any further drop in anxiety level causes the individual to switch from the lower fold surface to the upper fold surface where, because stimulus analysing efficiency suddenly increases, he begins to over-process information. This, in combination with a low anxiety level, leads to a euphoric or manic state, characterized by flight of ideas, fallacious 'insights', and all the other symptoms typical of a manic or hypomanic episode. However, the high level of processing causes the individual to commence attaching significance to events which, viewed objectively, have no real consequences for him: he thus starts to become anxious and, in so doing, moves back along the **x** axis of the cusp catastrophe surface towards the lip of the upper fold. A continued rise in anxiety leads to the individual passing over the catastrophe edge and switching suddenly to a low stimulus processing mode. Low processing efficiency in an individual showing simultaneously relatively high anxiety and low self esteem, will, it is suggested, present clinically as a depressive syndrome, with the individual appearing guilt ridden, self-reproaching, and both socially and physically withdrawn. The lowered stimulus processing efficiency does, however, have an adaptive function in that it allows the individual to cope with his anxiety which steadily drops. The cycle of manic and depressive mood swings is then repeated.

Evidence to support the model

It would be premature at this stage to advance supporting arguments too forcefully. If the catastrophe model has any value at the present time it is as a stimulator of ideas and new directions of research, rather than as an explanatory device drawing together previous findings. However, the model as applied to the phenomena associated with manic depression is not without some support in the psychological and psychiatric literature.

1. Anxiety: Considerable attention has been focussed in recent years on the close relationship which undoubtedly exists between anxiety and depression. Indeed, the term 'mixed anxiety-depression' has sometimes been used to refer to a special diagnostic grouping of patients to whom special treatment may be prescribed (8,9) and it seems not unreasonable to link anxiety with depression in this model. Such a link has been made more formally (4).

2. Self esteem: Whilst this is a difficult variable to operationalise and quantify, the justification for including it in the model stems from the recent work of Seligman (10) on learned helplessness in which it has been shown that a repeated history of failure may lead an individual to show symptoms which, if not identical to, are at least very reminiscent of, those found in states of depression. The conceptual jump from learned helplessness to a variable such as self esteem may not be such a great one, and it is taken here in order to make the model more acceptable in the clinical context.

3. Stimulus analysis efficiency: It has been hypothesized that one of the causative factors in the onset of depression may be an automatic adjustment of central stimulus analysing efficiency triggered by inbuilt mechanisms, the function of such mechanisms being to limit the experience of anxiety. These ideas are based upon studies of the effects of lithium carbonate (3). The reflex invokation of suppressive mechanisms, such as the sleep-controlling processes, to limit sensory analysis, can, it is claimed, account for many of the observed characteristics of depressive mood, such as concomitant sleep disturbances and the cyclical nature of mood swings (4).

The effects of lithium carbonate

The catastrophe model of manic depression can cope reasonably well with certain findings regarding the action of lithium carbonate in the clinical control of manic depression. In particular, it is able to throw light upon the fact that whilst lithium is apparently effective in the acute treatment of mania it is less evidently so against depression except prophylactically. Reference to figure 32.8 suggests why this might be so. Suppose that an individual in a manic state, as at point **f** on the cusp catastrophe surface, were given lithium carbonate. If, as has been suggested, this results in a lowering of the individual's stimulus processing efficiency, it is clear that this cannot occur in such a way as to lower point **f** to point **g**. Assuming that the administration of lithium does not affect ambient anxiety levels — and there is little or no evidence that it does — the only way in which a drop in stimulus processing efficiency can be reflected within the terms of the catastrophe model is by point **f** moving over the cusp catastrophe surface to point **h** which allows the stable coexistence of the unchanged anxiety level and the new level of stimulus processing. Such a move produces a change in the splitting factor, i.e. a rise in self esteem. At point **h** the individual is 'normalized' (the 'normothymotic' function of lithium) insofar as subsequent changes in anxiety level do not lead perforce to a resumption of the manic depressive cycle. In this way, lithium acts not only acutely against mania but also prophylactically against depression.

In contrast, lithium can do little that is effective against an existing depression. There is no simple meaning to be attached to a pharmacologically induced suppression of stimulus processing efficiency below the surface of the lower fold of the cusp catastrophe surface.

Predictions from the model

Catastrophe theory does not, by its nature, permit precise quantitative predictions to be made. The form of the cusp catastrophe surface is canonical: the disposition of quantitative measures along the three spatial axes is merely ordinal and it is not necessary for the axes to be strictly orthogonal with respect to each other. Such predictions as can be made from the model are in terms of an increase or decrease in one or other of the variables, but the magnitude of such changes cannot be specified: the predictions are testable only within a general descriptive framework.

Having said that, it is clear that the model as proposed here produces at least three fairly strong predictions. In the first place it follows from the model that it ought to be possible to alleviate depression by raising self esteem (by assertion training or some similar device). This is not tautologous provided that depression is not equated with low self esteem but defined instead as a complex condition in which self esteem or related effects are partly involved. Secondly, and clearly related to the first, is the prediction that any treatment for depression which acts by raising stimulus processing efficiency, or any anti-manic treatment which acts (like lithium carbonate) by lowering it, should result in a raising of self esteem. Thirdly, contrary to common (but possibly superficial) experience, mania may be associated with low levels of self esteem. The expansiveness and grandiosity sometimes exhibited in the manic or hypomanic state may reflect an attempt on the part of the patient to offset, by overt behaviour, covert low levels of self esteem. All three predictions are broadly testable but have not, so far, been put to any empirical test.

Catastrophe models in psychiatry

Given the present state of our knowledge about any major psychiatric illness, it would be surprising if the catastrophe model of manic depression, which has been put forward here, did not turn out to be unsupportable in one or more of its major tenets. That, in a way, is of no great importance. Catastrophe theory is extraordinarily resilient and may still provide a viable basis for a model of manic depression even though the natures of the underlying continuous variables are changed. Indeed, Zeeman (6) has already proposed a quite different style of manic depression model based on the cusp-catastrophe surface. Zeeman suggests that with mood as the behavioural factor an appropriate normal factor might be environmental (though he does not specify this more closely) with the splitting factor being something along the lines of a chemical imbalance in the brain. A model based on these or other underlying continuous processes, whilst not necessarily incompatible with the model presented here, may yet be preferable. The aim here is less to postulate a model of manic depression which provides a complete description of all the various phenomena associated with that condition, than to indicate how the notions of a catastrophe theory in its simplest form (and there are more complex variations which may have greater utility, given the complexity of most psychiatric syndromes) can be applied to abnormal behaviour and thought.

At the present time the cusp catastrophe model may be no more than an informative plaything which enables the research worker to make theoretical manipulations of putative causative factors, and to see how, out of fundamental biological continuities, it is possible to derive the discontinuities of behaviour which are frequently, in more than a mathematical sense, catastrophes.

Models at the organism system level

It is possible to go beyond the level of the individual organism in the search for a model of lithium action. There is already considerable evidence that lithium affects the response of one organism to another: thus Weischer (11) and Sheard (12) have reported on the inter-individual aggression reducing effects of lithium, whilst the Symes (13) have found that the effects of lithium on activity levels in rats depend upon the social conditions under which the rats were tested, and they comment that 'animal data must be obtained in a social setting if we wish to relate such studies to those using human subjects.' This, of course, is a thoroughly sensible statement, particularly if we accept that the definition of mood disorders depends — at least in part — on the effects which such conditions have upon other individuals (friends, members of the family, and so on), and on the experiences which the depressed or manic individual has in relating his behaviour to that of others.

With sentiments such as these in mind, we have recently diverted our attention to studies of the effects of lithium on social behaviour in animals. Here, instead of taking as our unit of study the environment — organism—behaviour system, we adopt the environment—(social group)—behaviour system, recognizing that the abstraction of a single animal from its social setting does just as great a violence to biological normality as does the removal of an organ from an intact animal.

The effects of lithium on social aggregation in goldfish

We observed goldfish in an apparatus which is illustrated diagramatically in Figure 32.9. This consisted of three glass tanks, 18 cm long × 12 cm wide × 12 cm deep, one mounted above the other two, and all three screened from each other. Each tank was marked externally in such a way as to indicate three equal-sized sections (A, B, C and D). In the upper tank were placed two fish, whilst each of the lower two tanks contained a single fish. Observations were made every 20 s for a total of 5 min (15 observations in all) and the compartments occupied by all four fish on each occasion were recorded.

Taking the upper tank first, the fish were scored for social contact in the following manner: if both occupied the same compartment (AA, BB, CC or DD) a score of 3 was recorded; if they occupied adjacent compartments (AB, BC, CD) the score was 2; for a gap of one compartment between fish (AC, BD) the score was 1; and for fish at maximum separation (AD) a zero (0) score was recorded. Thus a maximum social contact score of 45,

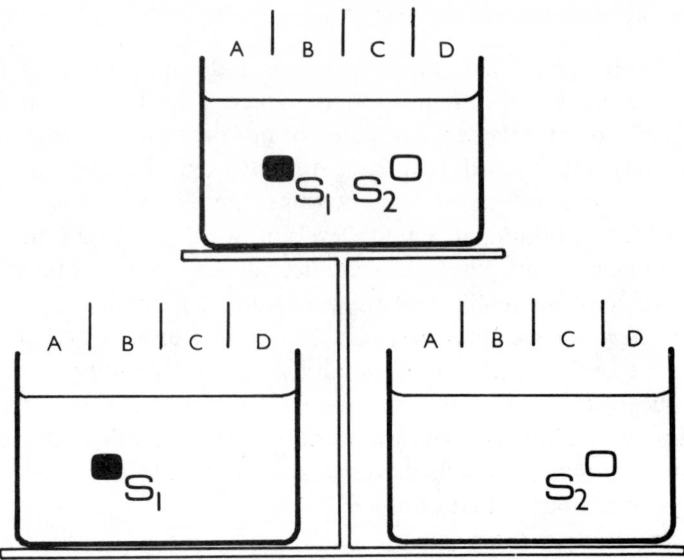

Figure 32.9. Diagrammatic representation of the apparatus used to investigate the effects of lithium chloride on social behaviour in goldfish: in the upper tank two fish are placed together, whilst in the lower tanks one fish is put into each tank. S1 is placed in the apparatus 5 min before S2. A, B, C and D are four equal-sized compartments indicated by external markings on the tanks.

and a minimum of 0, were possible. The two lower tanks were scored in exactly the same way, being treated as though they were a single tank: in this way the degree of social aggregation in the top tank could be directly compared with a situation in the lower tank where the fish were unaffected by social stimulation.

The fish were distinguished (using their natural markings as indicators) as S1 and S2 (see Figure 32.9), S1 being placed in the apparatus 5 min before S2.

In order to examine the effects of lithium on social behaviour, the following procedure was adopted. Fish being treated with lithium were allowed to swim in a tank containing lithium chloride solution for a total of 6 h before being placed in the test apparatus (the latter contained de-chlorinated tap water at room temperature). The 6 h exposure to the lithium chloride solution allowed the body fluids time to equilibrate with the concentration of the surrounding medium. Three concentrations of lithium chloride solution were used: 10, 20 and 30 mmol/l. Control animals were subjected to exactly the same procedure, but sodium chloride solutions, at the same concentrations as the lithium chloride solutions, were used instead. Goldfish are naturally brackish water animals and osmoregulation problems were therefore regarded as likely to be minimal.

Either S1 or S2 or both received treatment with lithium chloride; an animal not treated with lithium chloride received treatment with sodium chloride.

The experimental design was a 4(drug combinations: Na/Na; Na/Li; Li/Na; Li/Li) × 3(Doses: 10, 20, 30 mmol/l) × 2(Social conditions: Alone, in the lower tanks; Together, in the upper tank) factorial. Five pairs of fish were tested in each of the 4 × 3 × 2 = 24 conditions, i.e. 120 pairs or 240 fish in all.

An analysis of variance carried out on the results revealed a marked social aggregation effect. $F(df\ 1, 96) = 56.45$; $p < 0.001$, indicating that goldfish tend to school when placed together; there was a significant effect of the drug combination used, $F(df\ 3, 96) = 4.15$; $p < 0\ 01$, and a significant interaction between the drug combination and social condition, $F(3, 96) = 5.04$; $p < 0.001$. There was no significant effect of drug dose.

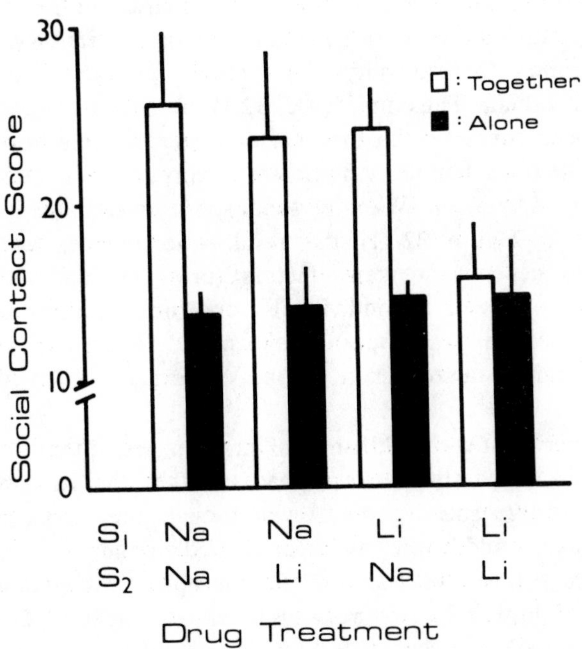

Figure 32.10. Results of the experiment on lithium effects on social aggregation in goldfish; only when both animals in the social situation had been treated with lithium chloride did they behave as though not in a social situation. Treatment of just one of the fish, either S1 or S2, had no effect on social aggregation

The most interesting finding here is the statistically significant interaction between drug combination and social condition, and this is illustrated in Figure 32.10. It can be seen from this figure that when neither, or only one, of the fish in the upper tank has received prior treatment with lithium, they show marked social aggregation responses as compared to the fish in the lower tank. When, however, both fish in the upper tank have received lithium treatment, they behave in exactly the same manner as the fish in the lower tanks: social aggregation is eliminated and they behave as though they are in separate and independent tanks.

A model of lithium action based on personal space

What kind of model of lithium action can be developed on the basis of the findings from the goldfish experiment described above? Many interpretations of the findings are, of course, possible. It may, for example, simply be that the fish were disorientated by the lithium, or that they swam more erratically, and so on. A rather more elaborate hypothesis can be constructed using a rather old-fashioned, but still attractive, notion, namely the concept of 'personal space'. This is based on the idea that each individual is surrounded by a personal volume, or territory, the size of which determines the proximity of any social approach made to, or by, another individual. Thus in Figure 32.11 individuals A and C make effective social contact when their personal spaces come into contact; A and B, on the other hand, are not in social contact, their personal spaces being separated by a gap. When personal spaces overlap (as in the case of A and D in Figure 32.11) the result — acceptance, aggression, or withdrawal — depends on many factors (prior learning, the transient psychological states of the individuals concerned, relationships between the individuals, their sexes, attractiveness, and so on; and a number of non-psychological factors such as the context in which the meeting occurs).

In the experiment with goldfish it might be suggested that lithium acts as though it expanded the personal space so that the fish were able to maintain effective social contact even though they were more widely separated than would be the case for untreated animals.

But would such a model account for the apparent aggression-reducing properties of lithium as reported in other experiments? Expanded life space should make overlap of territories more likely to occur and hence lead to *more* frequent aggressive responses. If, however, we suppose that aggression elicitation is related to some additional factor, such as stimulation intensity based on the apparent size of an approaching animal,

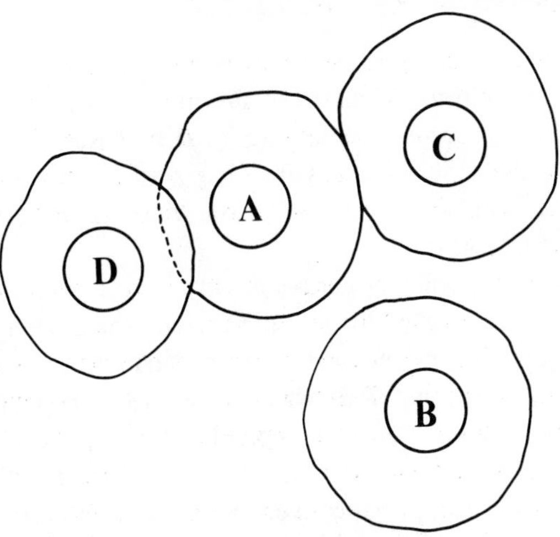

Figure 32.11. The concept of personal space. Individuals A, B, C and D may each be assumed to be surrounded by a personal space. Social contact is made when personal spaces meet (A & C). Overlap of spaces (A & D) may lead to withdrawal or aggression, but the precise response depends on many factors (see text)

as indexed by, for example, the angle subtended at the eye of the defending animal, then it would follow that expansion of personal space would lead to effective social contact being established at a distance which would be too great for the approaching animal to subtend an aggression-eliciting angle at the eye of the animal being approached. In the case of pathologically aggressive humans we would have then to postulate that their life space is, for one reason or another, contracted so that they are able to make social contact only at a distance which is so small that it automatically leads to a competing aggressive response. Lithium, by expanding the personal space, would allow social contact to be made at a distance too great to elicit aggression.

As in the case of the catastrophe model, the model of lithium action based on the notion of personal space leads to empirically testable (but, to my knowledge, so far untested) predictions, the most obvious of which is that lithium-treated individuals would be expected to engage in conversation, or other forms of social interaction, at greater distances than when untreated. Aggressive individuals should attempt to make closer approaches when initiating social contact, and this tendency should be reversed or offset by lithium treatment.

THE FUNCTIONS OF MODEL BUILDING

Models such as the catastrophe theory of manic depression or the personal space approach to lithium effects on social interaction, are of course very bold (some might say premature) attempts to pull together experimental findings within a theoretical framework. The process of model building is certainly great fun, but one is entitled to ask what *use* are such excursions into the realms of hypothesis.

I well remember the philosopher, A.J. Ayer, in a television interview, after first being asked to explain 'in words which the ordinary viewer will understand' exactly what he meant by logical positivism, being faced with the show-stopping question 'Well, what is the *use* of logical positivism?' Ayer did not even pause: 'Oh,' he replied, 'it's a great deal of use to people who are concerned with such matters'. That was exactly the right — indeed, the only — answer to have given, and it answers also the question of the usefulness of scientific models. Models are tools which facilitate our thinking about complex issues, and which lead us on to new questions — questions which may be framed and examined in an empirical manner. A model, once established, is independent of the experiments upon which it was based; it is a force in its own right. It is, however, dependent upon the outcome of experiments to which it gives rise. The failure to distinguish between experiments which lead to models and experiments which stem from models has led to much misplaced criticism of models of lithium action (14, 15).

It has been said that the main function of science is to limit its own pretensions; that, of course, is nonsense. The main function of science is to provide fuel for its pretensions, to lead on to new and, hopefully, better ideas.

Lithium has proved to be a prime stimulus for model building, and has provided us with an opportunity to observe models at all conceptual levels applied to the same set of issues. In this respect, its importance extends far beyond its use as a therapeutic agent. The models which are designed to encompass the many effects which lithium produces in biological systems, act as vehicles for our imagination, carrying our ideas beyond the confines of our particular experiments and leading towards different views about the nature of mental illness and possible new modes of treatment.

ACKNOWLEDGEMENTS

I am grateful to the publishers of IRCS Medical Science for permission to reproduce the arguments leading to the catastrophe model of manic depression, which previously appeared in *IRCS Journal of Medical Science,* **4,** 96 (1976).

References

1. Mellerup, E.T. and Rafaelsen, O.J. (1975). In: F.N. Johnson (ed.) *Lithium Research and Therapy,* pp. 381-389 (London: Academic Press)
2. Mandell, A.J. and Knapp, S. (1976). *Pharmakopsychiat.,* 9, 116
3. Johnson, F.N. (1975). In: F.N. Johnson (ed.) *Lithium Research and Therapy* pp. 315-338 (London: Academic Press)
4. Johnson, F.N. (1975). *Dis. Nerv. Syst.,* 36, 228
5. Thom, R. (1972). *Stabilite Structurelle et Morphogenese* (New York: Benjamin)
6. Zeeman, C. (1973). In: A. Hattari (ed.) *Manifolds.* p. 173 (Tokyo: University of Tokyo Press)
7. Isnard, C.A. and Zeeman, C. (1974). In: L. Collins (ed.) *Use of Models in the Social Sciences,* p. 242 (London: Tavistock)
8. Freeman, H.L., Bourne, M.S. and Schiff, A.A. (1974). *J. Int. Med. Res.,* 2, 107
9. Schiff, A.A., Murphy, J.E. and Anderson, J.A. (1975). *J. Int. Med. Res.,* 3, 125
10. Seligman, M.E.P. (1975). *Helplessness: On Depression, Development and Death* (San Francisco: Freeman)
11. Weischer, M.L. (1969). *Psychopharmacologia,* 15, 245
12. Sheard, M.H. (1970) *Nature,* 228, 284
13. Syme, L.A. and Syme, G.J. (1973). *Psychopharmacologia,* 29, 85
14. Smith, D.F. (1976). *Experientia, 32,* 1320
15. Johnson, F.N. (1976). *Experientia,* 32, 1350

Part V:
The Management of Lithium Therapy

Introduction

Even though we may not know exactly what lithium is doing biochemically or physiologically when it produces its therapeutic effects, produce those effects it does. No amount of physiological or biochemical investigation can change the now well-established fact that lithium, used therapeutically, works. Psychiatrists know that lithium is a powerful agent in the control of recurrent mood disorders and they therefore find it reasonable to use lithium even without any detailed rationale for doing so: such a situation is, indeed, the rule rather than the exception in the pharmacotherapy of psychiatric disorders and does, of course, reflect not only our lack of knowledge about the drugs but also our ignorance of the biological bases of the vast majority of psychopathological states.

Given such a state of uncertainty, it becomes all the more essential that empirically based guidelines should be established for the safe use of what is, after all, a highly toxic substance. Such concern for the patient's well-being, however, has not always seemed to govern therapeutic techniques, particularly where the manic patient is concerned. Dr Hes (Chapter 33) presents a brief summary of methods of treating mania down the ages which records some of the frightful things that were done in the name of medicine. Dr Kerry's detailed and clear exposition of the guidelines for safe lithium treatment (Chapter 34) comes as a breath of fresh air after Dr Hes's catalogue of barbarous techniques.

Choosing the correct dose of lithium for each patient and choosing the correct patient for lithium therapy, present two of the major issues for a psychiatrist contemplating the use of this form of treatment. Two chapters deal with such matters. In Chapter 35 Dr Hewick looks at the characteristics of patients which determine optimal lithium dose levels, whilst Drs Lee and Paschalis, in Chapter 36, consider the matter of patient selection based on predictive tests.

There are several types of lithium preparation available, the difference between them being based on the fluctuations in serum level which result from their administration. Dr Bennie and Dr Chalmers examine three proprietary preparations available in the UK (Chapter 37) and Dr Venkoba Rao (Chapter 38) examines in a rather different way the relationship between oral administered dose and serum lithium level. The theme is continued by Dr Tyrer who again examines a number of proprietary preparations of lithium carbonate (Chapter 39). It seems clear that this area is one which bears continuing investigation.

Dr Jerram and Dr McDonald reexamine established views about the minimum plasma lithium levels which are necessary for effective prophylaxis (Chapter 40).

The final two chapters in this section are concerned with the use of tissue level measurements in choosing patients for lithium therapy, with special reference to the difference between serum (extracellular) and intracellular levels. Dr Greil and Dr Eisenreid, in Chapter 41, consider the factors which may lie behind inter-individual differences in the uptake of lithium intracellularly. Miss Andrews (Chapter 42) casts doubt on the usefulness of erythrocyte/plasma lithium ratios in patient management, and this is a not inappropriate note of uncertainty on which to end the coverage of management techniques.

33

Treatment of Mania in Ancient Medical Sources

J. Ph. HES

Various empirical approaches exist in medicine from the beginning of medical thought.

1. One has to look for the 'cause' of a disease. Freudians look for psychotrauma in childhood; in cases of infection one looks for a bacterium or a virus; in cases of metabolic disorder one looks for a hyper- or hypo-production of some substance within the body.

2. One disease cures another. Examples are the observation that epilepsy cures schizophrenia, hence the application of electro-convulsive treatment to cases of schizophrenia; another example is that of von Wagner Jauregg's work on the administration of malaria to patients suffering from progressive paralysis, a work which gained him the Nobel Prize in medicine, the only time a psychiatrist ever received such a high award.

3. *'Similia similibus curantur'* or 'like cures like'—a principle we find in homeopathic medicine, but also, for example, in vaccination where a small dose of a disease generates immunity and thus protects the organism against the same disease.

The first of these approaches led to the establishment of lithium therapy: when John Cade, in 1949, was looking for the cause of manic depressive disorder, he was looking for a substance in the body which was produced to excess in cases of mania and in insufficient amounts in cases of depression.

Having an interest in the history of psychiatry I started investigating how our ancient preceptors approached mania. The first thing which becomes apparent in such a study is that we encounter various terms indicating a state of mania, such as 'insania', 'desipientia', 'delirium', 'furor' and 'rabies'.

A natural starting-point in any historical investigation into a medical topic, is an examination of the early Greek schools of Medicine—the schools of Knidos and of Kos, the latter being of greater interest in this instance. Hippocrates of Kos was a very conscientious physician and paid attention to the whole patient and not, as in the school of Knidos, to symptoms alone. In addition, Hippocrates searches for causes which could explain the aberrant behaviour of his patients. Current philosophy in those days postulated that the cosmos consisted of four elements: the warm *fire;* the cold *air,* the dry *earth* and the humid *water.* These four elements were reflected or represented in the four body fluids, the warm *blood* represents the fire, the *phlegm* of the brain represents the cold air; the yellow *bile* represents the dry earth and the black *bile* represents the humid water. Prominence of the various body fluids lead to the occurrence of body types: the sanguine type, the phlegmatic type, the choleric type and the melancholic type. Within the context of such notions, Hippocrates was able to discuss the causes of mood disorders. Thus, in the English translation of the Book of Epidemics (1) we read: If the brain is corrupted by *phlegma* the patients are quiet and silent; if by *bile,* they are vociferous, malignant and act improperly; if the brain is heated, terrors, fears and terrifying dreams occur; if it is too cool, the patients are grieved and troubled'.

Clearly, Hippocrates was capable of discerning manic and depressive states. The treatment of maniacal states did not essentially change from Hippocratic times until the 17th Century. We have this information from the ancient writers themselves and also from a recent work of Professor Diethelm (2) on old medical dissertations with a bearing on psychiatry. Diethelm's book deals with dissertations which appeared in Europe before 1750.

The Hippocratic treatment consisted of

1. Surgical measures: bloodletting by venesection and cupping in order to evacuate blood from the brain, to cool the brain.

2. The administration of drugs to evacuate bile (Rhubarb, senna, borage, bugloss). The use of bugloss is particularly interesting since it appears that this herb is still in use in Persian folk medicine today. The plant Anchousa Bouglosson is called, according to Linnaeus, *Borrago officinalis L.* In Persia to-day it is called gul-i-gavzaban, or 'ox-tongue

flower' and is used against headache and anxiety and as an antipyretic. This same Ancousa was used by Dioscurides and Galenus and also by the Jewish physician-philosopher Maimonides, who employed it as a sleeping pill as well as a euphoriant.

Information about psychiatric treatment procedures at the end of the 17th, and into the 18th Century has been provided by Kraepelin (3) who reports that laxatives were in common use against mania as well as against depression, their use in the latter condition apparently being indicated because of the concomitant constipation. At this time we find, as a new approach, the use of high dosage emetics. The purpose of this treatment was the generation of the new disease, nausea, which would, it was held, cure mania. Another approach to causing nausea was the use of a turning chair: a patient was put in a hanging chair and turned around with a speed of 50 to 100 revolutions per minute. Venesection, too was not neglected. As a rather new addition we find the sudden application to the patient of cold water, a procedure called 'bain de surprise' or also 'douche écossaise'.

Later, in the 19th Century we find the introduction of bromides (4-6 gram of natrium bromatum a day) and also the use of barbiturates as sleeping pills (trional and veronal). In the first decade of the 20th Century Ziehen (4) mentioned a new drug, duboisine, an alkaloid from the Australian shrub *Duboisia myoporoides,* and apparently very similar pharmacologically to scopolamine. Ziehan also prohibited sexual intercourse and smoking to his manic patients and believed a diet of milk and eggs to be beneficial.

Kraepelin emphasized the importance of removal from stimuli and was also a strong believer in hydrotherapy like Baruk (5). Kraepelin also advocated friendly conversation.

A brief review such as this cannot hope to cover the many forms of treatment which have, over the ages, been advocated for manic states. These were often cruel and bizarre and based on rationales which owed much to superstition and prejudice. There were, for example, psychiatrists who advocated flogging to get the devil out of the patients. Others advised the use of music to quiet the patients down and again others propagated the use of wine in mania.

In many ways, the reasoning behind the treatments which are applied today for many psychiatric disorders, bears a remarkable similarity to that which led physicians of earlier ages to introduce forms of therapy which we now regard as ill-founded or objectionable.

On the other hand, we have to recognise the vast strides which have been made in psychiatric treatment during the last 30 years when the phenothiazines, butyrophenones and lithium, have been introduced in the treatment of mania.

References

1. Hippocrates *Epidemiorum libri*
2. Diethelm, O. (1971). *Medical Dissertations of Psychiatric Interest,* Printed Before 1750 (Basel: Karger)
3. Kraepelin, E (1913). *One Hundred Years of Psychiatry.* Translated by W. Baskin (1962). (New York: Philosophical Library)
4. Ziehen, Th. (1908). *Psychiatric für Arzte und Studierende.* (Leipzig: Hirzel)
5. Baruk, H. (1950). *Précis de Psychiatrie.* (Paris: Masson)

34

Recent Developments in Patient Management

R. J. KERRY

INTRODUCTION

In this review it is hoped to give an up-to-date account of standard lithium practice and to introduce some general trends of the last few years.

Lithium was possibly first used in medicine in 1843 by Mr Ure, a London surgeon, for dissolving bladder stones and subsequently by Garrod in the treatment of gout. During the 1940s it became fashionable as a salt substitute for hypertensive patients but was discontinued in 1949 because of its toxicity. This was the year in which Dr Cade (1) introduced it into psychiatry and this 'foundation stone' of treatment has been highlighted for us by Dr Cade himself in Chapter 1. The second name that automatically comes to mind in the lithium field is that of Schou; we are greatly indebted to him for his early enthusiasm and for an early publication of the calibre of *Lithium in Psychiatric Therapy—Stocktaking after 10 Years* (2), published in 1959—almost unbelievably nearly 20 years ago.

Lithium is generally prescribed in psychiatry for the following reasons:

1. The treatment of acute mania;
2. The treatment of acute depression;
3. The prophylaxis of manic depressive illness;
4. Various other conditions including schizophrenia; childhood psychiatric disorders of a variety of kinds; hyperactive mentally retarded patients — both children and adults; patients with mild, but usually almost

subclinical, mood swings which cause social difficulties; periodic psychoses of a non-affective kind; premenstrual tension; mood disorders of old age; aggressive patients; alcoholism; drug addiction, etc.

Two points should be considered before we use lithium: the type of preparation to be used, and the state of the patient.

The choice of lithium preparation

We now have a wide range of lithium compounds available. It has been found that for prescribing purposes the carbonate is the most convenient salt and it has now been used for over 20 years without presenting any real difficulties. Some of the other lithium salts create problems; the chloride, for example, is one of the most deliquescent substances known, while the citrate is a little bulky for convenient use. Nevertheless, the sulphate, citrate, glutamate, gluconate, adipate and acetate are available commercially. The differential advantages of these salts are probably marginal, being related mainly to manufacturing and marketing pressures rather than therapeutic benefits, or to considerations of administration. However, the carbonate has gained almost universal acceptance because its high molecular ratio of lithium allows the smallest weight of the drug to be prescribed and its extensive use has shown it to be associated with very few problems. Dr Tyrer has taken a special interest in the choice and administration of lithium preparations and he deals fully with this topic in Chapter 39. There are something like 40 or more different preparations of lithium available, and it is advisable for the prescriber to know the characteristics of perhaps two or three compounds and use them confidently bearing in mind the small differences between them for most purposes. The main consideration nowadays is whether to use an ordinary preparation of lithium carbonate or one of its slow release rivals. The rationale behind the use of the latter has been the avoidance of serum lithium 'peaks' with their accompanying mild but unpleasant side effects. Whilst some early sustained release preparations were satisfactory, others did not have satisfactory absorption characteristics as their absorption curves varied from person to person, and in the same person from time to time, and several publications have appeared recently suggesting that there is little practical difference in the serum lithium curves obtained from conventional and sustained release lithium when they are correctly prescribed.

Considerable advantage can be gained if the prescriber 'tailors' the administration schedule to suit the needs of the individual patient, bearing in mind his personal and domestic circumstances.

The physical state of the patient

Twenty years ago the advice given about prescribing lithium was over-cautious, particularly if the patient was not physically fit. Since then its widespread use has shown that with careful use (and blood monitoring) it is much less risky for the patient than continuing manic depressive illness. But lithium ion is toxic and potentially dangerous if reasonable care is not taken over the clinical examination of patients before they receive treatment. In particular, it is essential to bear in mind the special risks undergone by patients with poor cardiovascular or renal function. Personal experience, and the experience of psychiatrists generally, suggests that patients who are physically fit when examined medically are not likely to be at risk when treated with lithium.

Where there are special risks, yet the danger of continuing manic depressive illness is high, we have found that smaller doses give sufficiently high therapeutic serum lithium concentrations (e.g. 0.8-1.0 mmol/l) and treatment has been safe for many years. We have, for example, treated a 60-year-old lady for 15 years with 500 mg of lithium carbonate daily, which has produced a serum lithium concentration of about 0.6-0.9 mmol/l. Before lithium treatment was started, she was severely hypertensive and had poor renal function. She has remained psychiatrically well since, although in her last year before starting lithium she had made two serious suicidal attempts during depressive illnesses.

Other reports suggest that in physical illness, low maintainance doses may be satisfactory. If the psychiatric indications are very strong but the physical state gives cause for concern, it is justifiable to begin prophylactic lithium with one tablet daily, increasing by one tablet daily after a week or so, having taken daily serum lithium estimations to determine when the serum lithium concentration reaches the lower limits of the desired prophylactic level (about 0.6-0.8 mmol/l). Obviously such 'at risk' patients will usually need a high degree of supervision, at least during the early months of their lithium treatment.

I now have a small series of patients all over the proverbial age of 'three score years and ten', who have been maintained very satisfactorily under these conditions. We should remember that there has been no precise serum lithium 'lower level' defined.

THE TREATMENT OF ACUTE MANIA

Historically, mania was the first condition to be successfully associated with lithium treatment and its use has been widely documented. In the actual attack of mania the usual dose range recommended is of the order of 1 000-2 000 mg daily (i.e. about twice the dose given prophylactically) depending on the body weight of the patient and the need to avoid toxic effects. Certain toxic reactions can be serious and even fatal and treatment can therefore only be justified when given in hospital with adequate clinical and biochemical supervision; it should never be started in the home.

Baastrup and Schou (3) suggest that the therapeutic dose is approximately 50 mmol of lithium per day, corresponding to 600 mg of lithium carbonate 3 times a day. It is fairly easy to reach the toxic serum lithium level of 2 mmol/l. It is felt that to obtain a satisfactory response the average serum lithium concentration throughout the day should be about 1.1 mmol/l. Schou and Shaw (4) feel that there is no therapeutic advantage in using serum lithium levels above 1.3 mmol/l and they recommend a range of 0.7-1.3 mmol/l. These concentrations are generally obtained with lithium doses of 25 to 60 mmol/l per day (equivalent to between 900 and 2 200 mg of lithium carbonate daily).

From the published clinical studies of lithium treatment in mania, it seems that fairly rapid control (within 5-10 days) may be, but not always, obtained over the manic state. Relapse occurs within about three days if lithium is stopped. During mania the patient tolerates, and indeed requires, higher doses than can be tolerated by normal people without toxic effects. The patient loses his high dose tolerance once the manic attack is under control and his pattern of lithium retention and excretion begins to resemble the normal. At this stage careful biochemical control is of added importance.

In view of the evidence so far available, certain conclusions about the use of lithium in mania can be drawn. It is not really suitable for use outside hospitals with special facilities, and few psychiatrists would disagree with the view that an acute attack of mania is usually best treated by the established methods of ECT and major tranquillizers such as the phenothiazines. Once the treatment of the acute attack is under way, it is usually appropriate to start lithium prophylactically.

Young people tend to excrete lithium more quickly than old people and the dose required may decrease with the age of the patient. Prien and his colleagues (5) consider that it is difficult to determine from the literature just what constitutes an adequate dose for acutely manic patients but all clinicians recommend that serum lithium levels do not exceed 2.0 mmol/l. Until the dose of lithium carbonate has been stabilised, it is better to use ordinary short-acting preparations rather than slow release compounds.

Short-acting compounds allow quicker effective dose reduction if the serum lithium concentration begins to rise too quickly; stopping a short-acting compound produces a more rapid fall in the concentration than would a long-acting compound. This is likely to be important if the patient is very disturbed and slow to respond. It may be desirable to stop lithium before giving an anaesthetic for ECT.

THE TREATMENT OF ACUTE DEPRESSION

In spite of an increasing number of enthusiastic reports about the effectiveness in mania, the evidence concerning the action of lithium in the treatment of an attack of depression is equivocal. Dr Bennie from Glasgow reports on lithium treatment in depression in Chapter 3.

There are certain dangers in giving lithium to depressed patients. For example, Allgen (6) reports a case in which the serum lithium rose to 3.6 mmol/l without toxic signs being recognized. A poor dietary and fluid intake during a depressive illness is likely to be accompanied by poor urinary excretion and a consequent rising serum lithium concentration. Under these circumstances there are extra dangers should an anaesthetic be given for ECT. The expected signs of lithium toxicity include somnolence, lethargy, muscle weakness and stupor. These signs are also seen with anaesthetic agents such as the barbiturates and an additive effect with lithium may be expected. Jephcott and Kerry (7) describe an incident in which a patient remained unconscious for over 2 h following an anaesthetic for ECT although all previous anaesthetics had been, and susequent anaesthetics were, followed by the normal recovery period of a few minutes. The patient's serum lithium had been monitored every week and was always in the accepted therapeutic range. On this occasion a serum lithium measurement was made during the period of unconsciousness and found to be 3.4 mmol/l. This suggests that an abnormally raised serum lithium concentration was responsible for this complication. These problems are likely to arise in depressive illness where there is an inadequate diet and therefore it is necessary for extra care and extra—often impracticable—lithium monitoring to be given before anaesthesia. We now simply omit lithium treatment during a course of ECT.

THE TREATMENT OF OTHER PSYCHIATRIC CONDITIONS

In view of its success in treating mood disorders where it modifies states of hyperexcitability and produces therapeutic benefit in a disorder which often runs a cyclical course, lithium has been tried in other psychiatric illnesses showing similar features. In particular it has been used in the various other conditions mentioned earlier. Although the results of lithium treatment have been disappointing in many patients with such disorders, our experience and that of others has been that it has been of benefit to a small number of patients.

In using lithium treatment with children it is important to relate the initial dose of lithium to the child's body weight. My practice (although my experience is limited) is to suggest a relatively low starting dose with serum lithium estimations about twice a week, gradually increasing the dose weekly until the serum lithium is in the range of 0.8-1.4 mmol/l. Rapid control of psychiatric symptoms is unlikely to be necessary and a regime such as this is safe and unlikely to alarm the child or his parents. The co-operation of the parents is essential and must include regular discussions and briefings.

THE PROPHYLACTIC TREATMENT OF RECURRENT AFFECTIVE DISORDERS

Many patients will have started prophylactic maintainance treatment with lithium in hospital during recovery from an acute psychotic illness. In the early days of the use of lithium in psychiatry, it was thought best to start treatment in hospital from the point of view of the patients' safety (1) but it is now considered safe to start prophylactic lithium in out-patients (6,8). In some areas it is found convenient and economical to have special lithium clinics (rather like diabetic clinics, etc).

The following general guide lines will be of help in choosing the correct dose of lithium for lithium prophylaxis. A normal healthy adult will need about 20-30 mmol of lithium ion daily to obtain a serum lithium concentration of 0.8-1.4 mmol/l. This corresponds to about 1000 mg of lithium carbonate daily (27.2 mmol/l of lithium ion). Depending on the stated lithium content of the preparation being used, a convenient starting dose expressed in mmol/l of lithium ion can be selected. Generally, and certainly where there is concern about the patient's physical state, about half the usual dose (e.g. about 500 mg of lithium carbonate or 10 mmol/l of lithium ion) can be chosen initially. In all cases the dose will have to be related to serum lithium estimations as one patient may need twice as much lithium as another to maintain the same serum lithium concentration.

There are probably advantages in using ordinary preparations of lithium (rather than sustained release preparations) during the stabilization phase of treatment. With the former it is easier to produce rapid changes in the serum lithium concentration by varying the dose and, more importantly, it is easier to obtain a rapid excretion of lithium by stopping treatment if toxic symptoms or dangerously high serum levels occur. The possibility of employing sustained-release preparations can be considered in each case once the patient is being maintained on a constant dose of lithium. Bearing in mind the advice which is given in Chapter 35 and 39, the following principles will be helpful:

1. It will be found that 1000 mg of ordinary lithium carbonate daily in divided doses will be appropriate for a normal, physically fit adult. As so many preparations of lithium are now available, it may be necessary to calculate a starting dose of the compound being used to give about 20-25 mmol per day of lithium. Smaller starting doses, e.g. 500 mg of lithium carbonate daily (about 10-12 mmol of lithium) should be used where the age or physical state of the patient suggests that the renal lithium clearance may be impaired. Since we are usually instituting prophylactic lithium in a patient who is well at the time of starting, it is obviously safer to begin a dose that is perhaps too small and then to increase the dose gradually.

In practice this procedure is probably more convenient and reliable than placing dependence on any form of test dose.

2. Some prescribers have found the patient's response to initial test doses to be helpful but the evidence to support the value of such procedures is still limited. Lithium metabolism is dealt with from this point of view by Drs Lee and Paschalis in Chapter 36.

Nevertheless, for general purposes, starting with smaller doses and the frequent monitoring of the serum lithium concentration will be found reliable in clinical practice.

3. The experience of most prescribers is that once the dose of lithium and the serum lithium concentrations have been stabilised for any one individual, they can both be expected to remain remarkably constant over many years unless something (such as the patient's physical or environmental circumstances) changes. It should be borne in mind that in exceptional cases there can be sufficient individual variation for one patient to need twice as much lithium as another to attain therapeutic serum lithium concentrations.

Patients very often do not take their tablets properly and the psychiatrist should look at these reasons first if there are irregular or abnormally low serum lithiums in his patient.

Fry and Marks (9) in the context of lithium treatment stress the need for doctors to use laboratory results in the management of their patients. They believe that more active supervision of patients taking drugs by measuring blood levels of the therapeutic agent will enable more of them to derive maximum benefit from the drugs they are prescribed. It is perhaps of doubtful value to measure blood levels every few months with a view to avoiding toxicity, but it is probably of considerable value in 'persuading' the patient to take his medication regularly.

LITHIUM ESTIMATIONS

The usual practice has been to measure serum lithium and to control the dose of lithium accordingly. It is generally considered that atomic absorption spectrophotometry is preferable to flame photometry. These methods are well documented and can be referred to in Coombs' chapter in *Lithium Research and Therapy* edited by Neil Johnson (10). Lithium estimation in several other tissues, instead of serum, has been investigated. These include:-

1. Urine: this appears to be technically more difficult and has been exhaustively reviewed by Amdisen (10).
2. Red blood cells (10);
3. Saliva; this may be a useful technique: Verghese and his associates (11) have published an interesting paper on the value of such a procedure in countries such as India where there are very few centres where serum lithium estimations can be conducted. A very high correlation is obtained between the lithium levels in serum and saliva. Verghese and his colleagues point out several practical advantages of saliva determinations. The patients are spared the discomfort of repeated venipunctures in a country where many are very frightened of blood loss. It avoids the need for trained technicians and sterile needles, and also saliva can be easily collected and mailed to the laboratory. However, a group in Edinburgh (12) has cast doubt on the value of saliva estimations until more is known about the saliva/serum ratio which may be affected by the saliva flow and consequently by drugs such as the tricyclics.

In spite of these other techniques, the determination of serum lithium is the standard practice in most places and it is found to be accurate, acceptable and convenient.

SOME PRINCIPLES IN THE SELECTION OF PATIENTS FOR PROPHYLACTIC LITHIUM

Each patient chosen for prophylactic treatment with lithium will need to be stabilised on his individual dose and then maintained on lithium, presumably for life, rather in the same way that a diabetic patient is stabilised and maintained permanently on insulin. Here also the physician will need to use clinical judgement as to whether stabilization of an individual needs to be carried out on an in-patient or out-patient basis.

Indicators of suitability for long-term treatment

1. Physical fitness: the contra-indications of lithium treatment arising from physical disorders such as hypertension, heart disease, kidney disease, and so on are relative rather than absolute. An important factor is the avoidance of toxic serum lithium concentrations by controlling both the dose of lithium and its concentration in the blood.

2. The frequency, nature and severity of previous psychotic attacks: the patient most in need of, and likely to benefit from, lithium treatment will have a long history of illness with many attacks. 'Psychosis rate' as described by Baastrup and Schou (3) is a useful concept when considering patients from this stand-point. Any patient who has had two or more manic-depressive episodes during one year, or has had one or more episodes per year during the last 2 years, is probably sufficiently ill to warrant serious consideration for treatment with lithium. It should also be realised that the frequency of attacks of manic depressive psychosis is likely to increase rather than decrease as the patient gets older (13).

The more classical the manic depressive history is, and the more severe the degree of psychotic disturbance shown, the better the patient is likely to respond. A history of more frequent manic than depressive phases also improves the prognosis, though it should be borne in mind that even classical recurrent depressives, if followed up for long enough, are often seen to have some degree of manic illness, and classical unipolar recurrent depressives can still show a good response to lithium.

Atypical clinical features in a patient's history of manic depressive illness worsen the prognosis for treatment with lithium. Schou (14) feels that unfavourable prognoses for lithium prophylaxis occur in about one-third of manic depressives where the manic picture is tainted with such atypical features as delusions without overt relation to mood, hallucinations of more than episodic character, periods with reticence and contact difficulties, and gross hysterical symptoms. On the other hand this observation confirms the opinion of most psychiatrists experienced in the use of lithium that such atypical features do not rule out a successful response in many cases. This is especially so in any episodic illness with a strong affective component. In fact it is probably true to say that the greater the mood swings during the course of a psychiatric illness, the better the chance is of a good response to prophylactic lithium (15). Misra and Burns (16) have recently shown that a group of lithium non-responders had severe bipolar illness with more than 4 cycles per year but otherwise no clear factors to separate them as a 'non-responder' group.

The concept of lithium responders

General principles

If we accept the evidence that prophylactic lithium is of considerable benefit to a large proportion of psychiatric patients, then identifying those likely to respond to lithium is important. The following guidelines will be found useful:

1. Most psychiatrists will be able to judge clinically those patients who are likely to respond, i.e. those patients possessing a large number of classical or typical features of manic depressive psychosis and a relatively small proportion of features atypical of this illness. As mentioned earlier, the stronger the affective component in the patient, the better is the prognosis for prophylactic lithium.

2. Even atypical cases should be tried since a small proportion of these do well. A trial of prophylactic lithium is ultimately the best way of separating the 'lithium responders' from the 'lithium non-responders'. Such a trial is reasonable as experience has shown that lithium is a safe long-term treatment. If the clinician feels strongly that the severity and number of psychotic attacks warrant a trial of lithium it is worth persisting for 1 or even up to 2 years, since the occasional patient responds only after about a year, perhaps having had two or three attacks whilst on lithium. Doctors should remember that the decision *not* to give lithium must often be made after considerable thought.

Lithium retention and response: e.g. Serry's Lithium Retention Test (17)

It appears that the lithium ion may be differentially retained in body tissues depending on the psychiatric state of the patient, i.e. whether manic, normothymic, or depressed. Unfortunately at this stage the different reports of the excretion and retention of lithium in various studies are sufficiently controversial to cast doubts on the idea of test doses as a guide to future clinical response. Schou (18) feels that there are several reasons that some clinicians have had difficulty with predictive tests, including the Serry test:

1. The absorption rate from the intestines not only varies from person

to person, but also in the same individual from time to time;

2. The rate at which lithium is distributed to the various tissues may vary;

3. The renal lithium clearance will affect the results of such a test. If there were a reliable predictive test in practice, one would use it, but at the present time one must repeat that the best procedure is to try each patient on lithium who is deemed sufficiently ill to be treated.

THE INTERVIEW WITH THE PATIENT AND HIS RELATIVES

It is essential to try to see both the patients and their relatives before starting prophylactic lithium. The importance of the family being involved over the following years of treatment cannot be over-stressed. Time spent with the patients and their relatives is associated with a greater chance of successful treatment. Repeated visits in themselves may be of great importance in obtaining the best response (8). Extensive experience in psychiatry with lithium has led Schou (18) to state quite definitely that unless the co-operation and support of the family are secured from the very beginning, lithium treatment is doomed to fail.

The patient alone

Briefly discuss with the patient the nature of his illness. The patient will understand the recurrent nature of his illness if the prescriber goes over his previous episodes with him. It can then be stressed that lithium is going to be prescribed to prevent attacks of illness that may otherwise occur in the future. At this stage it is important to gain his co-operation and for him to say that he is anxious to avoid further illness. Hypomanic illness, particularly if not too severe, is frequently a source of pleasure to the patient rather than a source of distress, and some patients are not prepared to give up their future expectations of mild periods of 'manic lift'. These patients should not be 'over persuaded' to undergo treatment. Once an agreement about treatment has been reached with the patient, the following issues should be discussed:

1. Stress dose control: i.e. the precise dose of lithium should be taken exactly as prescribed and the doctor should be told if the routine has been varied, particularly if any tablets have been forgotten. Whilst there is no need for special diets, he should be advised to avoid dramatic dietary changes, but should a special diet become necessary for medical or weight reducing reasons, the patient should be advised to maintain his normal sodium chloride intake (20).

2. Discussions of side effects: mild side effects may be expected in the first few weeks and can be regarded as a normal accompaniment of this new treatment but they will disappear of their own accord when the body has adjusted to the rising serum lithium levels.

Persson (19) has recently looked at the absorption curves and lithium peaks in relation to side effects. Tremor was related to high doses, to high serum concentrations, and to steep absorption curves. The latter was also related to nausea. Abdominal pain and loose bowels were not dose related. This is relevant to the comments of one of our patients who abolished tremor and nausea by taking her tablets before meals.

3. Explanation of possible weight gain: explain the gain in body weight that usually accompanies a successful response to lithium (21). It is important to point out that gain in weight usually accompanies successful treatment with lithium but that after a few months the weight stabilises at a somewhat higher level. Above all, appetite suppressing drugs must be avoided and a suggestion might be made that in about 6 months' time, weight stabilisation should have occurred.

The relatives

Go into the hopes of successful treatment for the patient; stress the importance of continuing the treatment on a permanent basis and go over some of the reasons frequently given by patients or by relatives for stopping the medication prematurely.

Introduce the idea of a 'mood normalizer'. The patient will eventually lose the characteristics and consequences of being a psychiatric invalid. It will help if the family is prepared for this change which is usually a happy event but which sometimes may create problems of adjustment in family relationships when the family has to readjust its behaviour to deal with an individual who is now in normal health. Previously there will have developed a peculiar psycho-social pattern in which patient, spouse, children, friends and associates all play special roles in a combined effort to mitigate the consequences of the patient's incessant mood changes (18). A degree of psychotherapy, such as that available through a lithium clinic, will probably be the best way of handling the problems raised by the changes brought about by recovery. Occasionally roles are reversed and the partner becomes the sick person.

SOME INDIVIDUAL PROBLEMS WITH PATIENTS ON PROPHYLACTIC LITHIUM

Various circumstances can arise which may interrupt an otherwise smooth programme of lithium maintainance. These should be anticipated and include the following:

Refusal of further treatment

The patient may refuse further treatment for one of several reasons:

1. Loss of hypomanic periods. In some individuals mild, but sub-psychotic, hypomania gives them drive and energy which is of considerable personal and professional benefit to them. Such patients can still be advised to start prophylactic lithium. Experience shows that their long-term productivity may be greater, particularly when they are likely to be protected from manic chaos when, although they may think they are doing well, they are nevertheless making a mess of their lives. In patients with frequent and predominantly depressive mood changes on the other hand, several months may pass before any relief is experienced and in such patients it is important to persist with lithium and to support them during their depressions, preferably without anti-depressants. Experience with such patients supports the advice given by Schou (14).

2. Experience of mild side effects during the early stages of treatment. These transient side effects, which may easily discourage a patient, are more commonly complained of by highly skilled people doing fine work and by some professional people who find a fine tremor especially disturbing.

3. Stigma of an incurable illness. The patient may have been well for years as a result of lithium therapy and may therefore decide to stop medication. The relapse rate is then high. Patients are often loath to accept lithium treatment as a lifetime need since this suggests permanent commitment to treatment and the stigma of an incurable illness which they prefer to deny by stopping lithium (22).

4. Persuasion by friends and relatives. Relatives and friends of the patient may persuade him to stop medication. After a few trouble-free years the patient may be told 'You are well now and you don't need tablets'. Again, in this context, relatives often take this opportunity of denying the presence of mental illness in the family and must be warned about the possible dangers if treatment is stopped.

Lithium in association with medical and surgical conditions

The key factors which should alert the prescriber towards extra care in the use of lithium are states which are likely to disturb the patient's electrolyte (notably sodium) balance. These include:

1. Surgical operations involving anaesthetics. The hazards of giving an anaesthetic with a very high serum lithium level are now recognized (7). The danger stems from the possible additive effects of lithium and drugs such as the barbiturates.

A recent paper from Finland (23) reports a study of the combined effects of lithium and methohexitone, and also of lithium and thiopentone. It showed that the barbiturates when given by injection to mice on lithium were associated with a prolonged sleeping time (although this did not happen if the mice were on long-term oral barbiturates). Interestingly, the sleeping times were shortened with rubidium.

The practical implication of this isolated clinical finding of ours has been supported by these animal studies in Finland and confirms the need for added caution when a barbiturate anaesthetic is given to a patient on lithium. It emphasises the point that, if possible, the patient should be off lithium for 24 hours, if not longer, when planning an anaesthetic.

2. Physical illnesses. Severe and acute illness may cause considerable metabolic upset. Fluid and salt balance may be disturbed. Then, although it may often be possible and always desirable to monitor the patient's serum lithium, it is better to stop treatment, for a time at least. The chances of the patient suffering psychiatrically over a short period are statistically remote.

Owing to the possibility of a sudden lowering of renal clearance at these times, there may be a sudden and unexpected variance in the patient's serum lithium concentration. The dangers if this happens are high, whereas the dangers of stopping treatment for perhaps a week or so, are very small. Physical illnesses, including Addison's disease, heart failure, treatment with diuretics, usually contraindicate continued lithium treatment. Any condition accompanied by sweating or diarrhoea could give rise to potentially dangerous increases in the serum lithium concentration.

The combined use of diuretics and lithium is rather topical at the present time. As is now known, in a small population of patients on prophylactic lithium, polyuria and a diabetis insipidus like state occurs. Paradoxically a diuretic decreases the output of urine and the following case report (24) highlights the features of their combined use. The combined use of lithium and diuretics has been said to be contraindicated (25,26). The dangers of prescribing lithium salts and diuretics together have also been stressed (27). In 1973 Levy and his associates (28), warned of rising lithium levels as the volume of urine falls. Bearing in mind these dangers the following case shows the salient points in the successful combined use of lithium salts and diuretics.

The patient, now 64 years of age, has been on lithium for 12 years (previously she had over 25 attacks of either mania or depression in 9 years, with an increasing frequency of attacks). During 1975 she started to complain of polyuria and thirst. She was admitted to hospital in 1976 for the investigation and treatment of this. Her urinary frequency was day/night = 15-20/5-7 and she was psychiatrically stable. She was started on bendrofluazide 5 mg daily and Slow-K 600 mg b.d. The graph shows the relevant changes in her serum lithium during the following weeks, i.e., the serum lithium rose steadily to 1.7 mmol/l when the dose of lithium carbonate was reduced from 250 mg q.d.s. to b.d. Following this the levels showed a slow decline and the dose of lithium was appropriately increased. On day 28 she was on her former dose of lithium with a symptomatic improvement in her urinary frequency to day/night = 3-4/0-2. She has remained well on this medication; her urinary complaints have ceased and she rarely gets up at night.

This case suggests that the following points should be borne in mind. when using lithium with diuretics: Close laboratory control, probably as an in-patient, is needed; an immediate increase in the serum lithium concentration should be anticipated; and restabilisation may be at a lower dose or, as in this case, at the original dose.

3. Simultaneous administration of other medication. Apart from the

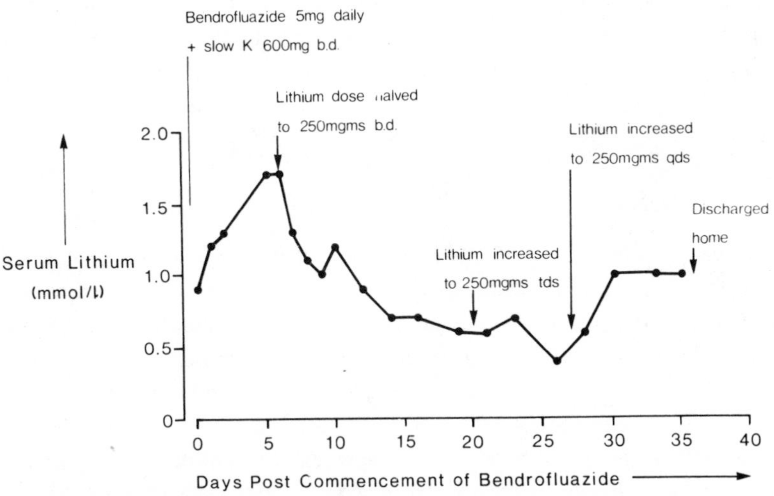

Figure 34.1. Serum lithium levels of a patient given concomitant bendrofluazide

emergency conditions described above, it seems that lithium is safe in combination with all drugs used by medical practitioners, enabling the use of lithium when there is a non-psychiatric illness needing medication. For general psychiatric management the patient should be encouraged to manage without any other psychotropic drugs — rather he should be helped with psychotherapeutic support during his adjustment to lithium.

4. The problems likely to occur when lithium is used during pregnancy have been dealt with comprehensively by Weinstein and Goldfield (26).

Travel undertaken during lithium treatment

Patients embarking on long journeys should be advised to keep to their dietary pattern. A proper fluid intake is important particularly when crossing time-zones.

Other factors

Patient factors are being most thoroughly covered in Chapter 35 but it is perhaps worth risking repetition to stress that general or localised climatic conditions may be very important.

Tropical climates and hot environments may lead to fluid and salt balance changes in patients who may lose both by sweating. In heavy industrial occupations, such as blast furnace work, the patient will be well advised to make sure that he maintains a normal diet. If a normal amount of salt is included in the food, a dietary supplement of salt tablets is unnecessary but it may be useful if mild lithium toxicity occasionally appears. It is more important to realise that frequent serum lithium monitoring in the early days of lithium prophylaxis tends to stabilise such workers at doses of lithium which are somewhat lower than average doses. In these cases alcohol intake should be restricted.

CONCLUSIONS

The value of lithium as a prophylactic against manic depressive illness has been established over a period of nearly 20 years. It is also often of value in the other conditions mentioned. It is still important to use adequate serum lithium monitoring combined with the continuing psychiatric support of both the patients and relatives, and this will increase the chances of a successful outcome of the treatment. Even though the mechanisms through which lithium treatment works are unknown, it does offer relief to many patients suffering from what would otherwise be crippling psychiatric illnesses.

References

1. Cade, J.F.J. (1949). *Med. J. Aust.,* **36**, 349
2. Schou, M. (1959). *Psychopharmacologia,* **1**, 65
3. Baastrup, P.C. and Schou, M. (1967). *Arch. Gen. Psychiat.,* **16**, 162
4. Schou, M. and Shaw, D.M. (1973). *Practitioner,* **210**, 105
5. Prien, R.F., Caffey, E.M. and Klett, C.J. (1972). *Br. J. Psychiat.,* **120**, 409
6. Allgen, L.G. (1969). *Acta Psychiat. Scand. Suppl.,* **207**, 98
7. Jephcott, G. and Kerry, R.J. (1974). *Br. J. Anaesth.,* **46**, 389
8. Kerry, R.J. (1968). *Br. Med. J.,* **4**, 187
9. Fry, D. E. and Marks, V. (1971). *Lancet,* **i**, 886
10. Johnson, F.N. (1975). *Lithium Research and Therapy.* (London; Academic Press)
11. Verghese, A., Indrani, N., Kuruvilla, K. and Hill, P.G. (1977). *Br. J. Psychiat.,* **130**, 148
12. Chick, J., Loudon, J. and Wilson, W. (1977). *Br. J. Psychiat.,* **130**, 524
13. Angst, J. and Weis, P. (1967). *Neuro-Psychopharmacology,* **129**, 703
14. Schou, M. (1968). *J. Psychiat. Res.,* **6**, 67
15. Levy, B.S. (1968). *J. Am. Med. Assoc.,* **206**, 1045
16. Misra, P.C. and Burns, B.H. (1977). *Acta Psychiat. Scand.,* **55**, 32
17. Serry, M. (1969). *Lancet,* **i**, 1267
18. Schou, M. (1973). (Personal communication.)
19. Persson, G. (1977). *Acta Psychiat. Scand.,* **55**, 208
20. Furlong, F.W. (1973). *Can. Psychiat. Assoc. J.,* **18**, 75
21. Kerry, R.J., Liebling, L.I. and Owen, G. (1970). *Acta Psychiat. Scand.,* **46**, 238
22. Polatin, P. and Fieve, R. (1971). *J. Am. Med. Assoc.,* **204**, 371
23. Manisto, P.T. and Saarnivaara, L. (1976). *Br. J. Anaesth.,* **48**, 185
24. Chambers, G., Kerry, R. J. and Owen, G. (1977). *Br. Med. J.* (in press)
25. Kerry, R. J. (1975). In: F.N. Johnson (ed.) *Lithium Research and Therapy,* pp. 143-163. (London: Academic Press)
26. Weinstein, M.R. and Goldfield, M.D. (1975). In: F.N. Johnson (ed.) *Lithium Research and Therapy,* pp. 237-264. (London: Academic Press)
27. Macneil, S., Hanson-Norty, E., Paschalis, C., Eastwood, P.R. and Jenner, F.A. (1975). *Lancet,* **i**, 1295
28. Levy, S.T., Forrest, J.N. (Jr.) and Meninger, M.D. (1963). *Am. J. Psychiat.,* **130**, 1014

35

Patient Factors Influencing Lithium Dosage

D. S. HEWICK

LITHIUM DOSAGE: ITS DEPENDENCE ON RENAL CLEARANCE

The lithium ion is not metabolised and therefore its pharmacokinetics are determined solely by the processes of absorption, distribution and excretion. With conventional lithium formulations the first two processes are not usually significant sources of inter-patient variation in dosage requirement. On the other hand, with sustained-release lithium preparations the possibility exists that inter-patient variation in the rate and extent of absorption could contribute to differences in the required loading and maintenance doses (1-3). Generally however, once therapeutic levels (0.7-1.3 mmol/l) have been obtained, the major factor influencing the dosage necessary to maintain the equilibrium state is the rate of excretion. Since lithium is excreted almost exclusively through the kidneys, the major determinant of dosage is renal lithium clearance.

RENAL LITHIUM CLEARANCE: THE INFLUENCE OF PHYSIOLOGICAL, PHARMACOLOGICAL AND PATHOLOGICAL FACTORS

The lithium ion is freely filtered through the glomerular membrane and normally about 80% is reabsorbed along with sodium and water in the proximal tubule. No further lithium reabsorption occurs in the more distal parts of the nephron and consequently lithium clearance (approximately 25 ml/min) is about 20% of the glomerular filtration rate. The clearance

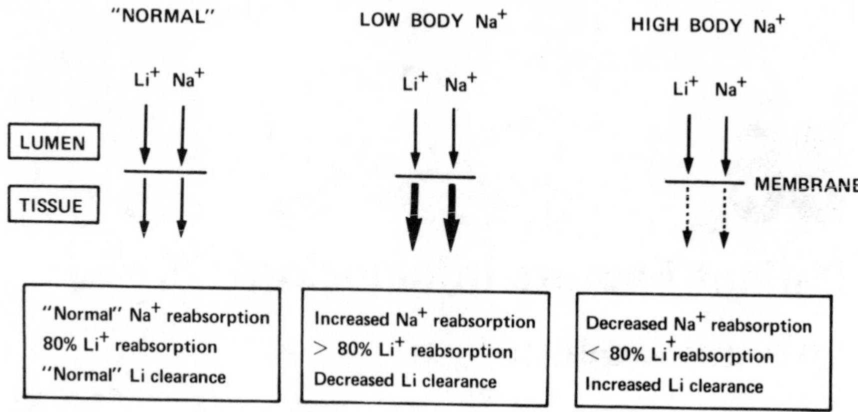

Figure 35.1. The influence of body sodium levels on Na^+/Li^+ reabsorption at the proximal tubule

therefore is governed by the glomerular filtration rate and the fraction of lithium reabsorbed in the proximal tubule. Under conditions of sodium deficiency increased lithium reabsorption occurs alongside the compensatory increase in proximal sodium reabsorption and conversely, when sodium levels are high, lithium reabsorption is decreased. Thus sodium balance is an important determinant of lithium clearance; low and high sodium levels reduce and increase lithium clearance respectively (4) (see Figure 35.1).

Although in many cases observed alterations in lithium clearance are probably due to changes in glomerular filtration rate and/or body sodium levels, there are some situations where the mechanism is unknown or has not been completely elucidated. In man in particular there is scope for further study on the factors that affect lithium excretion.

A number of physiological changes that alter lithium excretion have been demonstrated in rats by Smith (5-7). It was found that the rate of excretion was increased during the night (5) and on exposure to cold (6) but was decreased during strenuous exercise (7). The first of these changes was shown to be related to an altered glomerular filtration rate; the mechanisms for the other changes are not known. As far as the effect of strenuous exercise on lithium excretion is concerned it is difficult to extrapolate the findings in the rat to the human situation, since in man the possibility exists for lithium loss in the sweat (8). One of the few human studies relating physiological change to altered lithium pharmacokinetics was carried out by Schou and co-workers (9) who demonstrated that lithium clearance is increased during pregnancy and that this can be correlated with the increase in glomerular filtration rate that occurs during the second half of pregnancy. This knowledge is now of limited clinical value since it is generally accepted that lithium should not be taken during pregnancy due to the risk of teratogenesis. Variations in glomerular filtration rate also seem responsible for the changes in urinary lithium clearance associated with altered posture; a prompt fall in clearance occurs on changing from the recumbant to the upright position (10).

The critical role of sodium balance in lithium clearance was tragically demonstrated in the late 1940s by the fatalities occurring in patients on low salt diets given lithium chloride as a sodium chloride substitute (11). Lower lithium doses may be necessary in patients whose 'normal' salt intake is low (patients on 'slimming diets') and in those whose salt intake has been restricted as a therapeutic measure (patients with cardiovascular disease) (12). Altered sodium balance is also a major contributory factor in drug-induced changes in lithium pharmacokinetics. The drugs responsible are generally those that affect the sodium and/or lithium renal transport processes, with the most important group being the diuretics.

The effect a diuretic has on lithium clearance depends on its site of action within the nephron and the diuretic dosage regime. Many of the clinically-used diuretics (e.g. thiazides, frusemide, ethacrynic acid, mercurials, spironolactone) do not act on the proximal tubule, and therefore when given acutely have little effect on renal lithium reabsorption and clearance (4). However, as shown for the thiazides (13), prolonged diuretic therapy will decrease lithium clearance probably by reducing body sodium levels. A further study (14) has indicated that steady-state plasma lithium levels during chronic lithium therapy would rise by 25-30% if chlorothiazide therapy were given in addition. Himmelhoch *et al.* (15) have suggested that since thiazide diuretics are effective in treating nephrogenic diabetes insipidus, concurrent diuretic administration can be advantageous in patients with lithium-induced nephrogenic diabetes insipidus, providing a suitable lithium dosage reduction is made. These authors also noticed that patient mood control improved with the improvement of renal concentrating ability.

In contrast to the diuretics indicated above, those acting at the proximal tubule, such as urea and aminophylline will increase lithium excretion after single doses (4). However, part of the action of aminophylline could be due to its cardiostimulatory effect and a consequent increase in glomerular filtration rate. A similar mechanism involving cardiac stimulation may explain why adrenaline increases lithium clearance in rats (16).

Whether given acutely or chronically the mineralocorticoids have little effect on lithium excretion (17). The lack of an acute effect would be expected, since mineralocorticoids only act on the distal part of the nephron. The lack of a chronic effect (mediated through mineralocorticoid-induced sodium retention) may be due to the tendency of lithium to reduce the response of the distal part of the nephron to mineralocorticoids (18). No serious problems have been reported in the literature in patients receiving steroids in addition to lithium. In particular, there appears to be no interaction between lithium and the contraceptive pill (Schou, personal communication, 1976).

In line with the previous discussion, the main pathological interventions that alter renal lithium excretion are those that change the glomerular filtration rate and/or sodium balance. Thus a pathologically-induced reduction in lithium excretion may occur in cardiovascular and renal disease and in Addison's disease. On the basis of scattered clinical reports there is some indication that lithium clearance is also decreased during certain intercurrent infections such as influenza (19). Factors contributing to a possible reduced clearance in this case could be a decreased food (sodium) intake as well as increased salt loss if the illness were associated with vomiting and/or diarrhoea. After many years of controversy, the effect of manic episodes on lithium pharmacokinetics is still unresolved. Schou (20) considers that current evidence suggests a fall in steady-state plasma lithium levels occurring during manic attacks, possibly due to a short-lived increase in lithium clearance or a change in lithium distribution. An inevitable pathophysiological process and one that would be expected to alter lithium pharmacokinetics and present problems in patient management is ageing.

AGE AS A FACTOR IN LITHIUM THERAPY

It is generally assumed that elderly patients may require lower doses of lithium than their younger counterparts. Schou, in a number of review articles (8,19,21) has suggested that this is due to lower renal lithium clearances in the elderly. In support of this, Lehmann and Merten (22) comparing a small group of six 'middle-aged' patients (mean age 57.8 years) with 10 young subjects (mean age 25.2 years) reported a striking 60% decrease in renal lithium clearance in the older group. On the other hand, Fyrö and co-workers (23) in a study of 27 patients (aged 22-74 years) found no significant decrease in lithium cleance with age. In addition to this uncertainty over possible age-related changes in lithium pharmacokinetics there is virtually no information on lithium efficacy and lithium toxicity in the elderly compared with younger patients.

As a step towards clarifying the influence of patient age as a factor in routine lithium therapy, a preliminary study (24) was carried out at the Dundee lithium clinic. In this study information was extracted from the case notes of out-patients receiving lithium prophylaxis.

The 'Dundee study'

The case notes used in this study were from 82 patients who had been receiving the same dose of lithium for at least three months and had stable steady-state plasma lithium levels. The basic information used was age and weight of patient, lithium dosage, plasma lithium level, evidence of lithium side effects and clinical assessment; all of these were as recorded at the time of the last out-patient visit. Other information extracted was sex of patient, diagnosis, proprietary brand of lithium prescribed, other drugs prescribed. The clinical assessment had been recorded in the case notes according to the following rating; 0, no conspicuous affective disturbances; 1, mild mania or depression; 2, moderate mania or depression; 3, severe mania or depression.

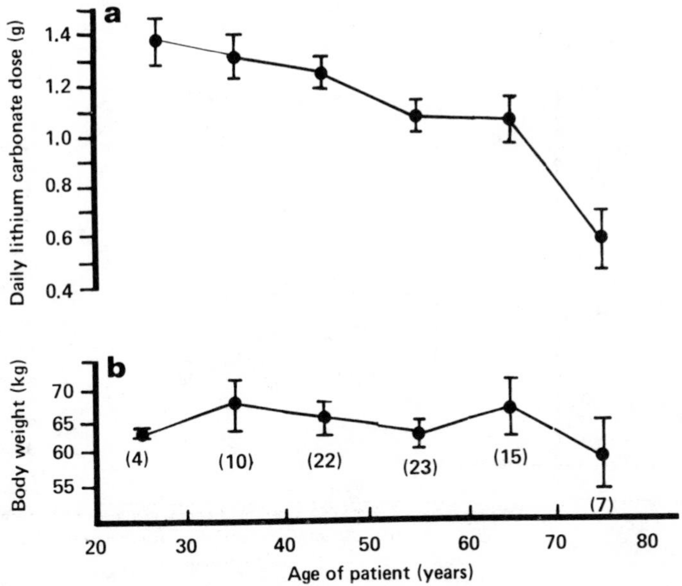

Figure 35.2. The relationship between lithium dosage and body weight versus age. The points are means of 10 year cohorts, the figures in parentheses giving the number of patients in each age group. The vertical bars indicate standard errors of the means. The data from one patient (aged 84 years) have been omitted

Changes in pharmacokinetics with age

As can be seen from Figure 35.2a the mean daily prescribed dose of lithium carbonate (in grams) fell by about 60% over the 20-80 year age range.

Since in this group of patients there was no marked decrease in body weight with increasing age (Figure 35.2b), the weight-related dose of lithium (mmol/kg) also fell significantly with increasing age (about a 50% decrease over the 20-80 year age range, (Figure 35.3a). There was however, a less marked decline in the corresponding steady-state plasma lithium levels; in fact the tendency for the levels to fall was seen only in the 7th and 8th decades (Figure 35.3b). To show more clearly that the age-related dosage reduction was not followed by a parallel decline in plasma levels,

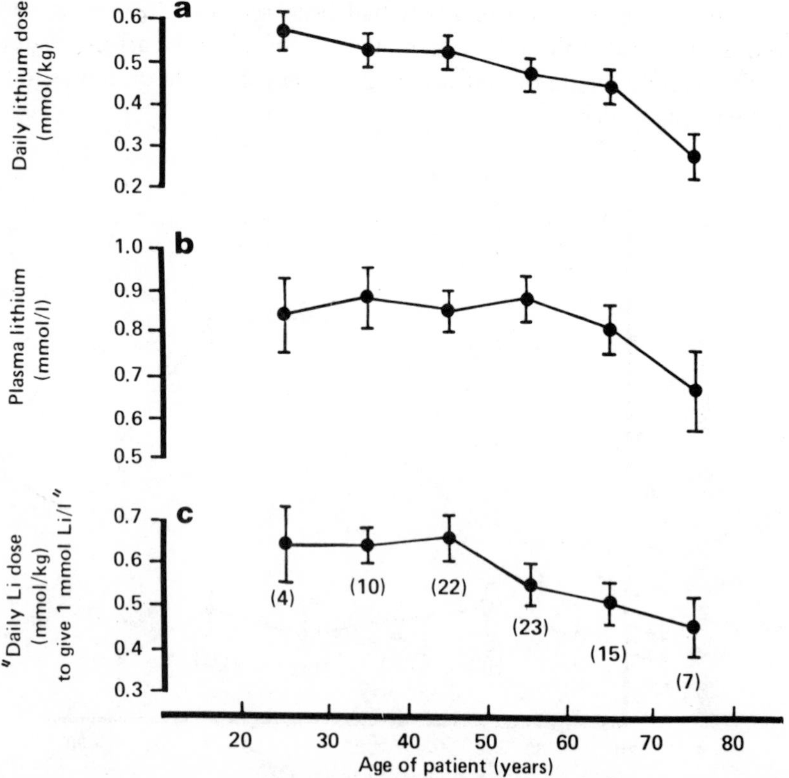

Figure 35.3. The relationship between the weight-related lithium dose and lithium steady-state plasma level versus age. The patient groups are identical to those in Figure 35.2. The data in (c) were obtained by dividing the weight-related doses by the corresponding plasma levels. The vertical bars indicate standard errors of the means. This Figure has already appeared in a modified form in the *British Journal of Clinical Pharmacology* (24)

these two variables were combined (dose divided by plasma level) to give a hypothetical lithium dose necessary to attain a plasma level of 1 mmol/l. This calculated dose remained constant over the third, fourth and fifth decades and then declined over the sixth, seventh and eighth decades (Figure 35.3c); it was about one-third lower in patients aged 70-79 years than in those aged 50 years.

The decline in the hypothetical dose required to give a steady-state plasma lithium level of 1 mmol/l in patients over 50 years of age is almost certainly due to an age-related deterioration in renal function, a lower lithium dose sufficing due to a lower lithium clearance. It is not unexpected that lithium excretion would be reduced in the elderly since an age-related decline in 'normal' renal function is well documented: for instance, a glomerular filtration rate and renal plasma flow fall by about 35% between the third and eighth decades, with the decline being most marked after the fifth decade (25). However, it must be borne in mind that the contribution of age to total inter-patient variation in lithium excretion is small. For instance, with the present data it was found that only about 14% of the total variance of the 'lithium dose required to give one mmol lithium/l' could be attributed to age. The large inter-individual variation in this parameter is probably due to the wide inter-individual variation in normal renal function (26) and lithium clearance (27).

Although the 82 patients were taking a wide variety of drugs in addition to lithium (e.g. other psychotropic drugs, hypnotics, thyroxine preparations) most of these were considered unlikely to significantly affect lithium pharmacokinetics. Only two patients were taking drugs that could have affected lithium handling; one (aged 58 years) was taking frusemide, the other (aged 43 years) was taking bendrofluazide. All patients were receiving lithium as the carbonate salt, mainly as Priadel (sustained release preparation) or Camcolit (conventional preparation). There was no clear association between age and the two main forms of lithium carbonate prescribed.

Possible increased susceptibility to lithium side effects in the elderly

Of the 36 patients under 50 years of age and the 46 patients of 50 years or over, the numbers with minor lithium side-effects (fine tremor of hands, polyuria, polydipsia, oedema, weight gain or diarrhoea) were 15 (42%) and 21 (46%) respectively. Thus at the time of the study the 'old' and 'young' groups had a similar incidence of minor lithium side effects. In no patient was there any indication of serious lithium toxicity (coarse tremor of hands, vomiting, dysarthria, vertigo, tinnitus). However, at out-patient visits prior to the time of this study, serious side effects (e.g. coarse tremor and marked unsteadiness) had been noted in some elderly patients. This had necessitated dosage reductions resulting in plasma levels at the lower end of the therapeutic range. These lower 'therapeutic' plasma lithium levels in some elderly patients probably account for the tendency for reduced mean steady-state plasma lithium levels in the seventh and eighth decades (Figure 35.3b).

Thus the dosage reduction in elderly patients may need to be greater than that required to compensate solely for age-related pharmacokinetic changes. The 'extra' dosage reduction may be required to reduce lithium side effects in the elderly patients to a level comparable to that acceptable in younger patients.

The clinical efficacy of lithium in the elderly

Of the patients under 50 years, 6 (16.6%) were not optimally controlled (clinical rating of greater than 0) while in the older group there were 13 (28%) such patients. The mean clinical rating for the younger group was 1.33 and 1.2 for the older group. However, it is not possible from these results to draw conclusions regarding the efficacy of lithium in young versus elderly patients for the following reasons. Firstly the steady-state plasma lithium levels were not comparable in the young and old groups; as indicated above the levels in the old group tended to be lower. Secondly the psychopathological profiles in the two groups were different. In the young and old groups respectively the diagnoses were: manic depression, 62% and 82%; recurrent unipolar depression, 19% and 9%. In the case of eleven patients the diagnoses were not clearly stated in the records.

Final comments on the 'Dundee study'

It must be remembered that the 82 patients used in this study were in effect the 'best' patients from the clinic, in that they attended regularly and had steady-state plasma lithium levels (indicating good drug compliance). There were about 40 patients recorded at the clinic who were not included in the study. Some of these patients never attended the clinic during the three month period of the investigation. This may have been due to a number of reasons such as, the patient may have moved away from Dundee, or may have become a psychiatric in-patient. Other reasons for not including a patient in the study were the patient having taken the last dose of lithium only a few hours before attending the clinic, and erratic plasma lithium levels. However, the fact that the mean age of the patients not included in the study (42.8 years) was significantly lower ($p < 0.005$, Student's t test) than that of the patients included in the study (51.6 years) indicates that old age as such was not a major factor influencing whether an out-patient was 'unreliable' or not.

The present investigation, which was essentially cross-sectional and retrospective in design, clearly indicates that patient age is a factor that must be considered during lithium therapy and that lithium dosage may need to be markedly reduced in old patients. It is obvious however, that more information is required particularly on the age-related incidence of lithium side-effects and the efficacy of lithium in elderly patients. To this end we are currently carrying out a detailed longitudinal prospective study at the Dundee lithium clinic.

References

1. Fyrö, B., Petterson, U. and Sedvall, G. (1970). *Pharmacol Clin.*, **2**, 236
2. Crammer, J., Rosser, R. and Crane, G. (1974). *Br. Med. J.* **3**, 650
3. Tyrer, S., Hullin, R., Birch, N. and Goodwin, J. (1976). *Psychol. Med.*, **6**, 51
4. Thomsen, K. and Schou, M. (1968). *Am. J. Physiol.*, **215**, 823
5. Smith, D.F. (1973). *Int. Pharmacopsychiat.*, **8**, 99
6. Smith, D.F. and de Jong, W. (1975). *Pharmakopsychiat. neuropsychopharmakol.*, **8**, 132
7. Smith, D.F. (1973). *Int. Pharmacopsychiat.*, **8**, 217
8. Schou, M. (1968). *J. Psychiat. Res.*, **6**, 67
9. Schou, M., Amdisen, A. and Steenstrup, O. (1973). *Br. Med. J.*, **2**, 137
10. Smith, D. and Shimizu, M. (1976). *Clin. Sci. Mol. Med.*, **51**, 103
11. Corcoran, A., Taylor, R. and Page, I. (1949). *J. Am. Med. Assoc.*, **139**, 685
12. Demers, R., Heninger, G. (1971). *Am. J. Psychiat.*, **128**, 100
13. Petersen, V., Hvidt, S., Thomsen, K. and Schou, M. (1974). *Br. Med. J.*, **3**, 143
14. Poust, R., Mallinger, A., Mallinger, J., Himmelhoch, J., Neil, J. and Hanin, I. (1976). *Psychopharmacol. Commun.*, **2**, 273
15. Himmelhoch, J., Forrest, J., Neil, J. and Detre, T. (1977). *Am. J. Psychiat.*, **134**, 149
16. Zvolsky, P. and Krulik, R. (1972). *Act. Nerv. Super.*, **14**, 207
17. Baer, L., Platman, S., Kassir, S. and Fieve, R. (1971). *J. Psychiat. Res.*, **8**, 91
18. Thomsen, K., Jensen, J. and Olesen, O.V. (1976). *J. Pharmacol. Exp. Ther.*, **196**, 463
19. Schou, M. (1973). In: Gershon, S. and Shopsin, B. (eds.) *Lithium: Its Role in Psychiatric Research and Treatment* pp. 189-199 (New York: Plenum Press Inc.)
20. Schou, M. (1976). *Ann. Rev. Pharmacol.*, **16**, 231
21. Schou, M. (1969). In: Cerletti, A. and Bove, F. (eds). *The Present Status of Psychotropic Drugs* pp 120-122 (Amsterdam: Excerpta Medica Foundation)
22. Lehmann, K. and Merten, K. (1974). *Int. J. Clin. Pharmacol. Biopharm.*, **10**, 292
23. Fyrö, B., Petterson, U. and Sedvall, G. (1973). *Acta Psychiat. Scand.*, **49**, 237
24. Hewick, D.S., Newbury, P., Hopwood, S., Naylor, G. and Moody, J. (1977). *Br. J. Clin. Pharmacol.*, **4**, 201
25. Davies, D. and Shock, N. (1950). *J. Clin. Invest.*, **29**, 496
26. Rowe, J., Andres, R., Tobin, J., Norris, A. and Shock, N. (1976). *J. Gerontol.*, **31**, 155
27. Fyrö, B. and Sedvall, G. (1975). In Johnson, F.N. (ed.) *Lithium Research and Therapy*, pp. 287-312 (London: Academic Press Ltd.)

36

Lithium Metabolism as a Guide to the Selection of Patients for Lithium Therapy

C. R. LEE and C. PASCHALIS

INTRODUCTION

Although lithium is often therapeutically effective within one or two weeks, its beneficial effects sometimes take longer to become apparent, especially when it is given as a prophylactic (1,2). Because of its relatively slow action, lithium is frequently supplemented in the early stages of treatment by other drugs, so that when an acute psychotic episode is over there may be some doubt whether lithium should be continued. Nosological criteria can be used to select a group of patients in which there would be relatively few treatment failures (1) but there are no satisfactory criteria for predicting the response in many cases where the diagnoses are not clear cut.

The need to control blood levels of lithium with an accuracy unprecedented in routine drug therapy drew attention to wide inter-individual variations in the distribution and excretion of lithium, and attempts have been made to relate differences in lithium metabolism to diagnosis, mood and response or lack of response to lithium.

Some methodological problems

Initial investigations were of lithium balance and renal clearance; more recently, efforts have been directed towards the distribution between cells and plasma. Although these two aspects will be considered separately, a number of methodological difficulties are common to both.

Firstly, as was recently pointed out by Naylor (3) and ourselves (4) it is difficult to distinguish between a remission due to lithium and spontaneous remission. A patient whose illness has been documented for only a short time is very likely to improve while given a placebo, thus it is not possible to designate a patient as a lithium responder unless there has been a long history of illness which has resisted other treatments. This is becoming more difficult nowadays, as lithium is sometimes the treatment of first choice.

An unequivocal response can sometimes be established by a relapse soon after withdrawal of lithium, but this is not often ethically possible except for the investigation of thyroid disorder, or diabetes insipidus. Sometimes patients provide their own evidence when they become careless about taking the tablets once they are well, but it is also possible that a patient who has relapsed might resume the full dosage for a few days before a blood sample is due to be taken, and thus present with a normal blood level. The effects of withdrawal are not always clear-cut. Two of our patients had well-documented histories of rapid mood swings which disappeared soon after lithium therapy was started. Lithium had to be withdrawn temporarily but one patient did not relapse for two years, and the other remains well after two and a half years.

Another problem is that psychoactive drugs may affect lithium metabolism. There seems to have been only one study (5) of the effect of a drug, chlorpromazine, but possible effects of other drugs must not be ruled out. Non-responders to lithium will inevitably need more of the other antipsychotic drugs, as well as ECT, than responders. Possible effects of under- and over-breathing and variations in activity have hardly been considered. Several workers have related lithium metabolism to the patients' mood at the time of study. This is a source of difficulty in devising a predictive test as the number of possible variables is increased.

Excretion and balance studies

Normal humans excrete ingested lithium almost quantitatively in the urine (6,7). Many workers have attempted to account for the inter-individual differences in plasma concentration produced by the same dose in terms of differences in kinetics of renal elimination. The results will be briefly summarised here, as the subject has been well reviewed by Fyrö and Sedvall (8). In normal volunteers and normothymic patients, lithium clearance is negatively correlated with plasma concentration strongly enough to account for the observed variability. Most interest has centred around changes in lithium excretion between psychotic and normothymic states. There are persistent reports (1,2) that manic patients require extremely large doses to achieve therapeutically effective plasma concentrations and that the dosage must be reduced when the mania has subsided. Paradoxically, some patients excrete abnormally small amounts of lithium in their urine. Serry (9) found that 70% of manic patients and 75% of depressed patients, but only 7% of normal controls, excreted less than 12 mg of lithium within 4 h of taking orally 1200 mg of the carbonate. When the patients had recovered, repeat tests gave normal results. Most of the 'lithium retainers' were said to be good responders to the drug and this test has been proposed as a means of predicting lithium responders. Several other workers have shown a negative lithium balance (as measured by urinary excretion) during mania, but there are some conflicting reports. Fyrö and Sedvall (8) emphasize the methodological inadequacies of most of the studies. The most serious problems are the use of psychotropic drugs and the need to control dietary intake of electrolytes, particularly sodium. It has been known for many years (10) that lithium clearance can be reduced by reducing the sodium intake and even in a metabolic clinic it is very difficult to ensure a reasonably constant diet. These objections would not seem to apply to a particularly well-controlled longitudinal study by Hullin *et al.* (6). The patients received a constant dietary intake of sodium and potassium and were given lithium while manic. All the patients excreted a smaller percentage of the ingested dose than a group of ten normal controls.

Although the experimental difficulties preclude the use of this type of test for routine screening of patients being considered for lithium therapy, these results nevertheless indicate an abnormality in manic patients which is reflected in their metabolism of lithium. The main interpretational problem, which also applies to another more limited study by Greenspan *et al.* (11), is to account for the accumulation of large amounts of lithium without a concomitant rise in plasma concentration. Hullin *et al.* (6) provide evidence that some may be stored in bone but it may be that in manic patients extra-renal routes of excretion are significant.

Studies of intracellular lithium

Following a suggestion by Maggs (12) lithium uptake by erythrocytes has been investigated by several workers in the hope that this might provide a measure of intracellular lithium generally. The most obvious reason for using erythrocytes is accessibility, but equally obviously they are poor models for excitable cells (13). However, this relatively uncomplicated type of cell, in which cation movements are slow, has been very convenient for study of the basic mechanisms of ion transporting systems. Until very recently the factors controlling lithium distribution were unknown so that nearly all the clinical investigations to-date were carried out in ignorance of them. If transfer were purely passive the intracellular concentration Li(in) would at equilibrium be greater than or equal to the plasma concentration Li(out) (14,15). For erythrocytes the ratio Li(in)/Li(out) is almost invariably less than unity (we have observed steady-state ratios greater than unity in a few patients, who were all receiving psychotropic drugs in addition to lithium), which implies an active uphill transport process. Very recently, a counter-current exchange process has been discovered (16,17), in which energy for the extrusion of lithium from the erythrocyte is provided by downhill flow of sodium from the plasma. For a discussion of the mechanistic factors controlling the erythrocyte-plasma lithium ratio, see the papers by Greil and his colleagues (14,18) and Chapter 41.

Mendels and Frazer (19) described the first controlled clinical study of lithium distribution between plasma and erythrocytes. This was a short-term (28 days) investigation of the effect of lithium on patients in the depressed phase of bipolar manic-depressive illness or recurrent unipolar depressive illness, as part of the extensive work on the nosology of depression being carried out by Mendels and his collaborators. A group of 13 patients who satisfied the criteria for the so-called Endogenous-Reactive Factor (20) and who had a score of at least 16 on the Hamilton Depressive Rating Scale were selected. Very seriously disturbed patients who could not take a reasonably well-controlled diet, or who required medication, were not included. (It is very interesting that few of the conflicting reports by other workers state explicitly that drugs were not administered). Of the 13 subjects (4 unipolar depressives, 9 bipolar) 7 showed substantial improvement within 28 days as measured by objective rating methods. The erythrocyte/plasma lithium ratios of the responders (0.56 ± 0.03 SEM) were higher than those of the non-responders (0.39 ± 0.02) (6–15 observations per subject). This difference was significant by the 7th day of treatment. Only one of the unipolar depressives responded. There is the posibility, acknowledged by the authors, that in a fairly short-term study a proportion of patients may improve as a result of a placebo effect, or a natural remission, but the careful selection to exclude patients with hysterical symptoms would be expected to minimize the possibility of a placebo effect, and such a high proportion of natural remissions seems unlikely. Nevertheless the subjects who recovered had markedly higher lithium ratios than those who did not.

Essentially similar results were obtained by Mendels' group in a long-term study (21) of the prophylactic effect of lithium in 31 patients with recurrent affective disorders. Unfortunately, it is not possible to withhold other drugs for long periods from non-responders to lithium, and it is not clear from this report whether the ratios for this group might have been affected by drugs.

Lithium-responders tend to have relatively high erythrocyte sodium levels before treatment and lithium caused the levels to rise still further (22), suggesting the possibility that the high ratios found in this group of patients could be due to abnormally low activity of the sodium countercurrent transport system. There is some evidence that (Na-K)-ATPase activity is slightly lower than normal in untreated patients with affective disorders and increased by treatment with lithium (23-25). The effect of altered (Na-K)-ATPase activity on lithium distribution would be difficult to predict; on the one hand, increased activity would lead to increased Li influx, but on the other, a decrease in intracellular Na causes increased efflux. Measurements of erythrocyte Na-K-ATPase must be interpreted with care, especially when attempts are made to obtain correlations with changes in clinical state, because erythrocytes survive for several months and they do not carry out protein synthesis. Naylor *et al.* (24) suggest that the enzyme may be regulated by a circulating factor, but Hesketh (25) considered that such a factor would be removed by the extensive washing of the *in vitro* preparations and suggested that the effect of lithium occurs during cell development. Recently, though, it has been shown that the increase in ATP-ase activity during lithium therapy occurs within 3 weeks of starting treatment (23). It was thought that the effect could be due to a relatively long-term alteration of the ATP-ase conformation, but it seems probable that washing would not remove a lipophilic steroid, for example, especially if it were bound to specific sites. Any irreversible effect of lithium, or of any other treatment, or a patient's clinical state on the erythrocyte might possibly account for some of the discrepancies in the literature, since it would persit for several months. In this context, it is worth noting reports (see later) that the erythrocyte/plasma lithium ratio appears gradually to increase for several months.

Other studies on lithium in erythrocytes

The paper by Mendels and Frazer (19) has aroused a great deal of controversy. It is difficult to make a critical review of the literature because most workers gave other drugs, at least to their 'non-responders'.

Attempts to distinguish responders from non-responders

A group from Milan (26,27) selected 50 patients with unipolar recurrent depressive and bipolar manic-depressive disorders by the criteria of Mendels and Frazer (19). Non-responders were identified by the use of a self-rating scale evaluated monthly for periods of 2-4 years, or by relapse requiring admission to hospital and/or high doses of drugs. Some of the patients classed as responders required low doses of additional psychotropic drugs. Preliminary results after one year were equivocal (26) but after a 2-4 year follow-up it was clear that the patients who relapsed had lower ratios (27). There was no difference between the results for unipolar and bipolar patients.

Casper *et al.* (28) studied 16 patients diagnosed as suffering from 'primary' affective disease or schizo-affective disease by the research diagnostic criteria of Spitzer *et al.* (29). The 7 responders (identified by good or excellent response to lithium, discharge from hospital without the need for other drugs, and successful maintenance for at least 6 months) had an average lithium ratio of 0.56 ± 0.04 (SEM), while the 9 non-responders had a ratio of 0.34 ± 0.05. The non-responders needed additional medication but it is not clear whether or not they were drug free when the lithium ratios were measured.

Lyttkens *et al.* (30) found a large difference between the ratios for healthy females (0.39 ± 0.03 SEM, n = 8) and manic-depressive females (0.50 ± 0.04, n = 23). The average ratio for manic-depressive males (0·38 ± 0.04, n = 14) was the same as that for the female controls, but their brief communication gives no information on the diagnostic criteria, whether drugs were used, or how many patients responded to lithium. A similar difference between males and females was found in a 12 month trial by Rybakowski and Strzyewski (31) of lithium prophylaxis in 14 male and 31 female patients with bipolar manic-depressive psychosis, but when sex difference was taken into account these workers found no difference between responders and non-responders. Patients classed as responders did not require additional medication or hospital admission for the 12 month period. Presumably the non-responders were given additional drugs. Other workers either found no such difference due to sex (27) or did not report any.

Mendlewicz and Verbanck, in a preliminary report (32), state that a homogeneous group of manic-depressive twins had a positive relationship between lithium ratio and long-term response, but the relationship disappeared in a more extended study of 42 pairs. However, the ratios of the responders had a smaller variance than those of the non-responders.

This study was carried out while the patients had been drug-free for 8 days.

There is strong evidence from studies on mono- and dizygotic twins that the lithium ratio in psychiatrically normal people is genetically determined (33). This result is of interest because there seems to be an hereditary element in bipolar manic depressive disease distinguishing it from unipolar depressions (34). Apart from the results of Lyttkens *et al.* (30) mentioned earlier, Mendels *et al.* (34) find a tendency for patients who are responders, and hence have high ratios, to be bipolar rather than unipolar. Elizur *et al.* (35) found no significant difference between drug-free patients in remission and a schizophrenic control subject. Demisch and Bochnik (36) could find no correlations with diagnosis when ratios were measured while the patients were in remission. The use of other drugs was not mentioned in this study. Albrecht and Müller-Oerlinghausen (37) in a study of depressed outpatients (who were receiving antidepressant drugs) found the same average ratio in bipolar and unipolar disorders.

Intra-individual variations in the lithium ratio

A number of conflicting reports suggest that the lithium ratio depends on the clinical state of the patient at the time the blood sample is taken. Elizur *et al.*, in the first study of this type (35), found that ratios were lower than usual in bipolar patients who were manic or depressed, with a tendency to increase during remission. Patients with recurrent depressive illness had higher ratios than normal in the depressed phase. All the ratios measured in this study were low compared to those found in responders by other workers (see later). This might have been due to the rather low average plasma levels, or possibly to the fact that the subjects were outpatients, and therefore probably not as seriously ill as those studied by others.

Other reports, in none of which the patients were stated to be drug-free, suggest that the ratio falls (38), rises (36) or does not change (39) during manic relapses. A fall in ratio could be due to the use of additional psychotropic drugs (37).

Rybakowski *et al.* (39) reported a positive correlation between the average lithium ratios of 37 patients and the corresponding average plasma concentrations. Lee *et al.* (40) found that the ratio increased with plasma level in five out of twelve acutely ill patients and decreased in two. There was only a slight positive correlation in some of the patients of Mendels and his colleagues (41), at least after the first week of treatment. This discrepancy will be discussed in the next section.

RECENT RESULTS FROM THIS UNIT

Introduction and methods

Research in this unit has been centred on the study of the predictably recurring psychoses, with a view to detecting periodic metabolic changes which might be associated with the course of an illness (42). Patients are referred to us by clinicians from various parts of the country, usually because of failure to respond to many years of conventional treatment, including, in some cases, moderate doses of lithium. They have in common a very severe affective or schizoaffective disorder whose periodicity is sufficiently marked in the environment of a general psychiatric ward to attract attention.

The study took place in a metabolic ward (Northfield Clinic, Middlewood Hospital) where facilities for extensive medical and nursing observation are provided. Constant dietary electrolyte intake is usually achieved (except in the most extreme mood states) by close supervision. All the patients spent sufficient time on the ward as inpatients for their clinical state to be assessed by several routine methods. Behaviour was monitored 6-hourly by experienced nurses using three-point charts for mood, speech and activity, and also by detailed written description. The activity of some patients who were able to co-operate was also recorded by a pedometer. The rating scores made by the nurse in charge correlated well with scores produced independently by other nurses, and with the pedometer readings. Ratings for a manic-depressive patient who did not respond to lithium are shown in Figure 36.1.

For each patient the average number of days in each mood state seems to be constant over a long period although the relative number of manic, depressed and normothymic days varies between individuals. Symptomatic treatment with large doses of drugs during severe manic episodes does not affect the overall course of the illness.

A total of 27 patients took part in the study of erythrocyte lithium; including the 12 reported previously, and a patient with a precise 48-hour cycle (43). Three of these were found after observation not to have affective or schizoaffective disorders. Of the remaining 24, 18 were female and 6 male. Two (1 male, 1 female) were periodic catatonic schizophrenics with pronounced mood swings and only 3 (1 male, 2 female) were unipolar depressives. One of the unipolar patients has a family history of manic-depressive disorder; he would probably be classed by Mendels and colleagues (34) as bipolar.

Comprehensive records like the case in Figure 36.1. were not obtained

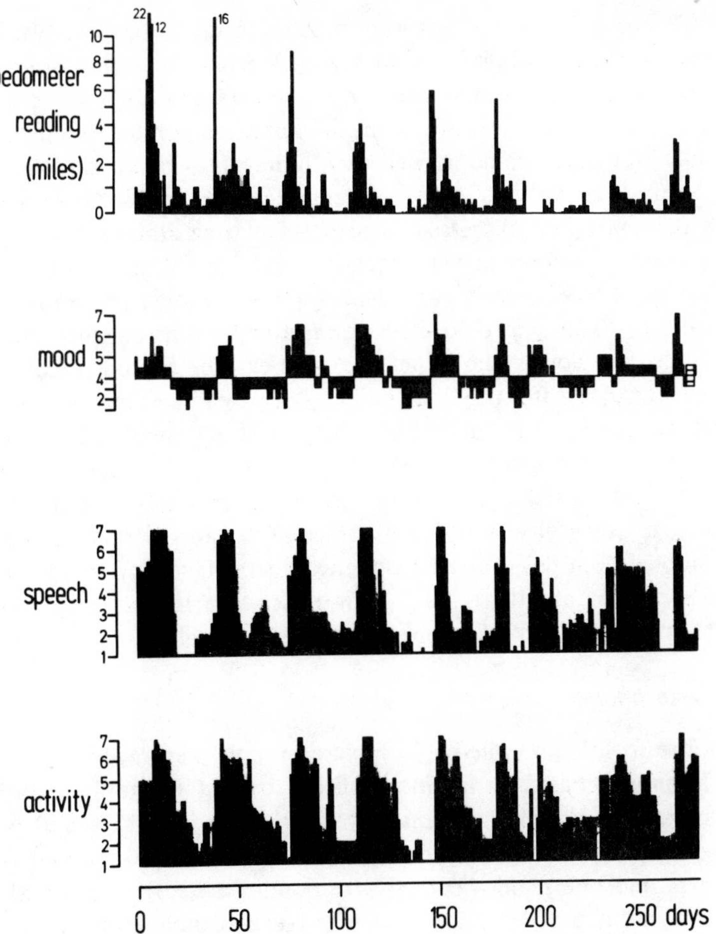

Figure 36.1. Comparison of nurses' ratings with activity recorded by a pedometer for a manic depressive patient

for all the patients, because most (18 out of 24) eventually responded well to prolonged treatment with lithium, usually at higher than usual plasma levels, and supplemented by other drugs. Somewhat lower plasma levels seem adequate for prophylaxis.

Results

Dependence of lithium ratio on plasma level

Initial studies of lithium distribution between plasma and erythrocytes revealed in some patients a strong dependence of the ratio on the plasma level (40). These determinations were made during the first few weeks of treatment. Recently, 12 patients, including 4 from the earlier study (40) agreed to reduce their lithium intake for a few days in order to alter their plasma concentrations. All are living at home on lithium maintenance; three take tranylcypromine as well as lithium. Two blood samples were taken from each patient. The quotients (change in ratio)/(change in plasma concentration) expressed as per mM plasma-lithium ranged from zero to 0·39, in agreement with Mendels and his colleagues (41), apart from two drug-free patients (who had not been studied previously) who had values of -0·59 and -0·20. The results for the four patients who had been studied previously show that the quotient for an individual varies from year to year. After the first few weeks of treatment the lithium ratio in most patients is not sufficiently influenced by small differences in plasma level to affect the interpretations which will be proposed later in this paper, but unless measurements are made at similar plasma levels, some patients may give misleading values. The ratio is said to stabilise within about seven days, apart from the general tendency to rise slowly over a period of months (22,28). Our experience is that with severely disturbed patients it can take somewhat longer to stabilise.

Response to lithium

A response to lithium, whether complete or not, was easily determined from the mood charts. In addition, all but two of the responders have been discharged, usually after many years (in one case 15 years) of illness, whereas the non-responders have not. One of the schizoaffective responders and one manic-depressive responder are given haloperidol in addition to lithium. One unipolar depressive and three manic-depressive patients who responded continue to take tranylcypromine. It was possible to obtain single blood samples from 12 responders and two non-responders after they had been taking lithium for at least 6 weeks but were otherwise drug free for a month (eight of the responders had been drug free for more than 6 months). The erythrocyte-plasma ratios for these patients, and the most recent values for patients who were also taking tranylcypromine and haloperidol are shown in Figure 36.2.

Interpretation is difficult when additional drugs were given. Tranylcypromine was used in some cases where the illness was predominantly depressive, and haloperidol where mania was predominant; thus these patients may not have been typical of the group as a whole. The three non-responders taking haloperidol were manic at the time of observation, but previous measurements showed no significant changes with respect to mood. In common with other workers we do not have a large group of drug-free non-responders, but it is clear that they cannot be distinguished from responders by their lithium ratios. The average ratio for all the drug-free patients was 0.63 ± 0.03 (SEM).

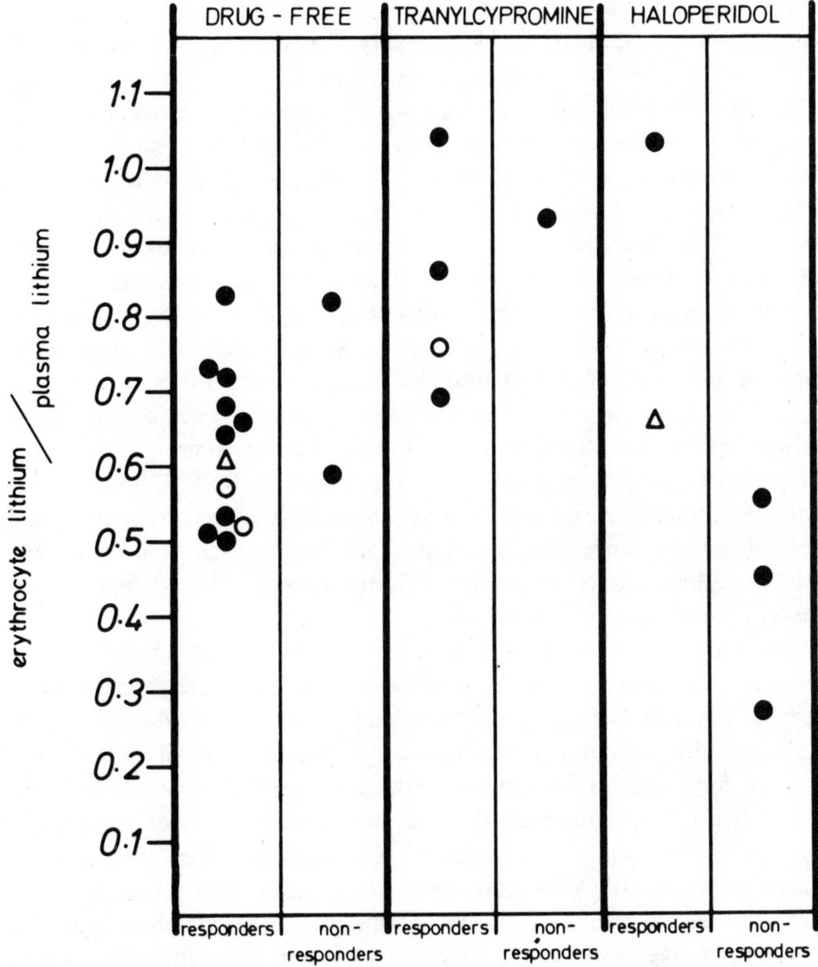

Figure 36.2. Erythrocyte-plasma lithium ratios for 24 patients
● Bipolar manic depressive
O Unipolar depressive
△ Periodic catatonic

DISCUSSION

In this study, it was not possible to distinguish responders to lithium from non-responders by means of their erythrocyte to plasma lithium ratios. However the average ratio for all our drug-free patients was, within experimental error, the same as that found for responders by other investigators. Results obtained by various workers from subjects who were said not to be taking psychotropic drugs other than lithium are summarized in the table. Strictly speaking, the average ratios are not comparable, as the values for each subject are means of differing numbers of samples, but this is not a serious problem as the variances are fairly small.

Patients classed as responders have with few exceptions markedly higher ratios than the normal controls. It is unlikely that the relatively short duration of treatment of the controls (1-2 weeks) could account for such a large difference, although a further longer-term experiment would be desirable. The only drug-free non-responders on whom data has been published are those of Mendels and Frazer (19). The average ratio for these six patients (0.39) was little higher than that of normals, whereas the ratio for our non-responders (0.7) was indistinguishable from that of the responders. We are confident that these two patients are bipolar manic-depressives, since they have been studied for many cycles of the illness (Figure 36.1), all attempts at treatment having been unsuccessful. Furthermore, both have been given prolonged trials of lithium in the metabolic clinic. The high ratio group cannot be predicted from the qualitative diagnosis, since Mendels and Frazer's group of non-responders with low ratios included a number of bipolar patients (19), whereas all our bipolar patients had high ratios. However, the subjects of these two studies were selected by different criteria: Mendels and Frazer (19) excluded patients who were too ill to co-operate, whereas our patients were referred to us because they had been unusually difficult to treat. Unfortunately, it is rarely ethically justifiable to withhold drugs from severely ill patients who have not responded to lithium. This ethical problem does not arise in the case of two of our non-responders, as the administration of remarkably large doses of major tranquillizers (for example over 100 mg/d of haloperidol) has little effect on their clinical state. This difficulty could have affected the results of two recent studies (31,44) which revealed no difference between responders and non-responders. Nevertheless, in agreement with our findings, all the groups of patients had fairly high ratios.

The data in Table 36.1 tend to support the hypothesis (19) that there exists a sub-group of patients with affective and schizoaffective disease who produce abnormally high erythrocyte-plasma ratios. According to our

Table 36.1. Distribution of lithium between erythrocytes and plasma of drug-free subjects.

	Erythrocyte Li × 100 ÷ plasma Li*	Sex	Diagnosis**	Ref.
	56 ± 4(3-6, 7)	-	'Primary affective and schizoaffective'	28
	56 ± 3(8-15, 8)	-	7BP, 1UP	19
	66 ± 3(-, 16)	-	'Recurrent depression and/or mania'	20
'Responders'	60 ± 3(5-20, 19)	F	BP	31
	45 ± 2(5-20, 6)	M	BP	31
	50 ± 4(1, 22)	13F, 9M	UP	44
	56 ± 5(1, 10)	8F, 2M	BP	44
	42 ± 7(1, 4)	2F, 2M	PC	44
	63 ± 2(1, 12)	9F, 3M	9BP, 2UP, 1PC	This paper
'Non-responders'	39 ± 2(6-12, 6)	-	3BP, 3UP	19
	70 (1, 2)	F	BP	This paper
Normal controls	39 ± 3(-, 8)	F		30
	28 ± 6(1, 9)	M		33***
	33 ± 2(5-6, 3)	M		20

* Mean ± SEM (number of samples per subject, number of subjects).
** BP = bipolar manic depressive, UP = recurrent depressive, PC = periodic catatonic
*** Values after 8 days' treatment for the first of each of 9 pairs of twins. The mean for 8 of the corresponding siblings was the same (30 ± 2), but the data should not be pooled as the subjects are not independent.

findings, this sub-group contains a very large proportion of those patients with severe affective disorder who exhibit fairly regular mood swings while under close observation in the stable environment of a metabolic clinic. Most, but not all, patients with high ratios respond to lithium, although in severe cases it may be difficult to maintain an adequate lithium intake for long enough to elicit a response, without close nursing supervision.

Suggestions that female manic depressives have higher ratios than male manic depressives (30,31) have not been supported by all other workers. The preponderance of females in our study is interesting, although we are aware that the patients were not randomly selected. There is general agreement that a smaller proportion of unipolar depressives than of manic depressives respond to lithium. The mood cycles of patients referred to us with a diagnosis of recurrent depression are rarely as regular and predictable as those of bipolar patients. Those who do have regular rhythms sometimes present episodes of slightly hypomanic behaviour which might be unnoticed in a different environment. From our observation of bipolar patients with regular cycles, a change of environment can disturb the cycles for a long period, and this may obscure the true clinical picture. It is possible that further studies on lithium metabolism might help to differentiate sub-groups among patients with endogenous depressive illness.

The lithium ratio seems to be under genetic control, at least in normals (33). The findings on drug-free patients described here invite comparison with the results of genetic studies, which indicate a strong hereditary element in a significant proportion of cases of bipolar manic depressive disorder. Of particular interest is the recent discovery of a possible genetic marker in about 30% of manic depressives (45).

CONCLUSIONS

Evidence from input-output studies, and studies of lithium distribution across the red cell membrane suggests that certain patients with affective or schizoaffective disorders may have abnormal lithium metabolism, which could be genetically determined. There is a great deal of disagreement in the literature, which seems to be due to the large number of variable factors which could be involved. These include the diagnosis and severity of illness, the clinical state at the time of investigation, variations in diet, and the use of drugs. The last two factors alone would render predictive tests unreliable except possibly in mild cases when control is possible. However, there is the prospect that work in this field may be useful in studies of the nosology of the affective disorders.

ACKNOWLEDGEMENTS

We are grateful to the nursing staff for their work during this study, and to Miss S.E. Hill and Mr G. Jennings for technical assistance. We also thank Professor F.A. Jenner and Dr R.J. Pollitt for reviewing the manuscript.

References

1. Schou, M. (1968). *J. Psychiat. Res.,* 6, 67
2. Kerry, R.J. (1975). In: F.N. Johnson (ed.) *Lithium Research and Therapy*. pp. *143-163* (London: Academic Press)
3. Naylor, G. (1976). *Lancet* ii, 749
4. Jenner, F.A. and Lee, C.R. (1976). *Lancet,* ii, 641
5. Sletten, I. *et al.* (1966). *Curr. Ther. Res.,* 8, 441
6. Hullin, R.P., MaDonald, R. and Dransfield, G.A. (1968). In: Ibor, J.J. Lopez (ed.) *Proc. 4th World Congr. Psychiat.* 1966 pp. 1900-1903. (Amsterdam: Excerpta Medica Foundation)

7. Kent, N.L. and McCance, R.A. (1941). *Biochem. J.*, **35**, 837
8. Fyrö, B. and Sedvall, G. (1975). In: F.N. Johnson (ed.) *Lithium Research and Therapy* pp. 287-312 (London: Academic Press)
9. Serry, M. (1969). *Aust. N.Z. J. Psychiat.*, **3**, 390
10. Talso, P.J. and Clarke, R.W. (1951). *Am. J. Physiol.*, **166**, 202
11. Greenspan, K., Goodwin, F.K. and Bunney, W.E. (1968). *Arch. Gen. Psychiat.*, **19**, 664
12. Maggs, R. (1968). In: Ibor, J.J. Lopez (ed.) *Proc. 4th World Congr. Psychiat. 1966* pp. 2211-2214 (Amsterdam: Excerpta Medica Foundation)
13. Richelson, E. (1977). *Science,* **196**, 1001
14. Duhm, J. and Becker, B.F. (1977). *Pflügers Arch.*, **367**, 211
15. Thomas, R.C., Simon, W. and Oehme, M. (1975). *Nature,* **258**, 754
16. Greil, von W., Eisenried, F. and Duhm, J. (1976). *Arzneim.-Forsch.*, **26**, 1147
17. Haas, M., Schooler, J., Tosteson, D.C. (1975). *Nature,* **258**, 425
18. Duhm, J. and Becker, B.F. (1977). *Pflügers Arch.*, **368**, 203
19. Mendels, J. and Frazer, A. (1973). *J. Psychiat. Res.*, **10**, 9
20. Mendels, J. and Cochrane, C. (1968). *Am. J. Psychiat.*, **124**, 1
21. Mendels, J. *et al.* (1976). *Lancet,* **i**, 966
22. Mendels, J. and Frazer, A. (1974). *Am. J. Psychiat.*, **131**, 1240
23. Hokin-Neaverson, M., Burckhardt, W.A. and Jefferson, J.W. (1976). *Res. Com. Chem. Path. Pharmacol.*, **14**, 117
24. Naylor, G.J., Dick, D.A.T. and Dick, E.G. (1976). *Psychol. Med.*, **6**, 257
25. Hesketh, J.E. (1976). *Biochem. Soc. Trans.*, **4**, 328
26. Cazzullo, C.L. *et al.* (1975). *Br. J. Psychiat.*, **126**, 298
27. Sacchetti, E. *et al.* (1977). *Lancet,* **i**, 908
28. Casper, R.C. *et al.* (1976). *Lancet,* **ii**, 418
29. Spitzer, R.L. *et al.* (1975). In: A. Sudilovsky, S. Gershon and B. Beer (eds.) *Predictability in Psychopharmacology: Preclinical and Clinical Correlations,* pp. 1-47 (New York: Raven Press)
30. Lyttkens, L., Soderberg, U. and Wetterberg, L. (1973). *Lancet,* **i**, 40
31. Rybakowski, J. and Strzyzewski, W. (1976). *Lancet,* **ii**, 1408
32. Mendelwicz, J. and Verbanck, P. (1977). *Lancet,* **i**, *41*
32. Dorus, E., Pandey, G.N. and Davis, J.M. (1975). *Arch. Gen. Psychiat.*, **32**, 1097
34. Mendels, J., Stern, S. and Frazer, A. (1976). *Dis. Nerv. Syst.*, **37**, 3
35. Elizur, A. *et al.* (1973). *Clin. Pharmacol. Ther.*, **13**, 947
36. Demisch, von L. and Bochnik, H.J. (1976). *Arzneim.-Forsch.*, **26**, 1149
37. Albrecht, von J. and Müller-Oerlinghausen, B. (1976). *Arzneim.-Forsch.*, **26**, 1145
38. Soucek, K. *et al.* (1974). *Activ., Nerv. Sup.*, **16**, 193
39. Rybakowski, J. *et al.* (1974). *Int Pharmacopsychiat.*, **9**, 166
40. Lee, C.R. *et al.* (1975). *Br. J. Psychiat.*, **127**, 596
41. Brunswick, D., Frazer, A. and Mendels, J. (1977). *Lancet,* **i**, 41
42. Lee, C.R. and Pollitt, R.J. (1974). In: A. Frigerio and N. Castagnoli (eds.) *Mass Spectrometry in Biochemistry and Medicine,* pp. 365-371 (New York: Raven Press)
43. Hanna, S.M. *et al.* (1972). *Br. J. Psychiat.*, **121**, 271
44. Knorring, L. *et al.* (1976). *Pharmakopsychiat.*, **9**, 81
45. Arnold, von O.H. (1976). *Arzneim.-Forsch.*, **26**, 1178

37

Serum Concentrations of Lithium after Three Proprietary Preparations of Lithium Carbonate

E. H. BENNIE and R. CHALMERS

INTRODUCTION

A number of investigations (1-5) have been carried out to monitor the fluctuations in serum lithium which occur in relation to dosing. The first experiments (6) showed that serum lithium was not at a constant level throughout, but tended to increase following gastric ingestion or oral lithium medication, and to subside following renal excretion. The precise shape and height of the lithium curve depends on gastric emptying which can be slowed with propantheline or speeded with metochlopramide (7).

Patient compliance on long term oral medication has been shown to be an important factor in determining the outcome of treatment and the fewer the number of doses to be taken each day the more likely is the patient to adhere to the prescribed regime (8). Lithium tablets given in small divided daily doses have been found to give serum levels from 0.6 to 1.3 mmol/l (6) and we have shown previously that a single dose of sustained release lithium can maintain the serum lithium from 0.6 to 1.2 mmol/l over a 24-hour inter-dose interval in those patients who have been on lithium for several weeks (2).

The objective of the present investigation was to examine the pattern of serum lithium over 24 hours in patients starting lithium and in those patients who had been on lithium for at least 2 weeks. Three lithium products were tested and two types of regimes examined. Although the emphasis of the study is on the blood lithium levels, in eight instances urine lithium findings are included.

METHODS AND PATIENTS

Camcolit contains 6.8 mmol of lithium carbonate in each tablet. Camcolit 400 contains 10.8 mmol of lithium. Each tablet of sustained release preparation Priadel contains 10.8 mmol and Phasal, a controlled release tablet, contains 8.1 mmol of lithium. Eight volunteers and seventeen male patients at Leverndale Hospital, Glasgow, gave informed consent to the study. Eleven patients selected for the study were suffering from schizo-affective psychosis and six from alcoholism. Six patients were examined following their first dose of 1200 mg lithium carbonate, three being given Priadel and three Camcolit 400. Fourteen experiments have been conducted on a variety of initial doses of lithium carbonate. Eleven patients received one of the three lithium preparations for at least ten weeks. During this time the dose was adjusted to bring the serum lithium within the accepted therapeutic range (0.6 to 1.2 mmol/l). In total, twenty experiments have been completed on subjects following their initial dose of lithium carbonate and thirty experiments on subjects who had serum lithium for at least two weeks. In all single daily dose studies the lithium preparation was given at noon; when a divided schedule was given the tablets were taken at noon, 6 p.m. and 8 a.m. These times were chosen to avoid interference with the patients' work and sleep.

Venous blood samples were collected and allowed to clot prior to the patients' being given medication and at 2, 4, 6, 8, 10 and 22 and 24 h after each preparation. In the three experiments where a thrice daily regime was given, blood samples were collected before the administration of lithium tablets, at noon, 6 p.m. and 8 a.m. After centrifugation the serum was diluted one in fifty (0.1 to 5.0 ml) in a suitable buffer (1% lanthanum chloride). These samples were assayed for lithium with an atomic-absorption spectrometer, PE 403, with an air-acetylene flame. A set of suitable standards (concentration range between 0.05 and 2.5 mmol/l) were diluted in the same buffer. The precision of this method was less than 3%. Although lithium remains stable in blood most analysis were performed within 24 h of sampling. In twelve instances a duplicate experiment was performed 2 weeks later. This was done to check that the patients took the prescribed medication.

RESULTS

Eight patients were examined on their first day of dosing with Priadel 800 mg and at the end of 24 h the average serum level was 0.18. Three subjects were examined on their 1st day of dosing with Camcolit 750 mg and the average serum level at the end of 24 h was 0.18 mmol/l. On the first day of dosing with lithium the percentage of lithium recovered in the urine varied from 40 to 70% and the half life of lithium in the body was calculated to be 11.4 h. When the experiments were repeated after intervals of fourteen days it was found that in three patients on Priadel the lithium level at the end of 24 h was 0.37 mmol/l and in two subjects given Camcolit the serum lithium level at the end of 24 h was 0.29 mmol/l. At this point the percentage of lithium recovered from the urine varied from 70 to 100% and the half life of lithium in the body had increased to 18.8 h. When the half lives of the two products, Priadel and Camcolit, were compared we found that in the seven Priadel subjects the average half life was 14.4 h and on four subjects given Camcolit the half life was 12.5 h

After 14 days it was found that the half life of a subject on Priadel had increased to 25.6 h, and for a subject on Camcolit the half life had increased to 19.3 h. It would appear that during the initial fourteen days of lithium experience the half life of lithium in the body increases, and that this increase is paralleled by increased recovery of lithium in the urine as can be seen from Figure 37.1. The percentage recovery of lithium increases from 60% to 100%. Lithium continues to be excreted beyond the point when the subject stops taking the lithium on day 11 and on day 14.

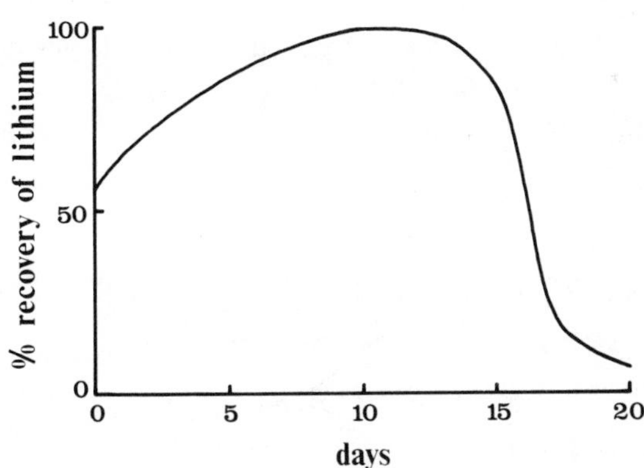

Figure 37.1. Percentage recovery of lithium in urine

Six subjects were given 1200 mg of lithium as a single dose, three being given Priadel and three being given Camcolit 400. The average values are expressed in Figure 37.2 and it can be seen that there is no meaningful difference between the two products at this stage.

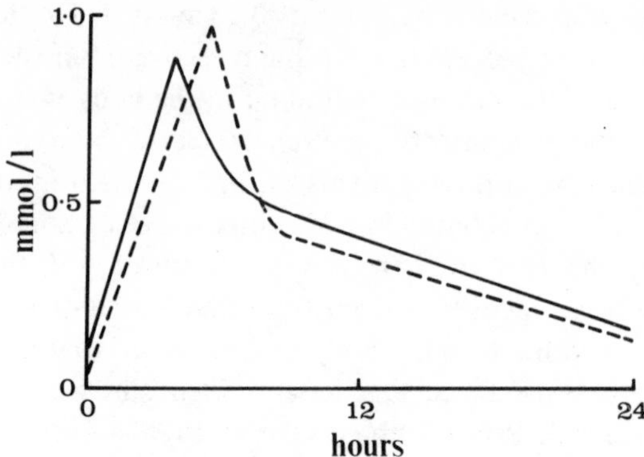

Figure 37:2. Serum levels of lithium following a single dose of Priadel (————) or Camcolit 400 (– – – – – – –). The curves represent mean values of three subjects for each preparation

Figure 37.3 compares the results of patients who have been on Priadel for at least ten weeks, with patients who have been on a single dose of Camcolit for ten weeks. The dose was individualised on each patient to give the serum level within the range 0.6 to 1.2 mmol/l. In the case of Camcolit subjects the dose derived during the time they were taking divided dose became the single daily dose. Figure 37.3 shows that ten subjects on Priadel had an average serum lithium from 0.6 to 1.2 mmol/l. The four subjects given Camcolit tended to have lower serum lithium levels and only for 12 h could one confidently say that the serum lithium level was within the therapeutic range.

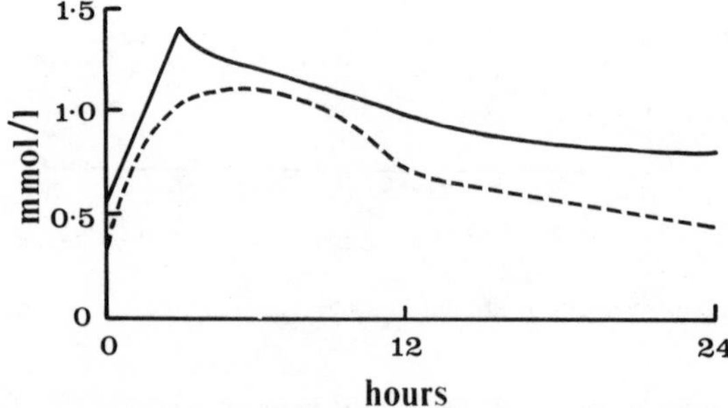

Figure 37:3. Serum levels of lithium following a single dose of Priadel (————) or Camcolit 400 (– – – – – – –) in subjects who had been treated with these products for 10 weeks. The curves are derived from the means of 10 subjects (Priadel) and subjects (Camcolit)

The eleven patients given Phasal for ten weeks had similar serum lithium levels to the ten patients taking Priadel. However, there was some fluctuation in the lithium levels on the patients on Phasal suggesting irregular absorption. Table 37.1 shows the standard deviation for each time that the serum lithium level was measured. We can see that the standard deviations are greater with Phasal than with Priadel or Camcolit.

Table 37:1. Fluctuations in serum lithium levels of patients receiving three proprietary lithium carbonate preparations

Preparation	Standard deviations							
Phasal	0.16	0.29	0.28	0.27	0.28	0.25	0.21	0.21
Priadel	0.12	0.35	0.25	0.16	0.13	0.12	0.10	0.11
Camcolit	0.13	0.11	0.22	0.21	0.16	0.20	0.16	0.15

The fraction of lithium absorbed by the subjects has been examined using the products Priadel and Phasal. When the subject is on repeated doses with regular intervals a steady state equilibrium will be attained where the drug is distributed throughout the body tissues. When this situation is reached, each dose will be in effect totally eliminated from the body during the interval between doses.

It is possible during one dosage interval to calculate the fraction of the administered dose which has been absorbed. The mean fraction absorbed for Priadel and Phasal are 0.203 and 0.184 respectively.

References

1. Amdisen, A. (1975). *Dan. Med. Bull.*, **22**, 277
2. Bennie, E.H., Manzoor, A.K.M., Scott, A.M. and Fell, G.S. *Br. J. Chem. Pharmacol.* (in press)
3. Coppen, A., Bailey, J.E. and White, S.G. (1969). *J. Chem. Pharmacol.,* **9**, 160
4. Shaw, D.M. Hewland, R., Johnson, A.L., Hiliary-Jones, P., Honlett, M.R. (1974). *Curr. Med. Res. Opin.,* **2**, 90
5. Tyrer, S., Hullin, R.P., Birch, N.J. and Goodwin, J.C. (1976). *Psychol. Med.,* **6**, 51
6. Amdisen, A. and Sjogren, J. (1968). *Acta Pharmaceut. Suecica,* **5**, 465
7. Crammer, J.L., Rosser, R.M. and Crane, G. (1974). *Br. Med. J.* **3**, 650
8. Willcox, D.R.C., Gillan, R. and Hare, E.H. (1975). *Br. Med. J.,* **2**, 790

38

Some Observations on Serum Lithium and Clinical Response in Manic-depressive Psychosis

A. VENKOBA RAO and N. HARIHARASUBRAMANIAN

INTRODUCTION

Lithium has been in use in the Department of Psychiatry, Erskine Hospital, Madurai for the last 5 years or more. Certain observations made on patients treated with lithium in this Department during the period July 1976-April 1977 are presented in this chapter.

PURPOSE OF THE STUDY

The principal aim was to ascertain whether, or to what extent, a correlation might exist between the oral lithium dosage on the one hand, and its serum levels and the extent of clinical response on the other.

MATERIAL

28 manic depressive psychotics (ICD 296) (18M:10F) formed the subjects for the study. Their age range was 17-56 years. At the time of commencing lithium therapy, ten of the patients were in the hypomanic or manic, and 18 in the depressive, phase.

METHOD

The patients who were attending the General Psychiatric Outpatient Department were selected for the Lithium Clinic. Some of them needed in-patient care when symptoms became aggravated. Psychometric assessment was carried out using Hamilton's rating scale for depression and Beigel's rating scale for mania.

Screening investigations included examination of urine including its specific gravity, estimations of blood sugar, urea and cholesterol, and recording of ECG prior to therapy. The weight of the patients was also recorded. Serum levels of sodium, potassium, calcium and magnesium were also determined.

Lithium tablets were administered at 450-1200 mg/day in two or three divided doses. The preparations used were Lithocarb (Merck) and Lithanate (La Medica). After 48-72 h of commencement of lithium treatment, blood samples were drawn, twelve hours after the last oral dose of lithium. The serum lithium levels were estimated by flame photometry.

Two or three estimations of serum lithium were repeated at weekly intervals and the dosage was adjusted suitably to keep the serum lithium levels in the accepted therapeutic range 0.6-1.2 mmol/l Thereafter for the first three months, the patients were reviewed once in 2-3 weeks and later at longer intervals. During each review, serum lithium levels and serum levels of sodium, potassium, calcium and magnesium were estimated. Routine urine examination and recording of body weight were also done. Clinical and psychometric assessment were done on each occasion.

Out of thirty-three patients who have been observed in the lithium clinic so far the findings on 28 have been analysed and are presented here. Five have been excluded from the study for such reasons as their inability to report periodically for review and discontinuation of medication and attendance at the clinic (these being felt by them unnecessary when they were symptom free).

RESULTS

The twenty-eight patients, on analysis, fell into three groups, which may be described as follows:

Group 1: 12 patients (43%) showed consistent clinical improvement, achieving an early remission any time between 30 and 50 days of medication and maintained a euthymic state at the time of the preparation of this chapter. At the time of setting in of clinical remission, the serum lithium levels continued in the range of 0.6-1.2 mmol/l. A good correlation was observed between oral dose and serum levels, which is illustrated in Figure 38.1.

While the patients were euthymic, the levels were above 0.8 mmol/l. The change in levels was due in some to an increase of oral dose consequent to

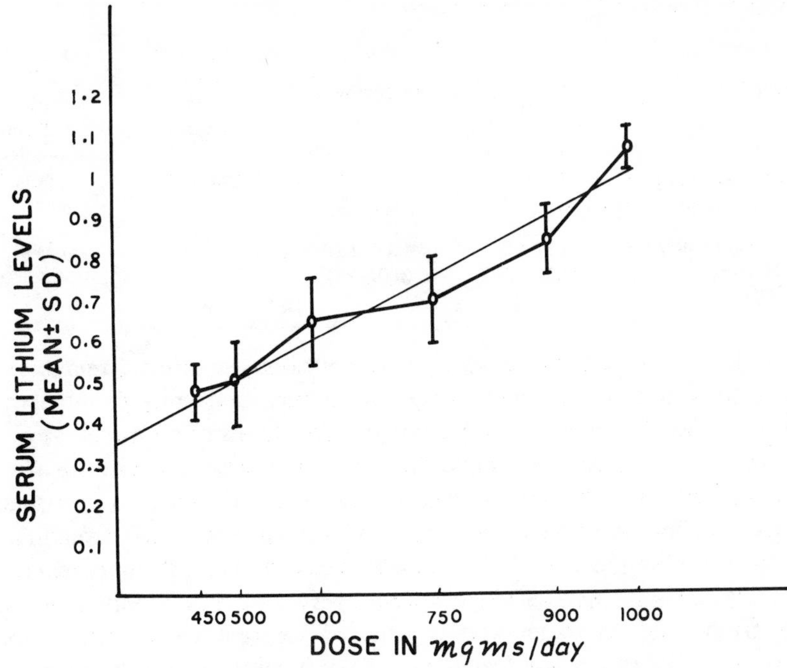

Figure 38.1. The relationship between oral dose of lithium and the serum level

cnanging over from one preparation of lithium to another, whilst in others it was a spontaneous phenomenon.

In this group, two patients have enjoyed a long remission while on lithium, beyond the intervals of euthymic state seen prior to lithium therapy. However, a statistical evaluation of this is not possible at present, since the patients need an extended period of follow-up.

Group 2: 11 patients (39%) had good clinical improvement, achieving remission between 30 and 60 days as in Group 1 but subsequently experiencing relapse. Relapses were noted more often in the depressives than in the manics. Relapses in six patients occurred when there was a failure of medication and consequently with very low serum lithium levels. In these 'defaulters', five had recurrence of mania and one of depression.

Five patients relapsed while they had been regularly taking lithium. In four of these, the relapses were 'mixed' (manic and depressive) while in the fifth a full manic picture was preceded by a sub-depression.

Clinical as well as psychometric assessment indicated that the severity of relapses in the 'defaulters' was more than in those on lithium.

Relapses in all these patients necessitated the use of ECT and

Table 38.1. Psychometric score during relapses

Category	Pre-treatment score	On recovery	Relapse due to with-drawal	Relapse while on lithium
Hypomania/mania (Manic score)	157 (10) (110-210)	34.2 (10) (24-46)	124.5 (6)	118 (3)
Depression (TSRQ) (Hamilton Scale)	0.32 (18) (0.24-0·38)	0.07 (18) (0.02-0·1)	0.3 (1)	0.25 (4)

phenothiazines or antidepressants besides lithium to achieve remission. The response to this combined therapy was better, supporting the observation of a synergistic action of lithium with other forms of chemotherapy.

In this group of patients, while they were on the same oral dose after achieving remission, the serum levels tended to fall. In those who relapsed while on lithium, the level at the time of relapse was less than 0.8 mmol/l.

Group 3: Five patients (11%) showed moderate clinical improvement, achieving remission in 60-90 days, a longer period than in Groups 1 and 2. The serum levels in these patients required frequent monitoring, being apparently unrelated to the oral dosage. Their symptomatology was marked by chronic hypochondrical features (in two) and an element of schizophrenic (schizo-affective) illness (in three).

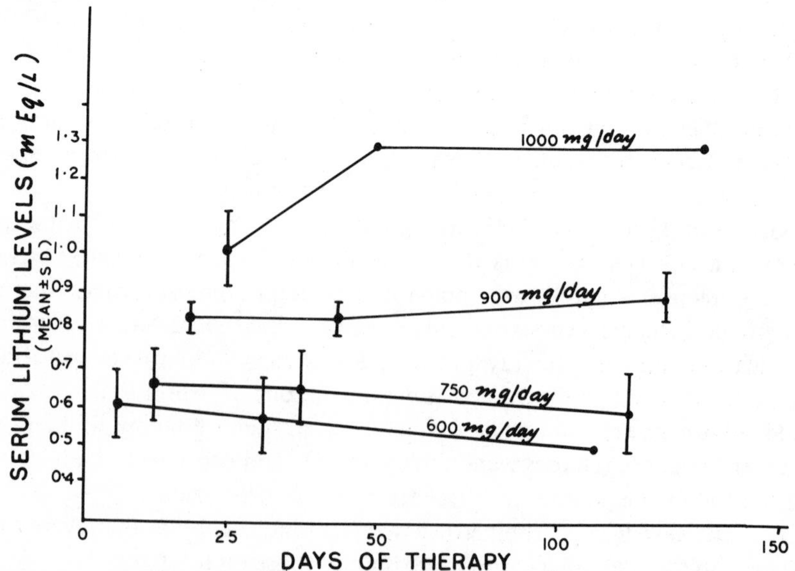

Figure 38.2. Change in serum lithium levels over time as a function of the daily oral dose

Side effects

The only side effects observed in this study include salivation, thirst, tremors and mild gastrointestinal disturbances which occurred early, and polyuria which occurred later, during the course of lithium therapy. No toxic effects have been seen. There was a solitary instance of a weight gain of 3 kg during 7 months of lithium treatment.

DISCUSSION

Serum levels of lithium and clinical response

The results indicate that the serum levels of 0.62-1.2 mmol/l when they were correlated with the size of the oral dose, are associated with favourable clinical response and remission. If a dose of 600-900 mg/day has brought in remission, a continuation of this dose is associated with a fall in serum levels. Relapses have been noted with serum levels falling well below 0.8 mmol/l. With serum levels of more than 0.8 mmol/l, a euthymic state has been maintained without relapses.

The tendency for serum lithium levels to fall may possibly be explained along the following lines. Orally administered lithium is taken up by all tissues, this uptake being of two types: firstly by neural and endocrine cells, involved in therapeutic action of lithium; and secondly by skin, gastro-intestinal tract, kidneys, salivary glands, bone, etc., which are involved in the storage and the elimination of lithium. A balance of these two uptake processes will ensure a stable blood level. The first type of uptake tends to decrease with time, consequent on the slow extrusion of lithium from neural cells by the 'lithium-pump', which may involve Na, K-ATP-ase (1); ATP-ase activity reported to be defective in manic depressive psychosis (2,3) is restored by lithium (4). The transport of lithium into the extacellular fluid results in a spontaneous rise in serum levels. The second form of uptake, involving the various excretory mechanisms is stepped up and elimination of lithium leads to a fall in serum lithium levels.

Increasing the oral dose will raise the serum levels and promote lithium entry into neural cells against the 'lithium pump' and facilitate its intracellular actions which may underlie the therapeutic effects.

Hence, it is suggested that in patients who have achieved clinical remission with serum levels of 0.6-0.8 mmol/l on a dose of 600-700 mg/day, the oral dose of lithium may then be raised in order to bring the serum levels to above 0.8 mmol/l especially in Group 2 patients in whom the serum level tends to fall. In Group 1 patients in whom the levels spontaneously rise, it may be desirable to raise the dose at the first recording of a fall in serum levels.

Relapses

Lithium appears to have modified the severity and symptom content of relapses in our patients, as indicated. This needs to be examined more closely, particularly in the light of the patients' previous clear-cut episodes prior to the institution of lithium therapy. The course of manic depressive illness with lithium in this group of patients will be compared to another group without lithium, which has been already reported from our department (5). The study is in progress.

CONCLUSIONS AND SUGGESTIONS

A predictable correlation exists between oral dose and serum levels of lithium before and until the onset of remission. This may be of help in selection of a dosage schedule for therapeutic purposes. In remission, serum levels tend to fall; this may well be a predictor of possible relapse. Hence, it is suggested that raising the serum lithium levels may forestall a relapse. Relapses in 'defaulters' are severe and resemble their previous episodes. Relapses with lithium are usually of the 'mixed' type.

A question that naturally comes up is whether frequent or occasional estimations of serum lithium are necessary at all. For therapeutic purposes, when it is known that a good predictable correlation exists between oral dose and serum levels, frequent estimations may not be necessary; however, in remissions, we have noticed a fall in serum levels which is a harbinger of possible relapse; this means, in remissions, estimations are necessary. Alternatively, one might choose to administer a higher dose in the range 900-1000 mg/day in remissions without serum estimations.

The fact that regular use of lithium has lessened the severity, modified the symptomatology, and increased the amenability to treatment of relapses justifies the usefulness of lithium in prophylaxis. However, it has to be borne in mind that in any culture in which drug-taking is considered to indicate evidence of ill health, prophylactic administration is beset with difficulties. In this respect, the patients in our study have done well, considering the fact that there have been only six defaulters, out of 29 who have been treated. The cost of the drug is as yet not as economical as it is supposed to be in a developing country. Improvement in this respect will be of help in extending the clinical use of lithium.

ACKNOWLEDGEMENTS

Grateful acknowledgements are due to Dr S. Gnanadesikan, Director of Medical Education, Government of Tamilnadu, Madras and Dr D. Bhupati, Dean, Madurai Medical College, Madurai for their kind permission for this presentation. Our thanks are due to Dr (Mrs) S. Parvathi Devi, Professor of Physiology, Madurai Medical College, Madurai for her valuable guidance and encouragement and to Drs Prakash Appayya, Vivekandan, Sukumar, Postgraduates, and Mr Nammalvar, clinical psychologist for all their help. We thank Dr Venkataramana Rao, C.M.O. and Mr Ramamoorthy, Lab. Technician TVS Hospital for their help in serum lithium estimations.

References

1. Thomas, R.C., Simon, W. and Oehme, W. (1975). *Nature,* **258**, 745
2. Dick, D.A.T., Naylor. G.J., Dick, E.G. and Moody, J.P. (1974). *Biochem. Soc. Trans.,* **2**, 505
3. Hokin-Naeverson, M. Spiegel, D.A. and Lewis, W.C. (1974). *Life Sci.,* **15**, 1739
4. Glen, A.I.M., Bradbury, M.W.B. and Wilson, J. (1972). *Nature,* **239**, 399
5. Venkoba Rao, A. and Nammalvar, N. (1977). *Br. J. Psychiat.,* **130**, 392

39

The Choice of Lithium Preparation and How to Give it

S. P. TYRER

INTRODUCTION

Lithium is one of the simplest drugs to administer in medicine. It is easily absorbed from the gut, is distributed readily throughout the body and is virtually entirely excreted in the urine. It is known that the lithium ion itself is the agent producing the wanted clinical effect in affective disorders and this is not broken down to any other constituent in the body. Yet in spite of its basically simple chemical nature large numbers of lithium preparations exist to tempt the patient receiving treatment with lithium. Why should this be so and what advantages do these preparations have over each other?

Originally the main reason for the search for the most appropriate lithium preparation was to produce a product that produced effective serum levels but yet remained free of toxic effects. This is particularly important with lithium because the therapeutic ratio is small. As lithium became prescribed more frequently as a prophylactic drug, attention was paid to producing a formulation that could be readily taken by the patient without side-effects, preferably on a simple dosage schedule. Finally it must be remembered that lithium is unpatentable and so there is no restriction to the number of drug companies that can produce products containing the drug.

Slow-release preparations of lithium have been marketed in order to fulfill the measures above. An ideal slow-release product can be taken every

24 hours, is free of severe side-effects because of the absence of sudden rises in the serum lithium level and is theoretically safer if swallowed as an overdose (1).

In Britain three lithium preparations are available. One of these is marketed as a standard preparation (Camcolit, Norgine Ltd.), whereas the other two are marketed as sustained-release preparations. Priadel (Delandale Laboratories) is termed a controlled-release preparation, whereas Phasal (Pharmax Ltd) is marketed as a prolonged-release product. Although Priadel originally had some slow-release properties (2) later work showed that the formulation of the drug had been changed (1). A recent study showed that Priadel has similar bioavailability to Camcolit whereas Phasal was ineffectively absorbed in some subjects (3).

In Scandinavia there have been encouraging results from two sustained-release preparations, Lithionit Duretter (4) and Litarex (5). Recent work has shown that these products are similar in their properties (6) although Lithionit Duretter consists of lithium sulphate whereas Litarex is a lithium citrate preparation.

The present study describes a comparison of the rate of absorption and excretion of Litarex with two of the British preparations, Camcolit and Priadel. An Australian quick-release preparation (Lithicarb) was also chosen for comparison. The main aim of the study was to see if Litarex differed substantially in its bioavailability from the other three products. It was also thought necessary to compare Camcolit and Priadel using a cross-over design as the previous study comparing these products was performed on separate subjects (3).

METHODS AND MATERIALS

The subjects chosen for the study were seven medical student volunteers, five males and two females. Seven subjects received Camcolit and Litarex, six Priadel and four Lithicarb. Camcolit was the first preparation to be given but the other three preparations were given in random order with at least 2 weeks drug-free interval between preparations. No subject was taking any other drug during the study apart from the two girls who were taking the contraceptive pill.

A single dose of 1000 mg of each lithium carbonate preparation (2550 mg of Litarex) was given to each volunteer on the day of the test. Each dose contained 27.2 mmol of lithium. Prior to this the subjects had nothing to eat or drink for 12 h before the dose of the drug apart from a standard metabolic breakfast of known composition, containing 500 mg of sodium. At 09.00 h the subjects swallowed the lithium preparation with 250 cc of water; 1.25 litres of water flavoured with lemon juice was drunk 2 h after taking the drug but no other food or drink was allowed in the four hours following administration of the drug. The water was to ensure an adequate urine flow and was also designed as a control for a separate experiment. After 13.00 h the subjects had an unstandardized lunch and further eating and drinking was allowed for the remainder of the test. Blood was drawn at intervals of 1, 2, 3, 4, 6, 8, 12 and 24 h after the lithium dose and all urine passed was collected for 24 h after the dose. The 0-12 and 12-24 h specimens were pooled.

Lithium was determined in duplicate samples of serum and urine using an Instrumentation Laboratories 151 Atomic Absorption Spectrophotometer at a wave length of 670·6 nm. The serum samples were diluted 50 times with deionized distilled water, the urine samples 200 times. The variation between the two duplicate samples was 1.27%.

RESULTS

All the preparations were well tolerated and no subjects had to be withdrawn from the test because of side-effects. The mean serum lithium levels for the four preparations are illustrated in Figures 39.1, 39.2 and 39.3. The mean serum lithium values for the four products at the times samples are indicated in Table 39.1.

Table 39.1. The mean serum lithium concentrations with the four preparations

Preparation	Serum levels (mmol/l)							
	Hours after dose							
	1	2	3	4	6	8	12	24
Camcolit	0.45*	0.75*	0.73*	0.67*	0.50	0.39	0.30	0.19
Lithicarb	0.61	0.72	0.75	0.68	0.52	0.42	0.33	0.22
Priadel	0.33*	0.53*	0.72	0.78	0.59	0.47	0.35	0.22
Litarex	0.29*	0.47*	0.51*	0.54*	0.46	0.40	0.31	0.21

*Significant differences ($p = 0.01$) are shown between Camcolit and Litarex at 1, 2, 3, and 4 hours, and between Camcolit and Priadel at 1 and 2 hours by the Orthogonal Comparisons Method

Although there are no significant differences from the sixth hour following ingestion of the drug to the end of the study there is significant variation between the 1st and 4th hour in some products. Camcolit and Litarex differ significantly on every occasion between the 1st and 4th hour and these differences are also shown between Litarex and the other preparations although the differences are more marked between the 3rd and 5th hour with Priadel. Camcolit and Priadel show significantly different serum levels at the first and second hour following ingestion of the drug and this is because Priadel has a slower release. Lithicarb is similar to Camcolit in the shape of its absorption and excretion curve and there were no significant differences at any time. The area under the blood level curves show Litarex to have the lowest net bioavailability whereas Priadel and Lithicarb demonstrate the highest values (Table 39.2).

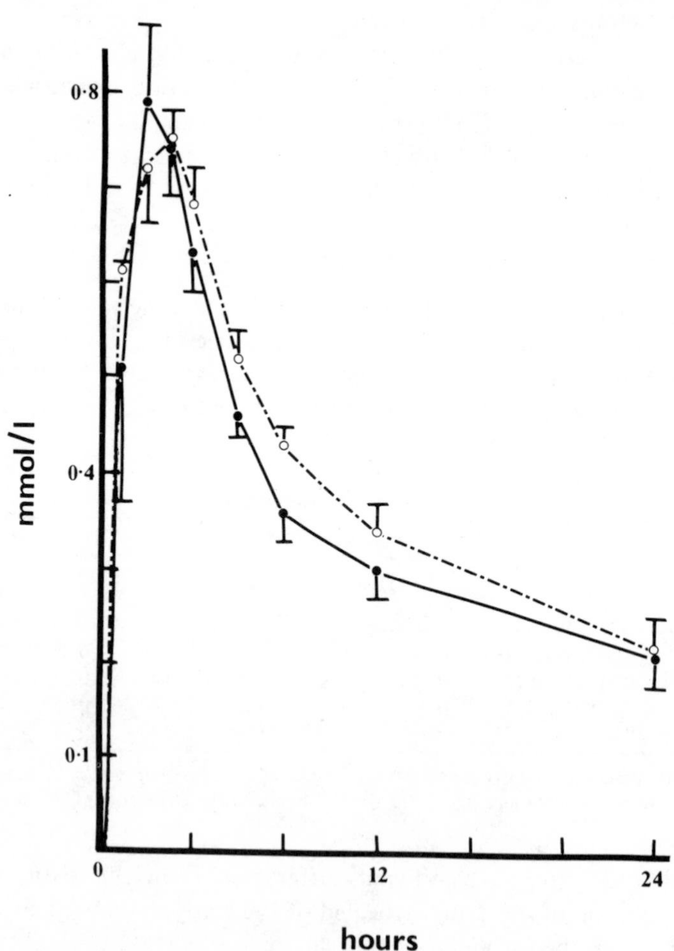

Figure 39:1. Mean serum lithium concentrations following a single oral dose of 1000 mg of Camcolit and Lithicarb in the same four subjects. Camcolit ———————; Lithicarb –·–·–·–·–·.'

Table 39.2. Bioavailability of the four preparations

	Camcolit*	Lithicarb	Priadel	Litarex
Area under 24 h blood level curve (mmol/l.h)	8.65	9.47	9.40	7.64**

*mean of three curves
**significantly different from the other three preparations

Figure 39.1 shows that there is an early peak lithium with Camcolit and this is higher than for the other products. There is a relatively quick excretion of lithium in the urine. The blood absorption and excretion curve for

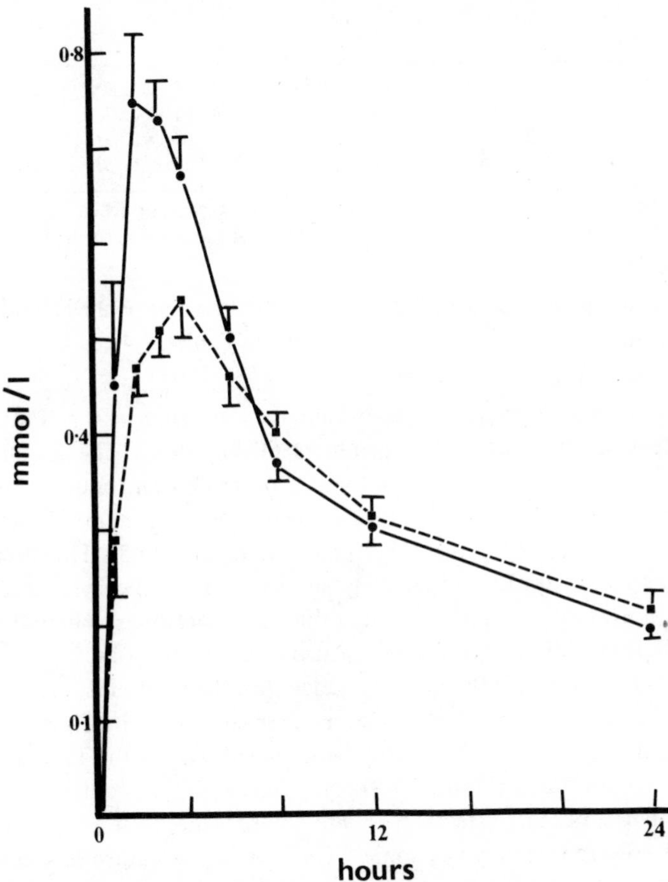

Figure 39.2. Mean serum lithium concentrations following a single oral dose of 1000 mg of Camcolit and Priadel in the same six subjects. Camcolit ———————— ; Priadel - - - - - - - .

Table 39.3. Time and height of mean peak serum lithium

Preparation	Time of peak (h)	Height of peak (mmol/l)
Camcolit	2.5	0.91
Lithicarb	1.75	0.80
Priadel	3.2	0.83
Litarex	2.8	0.60

Table 39.4. Mean urinary lithium excretion following administration of the three preparations.

	(Lithium in urine (mmol)			
Preparation	0-12 (h)	12-24 (h)	0-24 (h)	% of dose (excreted in 24 h)
Camcolit	9.82 ± 1.45*	4.37 ± 0.41	14.19 ± 1.66*	52.17
Lithicarb	9.13 ± 1.89	3.48 ± 1.11	12.61 ± 2.67	46.36
Priadel	14.22 ± 4.74*	4.74 ± 1.64	18.96 ± 3.57*	69.71
Litarex	7.91 ± 1.66	4.27 ± 0.78	12.18 ± 1.95*	44.78

*Significant differences ($p = 0.01$) are shown between the 0-12 h and 0-24 h excretions of Camcolit and Priadel and Camcolit and Litarex (Orthogonal Comparison Method)

Lithicarb is not dissimilar from that of Camcolit (Figure 39.1) and the urine results do not show significant differences (Table 39.4).

Priadel has a more delayed peak than Camcolit (Figure 39.2; Table 39.3). There is greater excretion of lithium in the urine in the first 12 h with Priadel than with the other products (Table 39.4). The graph for Litarex is of a different shape than for the other three products (Figure 39.3). There is a much flatter initial peak serum lithium which is considerably lower than for the other products (Table 39.3). However by the 6th hour the serum lithium level is similar to the other preparations and the rate of excretion resembles the other three products. There is also significantly less lithium excreted in the urine during the first 12 h of the test with Litarex than with the other products (Table 39.4) and this corresponds with the lower serum lithium levels over the first 4 h. There is less variation in the serum levels of lithium between subjects at the 1st and 2nd hour after taking Litarex (Figure 39.3) compared with Camcolit.

The incidence of side-effects was similar for the four preparations (Table 39.5). There was however some difference in the nature of the side-effects. There was more nausea experienced with Camcolit than with the other three preparations. Light-headed feelings and occasional diarrohea were noted with Litarex.

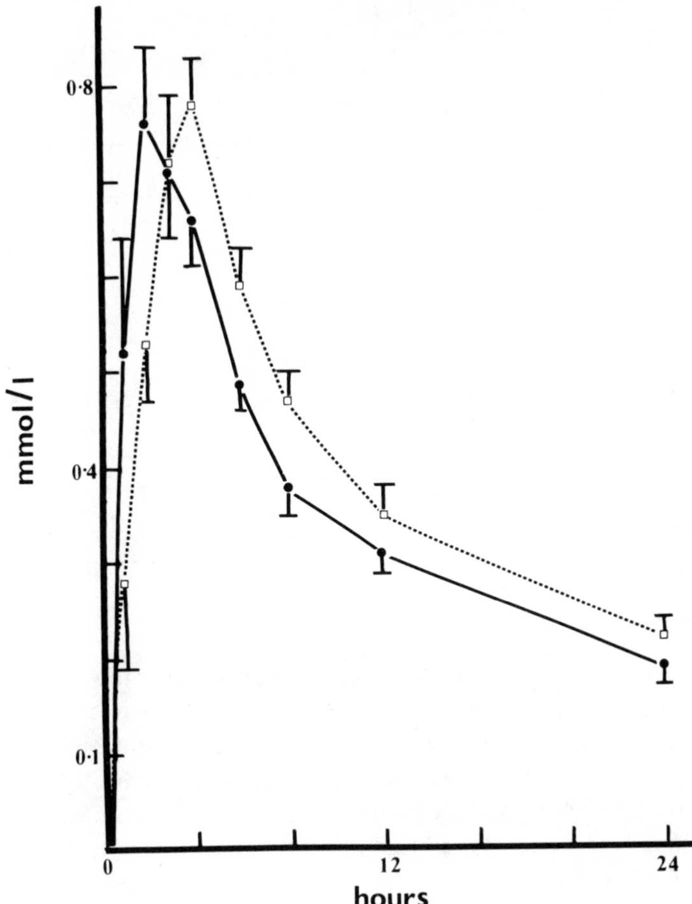

Figure 39.3. Mean serum lithium concentrations following a single oral dose of 1000 mg of Camcolit and Litarex in the same seven subjects. Camcolit ———— ; Litarex ....

Table 39.5 should be interpreted with some caution. It is known that subjects experience less side-effects during the progress of an experiment of this nature (7). All subjects initially took Camcolit and one would expect that the incidence of side-effects with the first product would be greater than with subsequent preparations because of familiarity.

It has also been pointed out that volunteers do not complain of side-effects so readily as patients (8) and it may be that the product under test would be differently tolerated by patient subjects. Furthermore the products were not administered blind to the subjects.

Table 39.5. Nature and frequency of side-effects

Symptoms	Number of Subjects	Frequency with different products (% incidence) Camcolit	Lithicarb	Priadel	Litarex
Tiredness	14	67	67	50	67
Nausea	9	67	50	17	33
Light-headed	9	17	50	33	67
Dry mouth	8	50	50	33	17
Headache	4	33	0	33	0
Diarrhoea	3	0	0	17	33
Abdominal fluttering	2	0	0	0	33
Sweating	2	0	25	0	17
Trembling	1	0	25	0	0
Total number of side-effects per Subject		2.5	3.0	1.9	3.0

One subject complained of yawning and frequent eructations with all four preparations

DISCUSSION

There are measurable differences between three of the four products tested. Litarex differs most widely largely because there is slower and lower absorption of this drug. This avoids the serum lithium peaks that the other products display but overall Litarex has lower bioavailability because of this. Camcolit and Lithicarb display similar blood level curves but Priadel is slightly delayed release leading to a similar curve to Camcolit but shifted further to the right.

In this study there was no significant difference in the side-effects between the four preparations. However it is now well established that the incidence and timing of side-effects is related to whether a lithium preparation is quick or slow-release (9,10) although this relationship is not invariably shown (11). The side-effects concerned have also been shown to be related to the gradient of the serum lithium level rise (10).

The bioavailability of Camcolit and Priadel is slightly different than suggested in a previous study (3). The present data are more accurate as a cross-over design has been used. This study shows clearly that Priadel has a delayed peak compared with Camcolit but the curves are not dissimilar otherwise. The difference may partly be due to the greater content of lithium in the Priadel tablet for experience with a 400 mg tablet of Camcolit shows some delayed release compared with the standard Camcolit preparation (Tyrer, unpublished work).

It is therefore accurate to describe Camcolit and Lithicarb as quick-release preparations, Priadel as delayed-release and Litarex as slow-release but not sustained-release. It is not possible from this study to determine precisely which preparation is preferable. It is not known how lithium should be administered to exert the maximum prophylactic effect, although it is prudent to choose a preparation that gives the least likelihood of toxic and side-effects. On this basis it is possible to recommend Litarex because of the fewer side-effects with this preparation and the smaller inter-individual variation between subjects. However it seems probable that the nature of the lithium preparation administered is not of vital importance in maintaining prophylaxis. For instance, many studies have indicated that Priadel is effective in prophylaxis even when administered in a once a day schedule (12-14). There are nevertheless good theoretical arguments for suggesting that lithium be administered on a twice-daily schedule as there is less likelihood of toxicity and variation in the 12 h lithium level with this procedure (1). It would therefore seem advisable to administer one's favourite lithium preparation in this manner to patients receiving prophylactic lithium. If side-effects occur, particularly within the first four hours, there are some arguments for changing to an adequate slow-release product, and Litarex and Lithionit Duretter can be recommended at present.

Procedure to determine adequate lithium dosage

Because of the wide differences in the way that subjects handle lithium (15) and because lithium is potentially a dangerous drug, a number of tests have been recommended prior to starting lithium particularly for prophylactic use. In the first instance, it must be established whether it is safe to give lithium to a particular patient and, if so, what is the appropriate dosage schedule. The basis of most of these tests is to determine the nature of the kidney function. Over 98% of the lithium in the body is excreted by the kidneys (16) and it is essential to determine that renal function is effective before starting lithium. To this effect it has been recommended that analysis of the urine for casts and formed products be carried out on all patients about to undergo lithium treatment and creatinine clearance estimations performed if there is any doubt about renal function (17). Lithium should be administered with caution to patients with a history of cardiac insufficiency, particularly if there is periodic decompensation and administration in the first 3 months of pregnancy is also not advised (18).

Once established that it is safe to give lithium it has to be established what is the most appropriate dosage for the individual. This can be determined if renal clearances are carried out on subjects about to receive lithium and a formula has been calculated to determine the most appropriate dosage once the renal lithium clearance is known (19). The lithium clearance test involves the patient taking a loading dose of a lithium preparation the previous night, coming up to the clinic the next day, collecting urine over a period of 7 h and performing a venepuncture at the beginning and end of the urine collection period. This is a time consuming procedure and the prediction of dosage is not always very accurate. It would therefore be advisable to have a test which is simpler to perform and which is more reliable.

Bergner *et al.* (20) showed that it was possible to predict subsequent lithium dosage following lithium kinetic studies on subjects. In his procedure blood was taken at regular intervals from the individuals in the study and it is impractical in practice to take multiple venepunctures in patients about to undergo lithium treatment. However, further work from the same unit showed that the 24 h lithium level following a loading dose of standard lithium carbonate was a very effective predictor in determining subsequent lithium carbonate dosage requirements (21). A recent follow-up study has confirmed the value of this and indicates that the test is reliable in the same individual over time (22). The test is also applicable with a slow-release product (23). All that is required for this test is for the patient to take a standard dose of lithium at a specified time and the concentration of lithium in the blood is measured 24 h later. The blood test can be taken at any time convenient to the patient who only needs one venepuncture and one visit to the clinic. The correlation between the serum lithium level determined in this way and the bioavailability of the particular lithium preparation has been shown to be very close (Tyrer and Hullin, unpublished work).

Once the loading dose has been determined it is rare to find that dosage requirements need to be adjusted within the first few months of treatment unless secondary medical conditions ensue. Virtually all discrepancies from the predicted dose level have been found to be due to non-compliance (22).

This test is both simpler and more reliable than previous screening tests for lithium requirements. One word of caution is that accurate laboratory determinations of the lithium levels are essential for the predicted dose to be determined precisely. Nevertheless no problems have so far been reported with its use and it should become a frequently used test in the armamentarium of the busy physician involved in treating patients with lithium.

ACKNOWLEDGEMENTS

My thanks are due to Dr Michael Peat and Mr Peter Minty for the standardization and analysis of the lithium samples. Considerable help in statistical analysis and artwork was provided by Miss Angel Luchini. The work would have been incomplete without the diligence and co-operation of the volunteers.

References

1. Amdisen, A. (1975). *Dan. Med. Bull.,* **22**, 277
2. Coppen, A., Bailey, J.E. and White, S.G. (1969). *J. Clin. Pharmacol.,* **9**, 160
3. Tyrer, S. *et al.* (1976). *Psychol. Med.,* **6**, 51
4. Persson, G. (1977). *Acta Psychiat. Scand.,* **55**, 147
5. Amdisen, A., (1975). In: Johnson, F.N. (ed.) *Lithium Research and Therapy,* pp. 202 (London: Academic Press)
6. Widerlöv, E. (1976). *Acta Psychiat. Scand.,* **54**, 294
7. Grof, P. *et al.* (1976). *Neuropsychobiology* (in press)
8. Otto, V., Paalzow, L. and Suren, G. (1972). *Acta Pharm. Suec.,* **9**, 595
9. Dick. P. (1975). *Ther. Umsch.,* **32**, 532
10. Persson, G. (1977). *Acta Psychiat. Scand.,* **55**, 208
11. Edstrom, A. and Persson, G. (1977). *Acta Psychiat. Scand.,* **55**, 153
12. Salkind, M.R. (1979). *J. R. Coll. Gen. Pract., 20,* 13
13. Coppen, A. *et al.* (1971). *Lancet,* **ii**, 275
14. Marini, J.L. and Sheard, M.H. (1976). *J. Clin. Pharmacol.,* **16**, 276
15. Fyrö, B., Petterson, U. and Sedvall, G. (1973). *Acta Psychiat. Scand.,* **49**, 237
16. Kent, N.L. and McCance, R.A. (1941). *Biochem. J.* 35, 837
17. Schou, M., Amdisen, A. and Baastrup. P.C. (1971). *Br. J. Hosp. Med.,* **6**, 53
18. Schou, M. (1976). *Curr. Psychiat. Ther.,* **16** 139
19. Schou, M. *et al.* (1970). *Br. J. Psychiat.,* **116**, 615
20. Bergner, P-E. E. *et al.* (1973). *Br. J. Pharmacol.,* **49**, 328
21. Cooper, T.B., Bergner, P-E.E. and Simpson, G.M. (1973). *Am. J. Psychiat.,* **130**, 601
22. Cooper, T.B. and Simpson, G.N. (1976). *Am. J. Psychiat.,* **133**, 440
23. Seifert, R., Bremkamp, H. and Junge, C. (1976). *Psychopharmacol.,* **43**, 285

40

Plasma Lithium Control with Particular Reference to Minimum Effective Levels

T. C. JERRAM and R. McDONALD

INTRODUCTION

The Regional Metabolic Research Unit situated at High Royds Hospital has now accumulated experience of managing patients on lithium for over a decade and we value the close co-operation that is possible between our scientific colleagues and the clinicians. The unit has 10 in-patient beds and in addition caters for just over 100 out-patients. These latter are seen at regular intervals on the Unit at a specifically organised lithium clinic such as has been proposed as a model for some forms of health care delivery (1). This allows both medical and nursing staff to gain expertise in managing such patients many of whom are happy to seek advice from nursing staff who, in turn, are confident enough in their own ability to deal with problems, being secure in the knowledge that they have laboratory and medical back-up facilities readily available. This association of in-patient and out-patient facilities permits easy care for the inevitable relapses that do occur; at any one time, between one and four beds will be occupied by patients who have been admitted for supplementary treatment of an affective relapse.

In addition to providing care for the patients, our main concern has been to preserve a cohort of subjects who have been well established on lithium for some time with a view to the early detection of possible side-effects and to the improvement and refining of our clinical management. In this last connection we would like to report some early results of a trial in which we set out to try to establish a minimum blood level for effective lithium prophylaxis.

In its original use as an anti-manic agent lithium was believed to be effective only at a plasma level just below the toxic level. As most patients develop some signs of toxicity when the plasma concentration approaches 2.0 mmol/l, a recommended level for the management of the acute manic episode would be a little way below this. This empiricial approach has been confirmed by the Veterans Administration study (2) which suggested that increasing the plasma level above 1.4 mmol/l does not increase effectiveness but does increase toxicity and that levels below 0.8 mmol/l are ineffective in controlling the acute episode. When lithium came to be used prophylactically and therefore for longer periods and in out-patients the recommended levels were slightly lower. Exactly how much lower the prophylactic level could be has, however, not been definitely established. It has usually been accepted that the level necessary for effective prophylaxis has been somewhere close to that effective in acute mania, although with other drugs such as anti-convulsants and antibiotics the prophylactic dose is often considerably less than the curative dose. Most authors (3) recommend that the level be maintained between 0.8 and 1.2 mmol/l, although it is recognized that lower levels may sometimes be sufficient and indeed be desirable for older patients, and others (4) have recommended that the level may be even lower than that.

Against this background three factors led us to study this problem further. Firstly, it was noted that many patients appeared to do well with blood levels which were consistently below the usually recommended range. Secondly, lithium takes weeks or even months to exert a full prophylactic effect and, therefore, the mechanisms of this action may be rather different from that of its anti-manic effect and may not necessarily require the same concentration of ion. Thirdly, while levels of 0.8-1.2 mmol/l do not give rise to acute side effects in most people, it is likely that lithium will have to be prescribed indefinitely, if not for life. Such long-term ingestion may have effects upon bone and upon the thyroid gland and it would appear logical that over a long period lower concentrations of lithium may be less harmful in these respects. These considerations led us to investigate what is the lower limit for effective use in preventing relapse and we accordingly designed a study in which a series of lithium-responsive patients currently taking the drug were allocated to one of three groups. In one group the mean 12-16 h plasma concentration was maintained below 0.49 mmol/l, in the second group the concentration was maintained between 0.50 and 0.69 mmol/l and in the third group it was above 0.70mmol/l and, therefore, in what is usually regarded as within the satisfactory range for prophylaxis. The particular levels of the groups were selected in the expectation that the last group would act as a control for normal use of lithium, that the middle group would demonstrate that levels below this were still effective, and that the first group would show that there was indeed a lower limit for effective prophylaxis, below which relapse would be frequent and would approach that of patients on placebo, as in earlier studies of lithium use.

PATIENTS AND METHODS

The general design of the study was similar to that of the earlier discontinuation studies of lithium except that in this case patients were allocated to different plasma levels instead of to a placebo regime. It was conducted at a well established lithium clinic as has been described above. Patients who (1) had a definite affective disorder (uni or bi-polar); (2) had consistent blood levels; (3) attended regularly; and (4) were currently in remission were selected, amounting to just over 80 patients.

It was explained to them that we were attempting to find the best way of achieving satisfactory blood levels and they were asked to co-operate in this. None refused and no further attempt was made to explain the procedure. The patients were randomly allocated to one of the three blood levels. The study was timed to run for one year including any time spent on restabilisation at the new level. This latter was achieved by substituting 250 mg for 400 mg tablets of lithium carbonate or vice versa and, in a few patients, by altering the total daily dose of tablets. The patients were seen at regular intervals by a psychiatrist, when blood was taken for lithium estimation 12-16 h after the last tablet had been taken and any necessary alterations in dose made by a biochemist. At the end of the study period the mean blood lithium levels were calculated (minimum of four readings), those with unstable blood levels (SD greater than 0.2) were discarded and the remainder compared as to outcome. Outcome was defined beforehand as the necessity for additional psychotropic medication and/or admission. In making this assessment the psychiatrist tried to be rigorous before accepting patients as relapsed, mainly to avoid rating as relapses those 'reminders' that have been described (5). Relapses were only accepted as such after at least one return visit and an interview with a close relative, unless immediate admission was necessary. The blood lithium was measured by laboratory staff experienced in the technique using an atomic absorption spectrophotometer.

RESULTS

73 patients completed the study period satisfactorily. Reasons for failure to complete included removal from area, reluctance to continue medication and unstable blood levels. So far as is known none of the excluded patients relapsed although one developed lithium toxicity. Details of the patients are shown in Table 40.1.

Table 40.1. Numbers of patients: sex ratio and diagnosis

Li (mmol/l)	n	Sex		Diagnosis	
		Male	Female	Unipolar	Bipolar
0.49	24	9	15	8	16
0.5-0.69	27	12	15	8	19
0.70	22	5	17	6	16

Table 40.2. Age and time on lithium in each group

Li (mmol/l)	Age in yrs. mean (range)	Mean time on Li (months)
0.49	49.5 (33-72)	56.2
0.5-0.69	56.8 (32-77)	59.6
0.70	55.2 (31-76)	64.6

Table 40·2 shows the mean ages and time on lithium for the three groups. Although the patients were all classed as lithium responders, several had had a relapse of some sort while on lithium (Table 40.3).

Table 40.2. Previous relapses on 'standard' regime

Li (mmol/l)	One episode	Two episodes	Three or more episodes
o.49	9	1	1
0.50-0.69	9	3	0
0.70	6	1	0

However, these had nearly all been in the first few months of treatment and the patients had since been well for a long time. There appears to be no significant differences in the constitution of the three groups.

The outcome variable was clinical relapse; the numbers and percentages of relapses that occurred are shown in Table 40.4.

Table 40.4. Relapse rate: all patients

Li (mmol/l)	No. relapsed	% relapsed
0.49	4/24	16.6
0.5-0.69	4/27	14.8
0.70	3/22	13.6

We wondered whether relapse at the lower levels may be more frequent in bipolar patients as it is possible that higher levels of lithium may be necessary to protect against manic episodes. However, Table 40.5 shows that bipolar patients were not over-represented among the treatment failures at lower levels.

Table 40.5. Relapse rate and diagnosis

Li (mmol/l)	Unipolar	Bipolar
0.49	0/8	4/16
0.4-0.69	1/8	3/19
0.7	0/6	3/16

and, if anything, manic relapses appeared commoner with higher plasma levels (Table 40.6).

Table 40.6. Form of relapse

Li (mmol/l)	Hypomania/ mania	Depression	Total
0.49	2	2	4
0.5-0.69	2	2	4
0.70	3	0	3

DISCUSSION

The results show surprisingly little difference between the groups, the relapse rate not being significantly different between individual groups, and several points need to be considered. Firstly, the patients were all lithium responders in that although some had relapsed previously while on lithium, most had remained free of further episodes and those who had had relapses were improved overall. Secondly, they had all been established on lithium for at least 6 months (and in most cases for much longer) so that it had had time to exert its full prophylactic effect.

Prien and Caffey (6) reported (after the beginning of our study) a series of 32 unipolar patients maintained on lithium for two years and noted that 10 out of 18 with a mean plasma level between 0.5 and 0.8 mmol/ relapsed while 2 of 14 whose mean level was above 0.8 mmol/l relapsed. They point out that they were treating a relatively high-risk group, and followed them up for 24 months, the median time of relapse being 17 months. It is possible that we may have missed some relapses by a shorter follow-up, and our group was a lower risk one, but our findings do suggest that patients, who have been stable for some time, may be maintained on rather lower levels of lithium than has been thought necessary. There is no evidence that the metabolism of lithium changes over such a time and it seems unlikely that there is any physical reason for any increased sensitivity to lithium.

Schou and Thomsen (5) have drawn attention to the possibility that patients on lithium complain of symptoms which are different from those experienced in previous episodes but we did not come across this, and they also mentioned that milder mood swings may occur on lithium and our criteria for relapse were made fairly strict so that such episodes would not lead to the patient being classified as a treatment failure. Similarly, there has also been described the "hypomanic alert"—the relatively minor upswing of mood which may progress to a major breakdown and which is regarded as an indication for increasing the dose of lithium. We found the minor mood swings to be rare and, like Prien and Caffey, found that relapse when it did occur was usually rapid and would not have allowed time to increase the dose effectively.

On the other hand, such mood changes as were seen were brief and resembled the reactions experienced by healthy individuals when exposed to psychological stresses both pleasant and unpleasant; indeed patients have often volunteered their relief at being able to express the extremes of emotion in the appropriate circumstances without they or their relatives immediately anticipating the onset of a relapse and Demers and Davis (7) have described the changing pattern of family relationships in patients who are maintained on lithium. As it is unlikely that the progress of manic depressive illness which has not been treated by lithium is towards longer and longer remission; and as there is no reason to expect the physical effects of lithium itself to change we must look elsewhere for an explanation of our findings. A possible model is in the hypothesis that lithium is fully effective as a prophylactic only after a period of months; that gradually following this the expectations of the patient and his family are improved to such an extent that the former is able to experience normal mood changes without necessarily developing an affective illness. Whether this is so or not it does appear that in many patients, especially in those who have done well on the drug for a prolonged time, lithium continues to be effective at a surprisingly low level and this has some implications for their future management.

References

1. Fieve, R.R. (1975). *Am. J. Psychiat.,* 132, 1018
2. Prien, R,F., Caffey, E.M. and Klett, J.G. (1972). *Arch. Gen. Psychiat.* 26, 146
3. Schou, M. (1968). *J. Psychiat. Res.,* 6, 67
4. Blachley, P.H. (1970). *J. Am. Med. Assoc.,* 212, 480
5. Schou, M. and Thomsen, K. (1975). In: F.N. Johnson (ed.) *Lithium Research and Therapy,* pp. 63-85. (London: Academic Press)
6. Prien, R.F. and Caffey, E.M. (1976). *Am J. Psychiat.,* 133, 567
7. Demers, R.G. and Davis, L.S. (1971). *Comprehens. Psychiat.,* 12, 348

41

Lithium Uptake by Erythrocytes of Lithium-Treated Patients: Interindividual Differences

W. GREIL and F. EISENRIED

INTRODUCTION

In Li-treated patients, the distribution ratio of Li between red blood cells and plasma shows marked interindividual differences. It has been reported that patients with high Li ratios, i.e. with high red cell Li concentrations, exhibit a better response to Li therapy and an higher incidence of Li side effects (1).

To determine the factors responsible for the interindividual differences in the Li ratio, we have studied Li transport *in vitro* on erythrocytes of healthy volunteers and of Li-treated patients (1-3).

In our first report (2), we demonstrated that Li can be transported out of the cells against an electrochemical Li gradient by Na-dependent Li countertransport. The *in vivo* Li ratios could be qualitatively reproduced *in vitro* (2). In a second paper (3), the countertransport system was characterized in more detail. In agreement with results of Haas *et al,* (4), it has been found that Na-Li countertransport mediates Li transport out of the cells and into the cells, depending on the Na gradient. At pysiological Na concentrations in red cells and in plasma, Li is transported out of the cells by this transport system (3). The Na-Li countertransport is ouabain-insensitive and does not depend on normal ATP concentrations (3). Finally, we could show that the *in vivo* Li ratios are related to the efficiency of the Na-dependent Li countertransport system: the more effective the countertransport, the lower the *in vivo* Li ratio (1).

Recent results demonstrated that the Na-dependent Li countertransport system is inhibited by phloretin (5,6) and it has been demonstrated that Li uptake by erythrocytes consists of at least three different components (5-8).

1. Ouabain-sensitive Li uptake due to the action of the Na-K pump (1,5,7,8);
2. Phloretin-sensitive Li uptake, which appears to be mediated by the Na-dependent Li countertransport system (5,6) and
3. Li uptake resistant to ouabain plus phloretin, which may be explained by leak diffusion (5).

In the present study, the three different ways of Li uptake were examined on erythrocytes from two groups of Li treated patients, namely from patients with high, and from patients with low, Li ratios.

METHODS

Patients exhibiting markedly different *in vivo* Li ratios (= red blood cell Li: plasma Li ratio) were selected. Blood was drawn into heparinized syringes. Li therapy had been interrupted at least 7 days before blood withdrawal so that red cell Li concentrations were below 0.01 micro mol/ml cells at the time of the experiments. Additional medication (antidepressants, neuroleptics) was maintained. The erythrocytes were washed three times in a five fold excess of media containing 20 mM tris-(hydroxymethyl-)aminomethane, 15 mM glucose, 1 mM $CaCl_2$ and 1 mM $MgCl_2$ (isotonicity maintained by choline chloride). Li uptake was initiated by adding washed erythrocytes to media containing 2.2 mM LiCl (without added Na and K, isotonicity maintained by choline chloride). In some experiments, 0.2 mM phloretin and/or 0.1 mM ouabain were present in the suspension media. Incubations were performed at 37 °C and pH 7.4 (haematocrit 10%). Analytical procedures are described elsewhere (1,3).

RESULTS

Li uptake by erythrocytes from patients with high and from patients with low *in vivo* Li ratios is compared in Table 41.4 and in Figure 41.4. The high ratio group consisted of patients with *in vivo* Li ratios greater than 0.60, the low ratio group of patients with Li ratios smaller than 0.35.

Table 41.1, shows Li uptake after 1 h of incubation (A) without the inhibitors, ouabain and phloretin, (B) in the presence of ouabain, and (C) in the presence of both, ouabain plus phloretin.

In high as well as in low ratio cells, Li uptake is inhibited by ouabain

Table 41.1. Li uptake by erythrocytes from Li treated patients with low, and from patients with high, in vivo Li ratios: effects of ouabain and of ouabain plus phloretin (means ± SD)

	Low ratio group (n = 5)	High ratio group (n = 5)	P(c)
In vivo Li ratio	0.28 ± 0.05	0.70 = 0.09	< 0.001
Li uptake (micro mol/ml cells) (a)			
(A) no inhibitors	0.39 ± 0.09	0.35 ± 0.03	NS
(B) ouabain 0.1 mM	0.17 ± 0.04	0.11 ± 0.01	< 0,02 (d)
(C) ouabain 0.1 mM phloretin 0.2 mM	0.07 ± 0.02	0.06 ± 0.01	NS
Nai (micro mol/ml cells) (b)	8.91 ± 1.40	9.22 ± 0.86	NS

(a) Li content as determined after 1 h of incubation of red cells in media containing 2.2 mM Li (see methods)
(b) Initial Na content of red cells (after washing procedure)
(c) Difference between high and low ratio group (Student's t test)
NS = difference not significant

(d) Li uptake in the presence of ouabain is lower in high ratio cells than in low ratio erythrocytes, as has already been reported in a previous paper (1). Under the experimental conditions applied in this study, variations of Li uptake in the presence of ouabain are essentially determined by phloretin-sensitive Li uptake

(Table 41.4, compare lines A and B). A further inhibition of Li uptake is achieved in the presence of ouabain plus phloretin (Table 41.1, compare B and C).

These results substantiate that Li uptake by red blood cells consists of different components: 1) ouabain-sensitive Li uptake, i.e. the difference of Li uptake in the absence and in the presence of ouabain (Table 41.1, A,B); 2) phloretin-sensitive Li uptake, i.e. the difference of Li uptake in the presence of ouabain and in the presence of ouabain plus phloretin (Table 41.1 B,C); and 3) Li uptake resistant to ouabain plus phloretin, i.e. Li uptake in the presence of these inhibitors (Table 41.1, C).

Figure 41·1 compares Li uptake by the three components (described above) for high and low ratio cells. Ouabain-sensitive Li uptake as well as Li uptake resistant to ouabain plus phloretin were not significantly different in both groups (Figure 41.1 a and c). In contrast, phloretin-sensitive Li uptake was significantly lower in high ratio erythrocytes than in low ratio cells (Figure 41.4b).

In Figure 41.2 the *in vivo* Li ratios observed in twelve patients are plotted versus the phloretin-sensitive Li uptake by erythrocytes of these

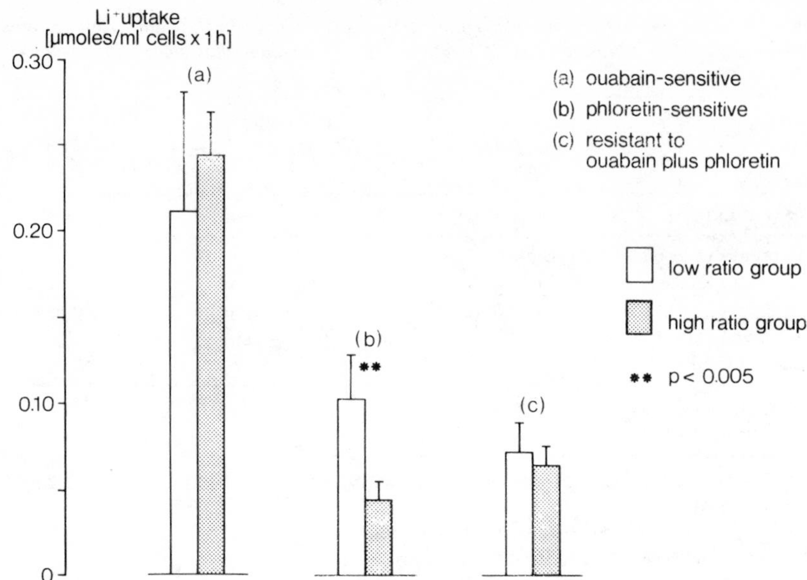

Figure 41.1. Components of Li uptake in red blood cells from patients wth high, and from patients with low, *in vivo* Li ratios. The data are derived from the results shown in Table 41.1.

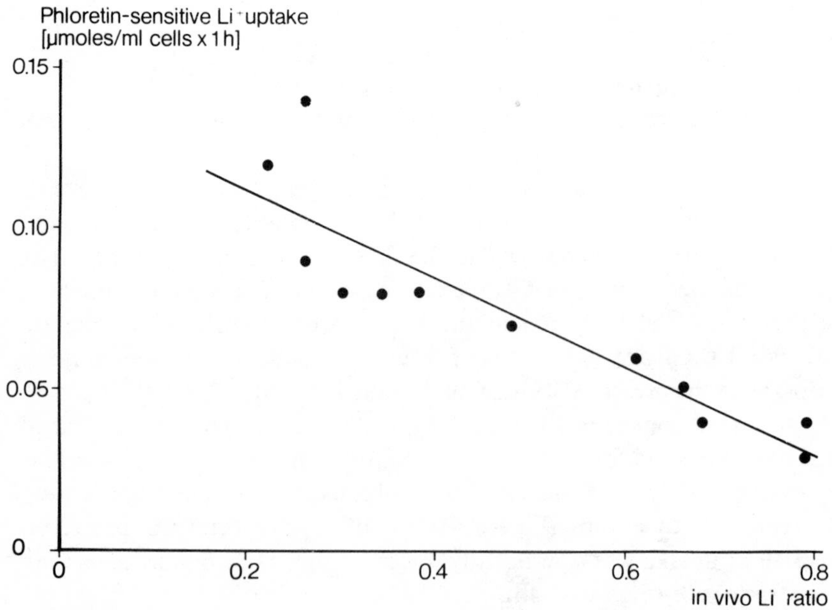

Figure 41.2. Correlation of *in vivo* ratios and *in vitro* phloretin-sensitive Li uptake of 12 Li treated patients.

patients. A high negative correlation has been found between the *in vivo* Li ratios and phloretin-sensitive Li uptake ($r = -0.896$, $r^2 = 0.80$). Hence, *in vitro* determination of phloretin-sensitive Li uptake may be used to predict the *in vivo* Li ratios. Li uptake in the presence of ouabain was also indirectly related to the *in vivo* Li ratios, but the correlation was less pronounced ($r = -0{\cdot}806$; $r^2 = 0{\cdot}65$).

DISCUSSION

Erythrocytes from patients with high, and from patients with low, *in vivo* Li ratios showed no significant differences in Li uptake by the Na-K pump and by leak diffusion. However, Li uptake by the Li-dependent Li countertransport system (i.e. phloretin-sensitive Li uptake) was markedly reduced in high ratio cells relative to low ratio erythrocytes although the internal Na concentrations were not significantly different. Furthermore, a highly indirect correlation has been found between the *in vivo* Li ratios and *in vitro* phloretin-sensitive Li uptake ($r = -0{\cdot}896$).

It is concluded that the interindividual differences in the *in vivo* Li ratios observed among Li treated patients are caused by interindividual differences in the effectiveness of the Na-dependent Li countertransport system of erythrocytes.

These results confirm our previous report (1), in which the Na dependent Li countertransport was investigated by different experiments, e.g. by determination of Li uphill transport out of Li loaded cells into media containing Li. Under such conditions, the *in vitro* ratios Li_i/Li_e obtained after 24 h of incubation were highly correlated to the *in vivo* Li ratios ($r = 0{\cdot}95$) (1). This relationship of *in vitro* and *in vivo* Li ratio has been confirmed by Frazer *et al.* (personal communication).

Based on these experiments, two *in vitro* tests that would predict the *in vivo* Li ratios can be proposed:

1. The determination of phloretin-sensitive Li uptake, presented in this study; and
2. The determination of the steady state *in vitro* ratio Li_i/Li_e as described in previous reports (1,2).

Both *in vitro* tests are measures of Na-dependent Li countertransport. These tests could be used to investigate the genetic control and the clinical significance of the *in vivo* Li ratio. Furthermore, they could help to test the membrane hypothesis of affective disorders (9), which has been derived from interindividual differences of the *in vivo* Li ratios. In a running study, we found similar interindividual variations of the *in vitro* Li ratios in erythrocytes from patients with affective disorders and in red cells from donors not suffering from affective diseases (1). Hence, high Li ratios, which are caused by a deficiency of the Na-dependent Li countertransport system, are apparently not restricted to erythrocytes of subjects with affective psychosis.

ACKNOWLEDGEMENTS

The work reported in this chapter was supported by the Deutsche Forschungsgemeinschaft grant for Research in Clinical Pharmacology.

References

1. Greil, W., Eisenried, F., Becker, B.F. and Duhm, J. (1977). *Psychopharmacol.,* 53, 19
2. Greil, W., Eisenried, F. and Duhm, J. (1976). *Arzneimittel-Forsch.,* 26, 1147
3. Duhm, J., Eisenried, F., Becker, B.F. and Greil, W. (1976). *Pflügers Arch.,* 364, 147
4. Haas, M., Schooler, J. and Tosteson, D.C. (1975). *Nature,* **258**, 425
5. Duhm, J. and Becker, B.F. (1977). *Pflügers Arch.* (in press)
6. Pandey, G.N., Javaid, J.I., Davis, J.N. and Tosteson, D.C. *Physiologist,* **19**, 321
7. Duhm, J., Becker, B.F., Eisenried, F. and Greil, W. (1976). *FEBS-Symposium on the Biochemistry of Membrane Transport,* Zürich, July 18-23, *Abstr. Vol.,* p. 342
8. Duhm, J. and Becker, B.F. (1977). *Pflügers Arch.,* **367**, 211
9. Mendels, J. and Frazer, A. (1974). *Am. J. Psychiat.,* **131**, 1240

42

The Intracellular Lithium Level: Is It of Any Use?

S. ANDREWS and E. CHIU

INTRODUCTION

Dr J.F.J. Cade (1) had observed that 80% of his manic patients responded promptly to lithium and 20% did not, so a series of single dose studies was started in 1969 in an attempt to find a method of recognizing those patients who would respond promptly (2). As part of these studies, the lithium levels in the erythrocytes were estimated on blood samples collected 2 hours after a single dose of 1200 mg of lithium carbonate. These estimations showed a similar range in the RBC lithium levels for both the patients who responded promptly and for those who did not, although the mean level appeared slightly higher for the group of patients who responded promptly in the first series tested (3).

Since then, other investigations of the RBC lithium levels have sought to establish a relationship between this level and the RBC Li/plasma Li ratio and the clinical improvement of the patient. Mendels and Frazer (4) tested a small group of 13 depressed patients and reported that clinical improvement in these patients' depression was associated with both a higher RBC lithium level and a higher RBC Li/plasma Li ratio (i.e. higher than 0.5). Some qualified support for this was given by Zerbi *et al.* (5) and by Cazzullo *et al.* (6) although the latter workers considered improvements in the manic phase as well as in the depressive phase, and they reported higher fluctuations in the ratios of individual patients as well as finding a considerable number of responders with ratios less than 0.5.

Other workers disagree with these findings. Rybakowski *et al.* (7) did not find this difference in the lithium ratio between the responders and non-responders in their series of 37 patients, but did find a positive correlation between the ratio and the intensity of the EEG charges. Lee *et al.* (8) considered the RBC Li/plasma Li ratio to be of no value for comparing individual response to lithium.

The above investigations were based on fairly small groups of patients of a similar nature. The Royal Park Psychiatric Hospital has many patients who have been on lithium therapy for long periods and who have been monitored regularly during that time. It was, therefore, decided to carry out a survey of the erythrocyte lithium levels in as many of these patients as possible without altering their treatment in any way, and to compare these levels and the RBC Li /plasma Li ratios with their clinical state at the time.

It was important to carry out this survey with the minimum of inconvenience to the patients concerned as blood collection is not usually a popular procedure with such patients. This imposed some limitations as the majority of patients studied were out-patients and those who usually attend in the evenings or at weekends could not be included. The need for prompt centrifugation at high speed for one hour also imposed some practical limitations on the number of samples which could be processed on a busy out-patients day.

PATIENTS AND METHODS

The samples estimated in 1969 and 1970 and a preliminary trial run of some 30 patients for this study (between April and June 1976) were performed by the indirect method of calculation from the values for the plasma and whole blood lithium levels and the packed cell volume (corrected for trapped plasma). The rest of the estimations were performed between November 1976 and April 1977 using a direct method similar to that of Frazer *et al.* (9) but without the special equipment. As the direct method is more time consuming, a series was performed by both methods to check on the agreement between them and to ascertain whether the direct method is really necessary.

A total of 350 estimations from 130 patients was performed. In 14 patients only one estimation was performed but the other 116 had from 2 to 9 separate estimations at different times during the test period. The majority of the patients included had been on lithium therapy for periods ranging from 2 months to 8 years beforehand and 20 were in-patients who had just been commenced on lithium therapy. The samples available during the test period were from 130 patients of whom 92 suffered from bipolar, 20 from unipolar affective illness, 12 schizo-affective patients, and 6 patients with Huntington's Chorea.

For both the direct and the indirect methods, 10 ml of venous blood was collected in a heparinized tube at the standard time (12 hours after the last dose of lithium). This blood was well mixed on a rotator and samples taken for the estimation of the packed cell volume. For the indirect method, whole blood samples were then taken out by pipette and diluted 1 in 10 with distilled water. The remainder of the blood was centrifuged immediately for 15 mins. and plasma samples pipetted out and diluted similarly.

For the direct method, after taking PCV samples, the blood was centrifuged promptly at 1600 g for 1 h. The top layer of plasma was transferred to another tube, and the remaining plasma 'buffy coat' and the top layer of packed red cells was removed by aspiration.

A pipette calibrated 'to contain' was used to measure the red cells by the wash-out method. The tip of this pipette was placed at the bottom of the packed cells, and 0.5 ml drawn up. The outside of the pipette was thoroughly wiped before running the 0.5 ml of cells slowly into 4.5 ml of distilled water. This water was then sucked up and down at least 20 times in the pipette until the red cells adhering to the inside walls were washed out. The diluted cells were thoroughly mixed on a vortex mixer so that they were completely laked.

A 1 in 10 dilution of the plasma was made with an ordinary 'to deliver' pipette. The lithium content of the laked cell dilution and the diluted plasma could be estimated by either an atomic absorption spectrophotometer or a flame photometer using standard solutions containing appropriate amounts of other cations. The whole blood dilutions could be estimated in the same way.

For the earlier work in 1969 an EEL flame photometer was used, and for the recent work a Varian-Techtron atomic absorption spectrophotometer. The standard solutions were checked against control sera of known lithium content and against one another on each run.

RESULT

The most obvious feature is the individual variation in the way lithium is handled by apparently similar patients. The long-term patients showed a surprisingly wide range of plasma lithium levels. Excluding two patients who were showing toxic symptoms at the time of testing, this range was 0.15-1.45 mmol/l. Nevertheless, 40% of these patients had average plasma levels between 0.8 and 1.2 mmol/l. with another 31.5% between 0.6 and 0.8 mmol/l. The mean was 0.74 mmol/l (SD ± 0·22).

Erythrocyte levels were much lower with a mean of 0·41 mmol/l (SD ±0.23). These covered a range of 0.1-1.6 mmol/l but 60% had an average erythrocyte lithium level between 0.2 and 0.5 mmol/l. The ratio of this RBC lithium was fairly evenly distributed above and below 0.5 with 63 of the patients showing an average ratio greater than 0.5 and 67 with a ratio up to 0.5. All diagnostic groups were evenly divided except the unipolar group with 6 ratios above 0.5 and 14 below 0.5. Of the total tests, 172 gave a ratio above 0.5 and 178 below 0.5. The magnitude of the ratio remained fairly steady and of the 116 patients tested more than once, 99 of these showed ratios which remained consistently above or below 0.5,and only 17 patients showed a movement in the ratio above or below 0.5. Some 41 patients did show a remarkable constancy in the ratio with a variation no greater than 0.05 in ratio levels despite considerable variations in lithium and erythrocyte levels between estimations.

The results were examined statistically to see whether there appeared to be any relationship between the plasma lithium and the RBC lithium; or the ratio and factors such as sex, total daily dosage, dosage considered as mg/kg body weight, diagnosis including polarity, and the mood and clinical condition of the patient at the time of testing. The statistical analysis included analysis of variance and test of linearity. The slightly higher mean levels found in female patients were not statistically significant.

Table 42.1.

		Plasma Li/RBC Li	Plasma Li	RBC Li
Females	83	0.54 SD ± 0.18	0.76 ± 0.24	0.43 ± 0.24
Males	47	0.50 SD ± 0.19	0.72 ± 0.17	0.27 ± 0.21
Total	130	0.53 SD ± 0.19	0.74 ± 0.21	0.41 ± 0.23

There was no correlation between the plasma lithium the RBC lithium or the ratio with the total daily dosage. When the dosage was considered as mg/kg body weight, the analysis showed a positive Pearson product-moment correlation. The total dosage varied between 500 and 2250 mg of lithium carbonate (mean 1146 mg) and the dosage/kg body weight varied from 8 to 25.4 mg/kg (mean 15.8).

Unfortunately the four diagnostic groups were not of similar size but the statistical analysis indicated that there was no correlation between lithium levels or ratios and the clinical classification.

Table 42.2.

Classification	n	Ratio (mean)	Plasma Li	RBC Li
Bipolar	92	0.54 ± 0.17	0.75 ± 0.22	0.41 ± 0.23
Unipolar	20	0.51 ± 0.26	0.72 ± 0.22	0.40 ± 0.30
Schizo-affective	12	0.49 ± 0.16	0.73 ± 0.17	0.37 ± 0.17
Huntington's Chorea	6	0.50 ± 0.18	0.80 ± 0.21	0.40 ± 0.24

No relationship was found between the mean lithium levels or ratios and the affective state of the patients during the study period.

Table 42.3.

Affective state	n	Ratio (mean)	Plasma Li	RBC Li
Sometimes depressed	15	0.48 ± 0.11	0.76 ± 0.17	0.38 ± 0.16
Remaining stable	96	0.52 ± 0.19	0.75 ± 0.21	0.41 ± 0.25
Sometimes hypomanic	19	0.59 ± 0.23	0.69 ± 0.26	0.41 ± 0.20

Although the total 350 tests show a similar distribution of mood at the time each test was done and similar Li figures, the analysis of variation suggests that there may be a significant variation (with a probability of less than 0.05) for the plasma Li and the ratio but not for the RBC Li.

Table 42.4.

Affective State	n	Ratio		Plasma Li		RBC Li	
Depressed	38	0.48	0.14	0.75	0.24	0.38	0.20
Stable	255	0.54	0.23	0.76	0.24	0.44	0.28
Hypomanic	57	0.62	0.26	0.67	0.28	0.41	0.23

None of the other analyses considering the 350 tests separately showed any significant variation.

The ratio does not seem to be of much use in the practical management of patients. Our series of 20 new patients showed 13 apparently responding to lithium therapy and 7 not responding. Of those responding only 2 had ratios above 0.5 and 2 of the non-responders also had ratios above 0.5.

Likewise with the 98 long-term patients who had multiple estimations, the range of clinical conditions among patients with ratios below 0.5 was similar to the range among patients with ratios above 0.5.

Table 42.5.

Condition during study period	Ratio up to 0.5	Ratio above 0.5	Changing ratio
Remained depressed	7	5	3
Remained stable	30	25	5
Remained high, hypomanic	4	11	4
Fluctuating	2	1	1
Totals	43	42	13

SINGLE DOSE STUDY

This study, completed in 1969-70, provides an interesting comparison. The 134 patients included had been divided (on the basis of the amount of lithium excreted in 4 h following a single dose of 1200 mg of lithium carbonate) into 'retainers' (with an excretion up to 15 mg), and 'intermediate' group (15-20 mg) and 'excretors' (over 20 mg). It should be emphasized that this division can be observed only for a short excretion period after an initial single dose and excretion values do not correspond with the lithium clearance values obtained when the same patients are stabilized on lithium. It was considered that 'retainers' are likely to respond promptly to treatment with lithium and excretors are not likely to respond promptly. It can be seen from the table below that RBC lithium levels and RBC Li/plasma Li ratios are generally higher at 2 hours after this single large dose than those found in patients on long-term treatment in our recent study.

Table 42.6.

Group		Number with ratio up to 0.5	Number with ratio over 0.5	Average Ratio	Average Pl Li	Average RBC Li
Whole group	134	17	117	0.77	0.78	0.60
Retainers	48	5	43	0.96	0.64	0.61
Intermediate	24	2	22	0.71	0.78	0.59
Excretors	62	10	52	0.66	0.89	0.59

This single dose study did not include any of the patients in the recent study but 23 of these did have a urinary lithium excretion test done between 1968-72. 12 were classed as retainers, 7 as excretors and 4 as intermediate. In the recent study these small groups of retainers and excretors now have very similar average RBC lithium levels (0.46 and

0.45) and ratios (0.57 and 0.58). This merely supports our previous observations that differences observed in the single dose studies occur only in the early stages after this initial dose.

CONCLUSION

It appears that RBC lithium estimations and RBC Li/plasma Li ratios are of very limited value in the management of patients but may be of value in further investigations into the way in which lithium works. It was found that the indirect method for estimating RBC lithium from plasma lithium, whole blood lithium and the packed cell volume gave very good agreement with the direct estimation from red blood cells. The indirect method would, therefore, be the method of choice because of its greater convenience and simplicity.

ACKNOWLEDGEMENTS

We would like to thank Mr Norman Carson for the statistical analysis, and Charge Nurse Ken Dixon, Sister Jan Williams and other staff members of the Lithium Clinic for collection of samples and assistance with the recording of patients' data. We also wish to thank the Mental Health Authority for permission to publish this paper.

References

1. Cade, J.F.J. (1968). Personal communication.
2. Serry, M. (1969). *Aust. NZ. J. Psychiat.*, 3, 390
   Aust. NZ. J. Psychiat., 3, 390
3. Serry, M. and Andrews, S. (1969). *The Lithium Excretion Test: Practical and biochemi-*
   Aust. NZ. J. Psychiat., 3, 395
4. Mendels, J. and Frazer, A. (1973). *J. Psychiat. Res.*, **10**, 9
5. Zerbi, *et al.* (1975). *Psychiat. Clin.*, **8**, 236
6. Cazzullo, C.L. *et al.* (1975). *Br. J. Psychiat.*, **126**, 298
7. Rybakowski, J. *et al.* (1974). *Int. Pharmacopsychiat.*, **9**, 166
8. Lee, C.R. *et al.* (1975). *Br. J. Psychiat.*, **127**, 596
9. Frazer, A. *et al.* (1972). *Clin. Chim. Acta.*, **36**, 499

PART VI:
Lithium Research in Prospect

Introduction

In the final chapter of this book, Dr Roy Hullin, Scientific Director of the Regional Metabolic Research Unit which is based at High Royds Hospital, at Menston in West Yorkshire, looks at the advances which have been made in lithium research to date, and speculates on the directions which future research might take. He also outlines work being done in his unit which is in the forefront of lithium research in the UK. In particular he refers to studies on thyroid function in patients undergoing lithium therapy; this issue, not dealt with in earlier chapters, is of considerable interest and potential importance.

There can be no doubt that lithium will be a very influential guiding force in research on many aspects of psychiatry for a long time to come. Work in this area has already led to new insights into the mechanisms underlying psychiatric disorders and the large numbers of talented research workers who are being attracted to this topic will certainly uncover new information which will help in the fight against mental suffering.

43

The Place of Lithium in Biological Psychiatry

R. P. HULLIN

INTRODUCTION

When I was invited last autumn to give the closing address at the First British Lithium Congress, I was greatly honoured. In accepting the invitation, I was conscious of this honour but I was also attracted irresistibly by that rare prospect, professionally and domestically, of having the last word.

If anyone should be expecting me to tie up the confusion of hypotheses regarding the effective disorders, or to tell which of the haystack of needles (to use one of David Shaw's apt phrases), that is, which of the large variety of metabolic and endocrinological effects of lithium is responsible for its therapeutic and prophylactic effects in manic depressive psychosis, they will be disappointed. It would require someone with greater intellectual abilities than I possess to do either of these tasks. Indeed, I think it would require supernatural insight or second sight. I therefore propose to approach my task in five stages. Firstly, I will make some observations on the place of lithium in biological psychiatry, as I see it. Secondly, I will make some observations on the proceedings of the Congress. Then I will describe two areas of research in this field which have been carried out in our unit. Finally, I will briefly indicate areas of research which I believe may be productive in clarifying the mechanisms and management of lithium treatment.

In this Silver Jubilee year we, in the United Kingdom, have been looking back at the last 25 years from many different aspects. It is therefore appropriate to look back to the position of biological psychiatry and the treatment of mental illness in 1952. Already, 3 years had passed since Professor Cade's report of the anti-manic effect of lithium salts. 1952 was also the year that reserpine was isolated from Indian snake root which led to its use as an anti-hypertensive agent. It soon began to be appreciated that reserpine was also useful as an anti-psychotic drug. Reserpine, however, because of its limited effectiveness and serious side-effects, was soon replaced by the phenothiazines. Nevertheless, the occurrence of depressive reactions in patients receiving reserpine for hypertension had a major impact on the development of biogenic amine hypotheses for the affective disorders, since reserpine and related compounds produced depletion of serotonin, noradrenaline and dopamine in peripheral tissues and in the brain.

No substantial development of John Cade's observation took place for approximately a decade, due, no doubt, to the fatalities reported in the United States when lithium chloride was used as a salt substitute under conditions and in patients which, in the light of hindsight, were peculiarly unfortunate. There may be a lesson for us in this fallow period when an original discovery was not exploited for benefit because of the fears of harm. I would like to add my voice to those of Mogens Schou and Alec Jenner, that reports of nephrotoxic effects of long-term lithium be put in proper perspective so that undue, and maybe unnecessary, fears do not inhibit the further development of lithium treatment. It is clear that this matter must be investigated and assessed as quickly as possible, possibly by means of international co-operation between groups active in treating patients with lithium. It should be possible to assess the significance of the finding quite soon, but since it is my impression that, generally, prophylactic lithium is used at lower serum levels in the United Kingdom than in Scandinavia, it is important to include groups from this country in any study, since the effects, if substantiated, may be dose-related. Thus lower levels of lithium sufficient to maintain the prophylactic effect might avoid unwanted effects of this nature. In the meantime, judgement should be reserved.

The prophylactic use of lithium salts, and the demonstration of their beneficial effects, did not commence until the middle sixties. Since then, interest in lithium has been reflected in an almost exponential growth of the literature culminating in the First British Lithium Congress which has attracted 250 delegates from all over the world and which has involved scientific sessions, some running in parallel, of over 20 hours duration.

There is no doubt that lithium treatment has conferred great benefit upon thousands of people who formerly spent their lives either in hospital permanently, or with frequent admissions for affective disturbances. Unlike anti-depressants and neuroleptic drugs which have changed the type of treatment and reduced time in hospital following acute admission, lithium salts have kept responsive patients out of hospital altogether. Many of the unfortunate consequences of recurrent illnesses, such as unemployment, promotion prospects, marital difficulties and much unhappiness, have thus been avoided. Patients have been enabled to resume a life of a worthwhile quality with consequential social and economic gains for themselves and the community as a whole.

I have recently been seeking information in order to estimate the number of patients receiving prophylactic treatment. In 1976, 136 000 prescriptions for lithium carbonate were dispensed by general practitioners in the United Kingdom, amounting to a total of 6700 kilograms. Hospital dispensing would probably add a further 15% to this total. Assuming that all the lithium carbonate is used for prophylactic treatment and the average daily dose is 1 g, these calculations suggest that 20-25 thousand patients are receiving treatment or approximately 1 per 2 000 of the population. The figure of 1 per 1000 in Edinburgh cited by Dr Glen is of interest in this connection. Whilst I recognize that this higher value probably reflects the greater enthusiasm for this treatment in Edinburgh, is it pertinent or impertinent to ask whether this is responsible for Scottish Nationalism? Only a Welshman could ask such a question and hope to get away with it. The number of people who could benefit from lithium treatment will obviously depend upon the criteria adopted for its use. Statistics from the Camberwell register suggest that 50-100 thousand people might benefit. There is therefore quite a long way to go in the United Kingdom before the drug is given to all who might benefit.

In addition to the direct role of lithium in treatment, the demonstration of its usefulness in therapy has provided a major stimulus to research into affective disorders as shown by the literature and by the British Lithium Congress.

I hope our overseas visitors will not regard it as scientific chauvinism if in Jubilee Year I draw attention to the contributions of British workers to lithium research. Whilst the pioneering work of Cade, Schou and the Scandinavians can rightly be regarded as playing the major initiatory role, contributions have been made by workers in Hellingly, Sheffield, Cardiff, Edinburgh and Dundee. The Maudsley Hospital should also receive recognition, since although lithium is not a therapeutic myth in recurrent unipolar depression, this suggestion stimulated much useful work which confirmed the efficacy of lithium salts in this condition. I hope also that our small contribution in Leeds is worthy of mention. It is easier for me, as one fortunate to be born in the principality of Wales, to take part in a little trumpet blowing, however muted, since, unlike our English conquerers with their stereotyped reserve and understatement, and the dourer qualities of our Celtic cousins north of the border, the Welsh are not expected to refrain from hyperbole and certainly on the rugby field this is well justified.

Turning next to the Congress, the proceedings of which are recorded in this book; we heard during the various sessions about the clinical uses of lithium which are extensions of its established role in recurrent affective disorders. We heard a paper on its acute anti-depressive effect, but this must be weak if it exists, since this role has not been obviously recognized by groups with a long and wide experience of lithium treatment. Interesting papers were also given on the use of lithium in alcoholism, drug addiction in rats, as an anti-aggressive agent and in schizo-affective disorder and emotional disturbances in children.

Nothwithstanding these extensions, I find it reassuring that the dominant clinical effect of lithium still remains on mood or conditions where mood might play a part. This indicates a degree of specificity in its effect and not the well-known panacea syndrome.

Reports were also presented of a very wide range of metabolic and endocrinological effects of lithium ranging from effects on magnesium-containing enzymes, adenylate cyclase, calcium, magnesium and bone and on carbohydrate metabolism, the latter arising from weight gain experienced by some patients on lithium. There were also papers demonstrating effects of lithium on 5-hydroxytryptamine metabolism, prostaglandins and transport processes for choline and sodium in erythrocytes and platelets. The irreversible effect of lithium on choline transport in red cells is of particular interest. Dr Greil's paper elegantly clarified the processes involved in the inter-individual differences in red cell: plasma ratios of lithium, and there was a fascinating symposium on model systems of various kinds ranging from the theoretical through bio-chemical to behavioural models in animals.

Finally we came to the nitty-gritty of the management of patients on lithium. Even if work in this area is not as high flying as some fields, it is certainly very important to the patients. In any event the therapeutic effect on patients has provided the motivation for all the other fields of investigation.

The papers were so wide-ranging that it would not only be inappropriate, but impossible, to make other than selected comments. One general comment I would make is for an awareness of the balance of advantage and disadvantage of investigations as the degree of disorganisation increases from studies in human subjects and whole animals, especially the rat (which may not be the ideal species), to investigations on organs, tissues, organelles and finally to isolated enzymes. There are gains and losses at each stage. The more the system used is isolated from other influences, the easier it is to reproduce and interpret the results. However, this is also the situation furthest removed from clinical studies of patients. We must take care not to let the gap in thinking become too wide. It is also important to differentiate and define carefully whether investigations are of acute or long-term effects of lithium remembering that the locus of the anti-manic and prophylactic effect may not necessarily be the same. Dosages used in certain *in vitro* investigations often bear little relationship to therapeutic levels in man.

Regarding patient management, it seems to me that, in the light of possible dose-related, unwanted, side-effects of lithium, it is preferable, whichever lithium preparation is used, to administer it in divided dosage, not in a single daily dose. There is little reliable evidence that any commercial preparation is slow, or sustained, release as opposed to delayed release *in vivo*. Thus a divided dosage schedule would avoid large peaks in serum levels and hence reduce the likelihood of toxic effects. The argument that a single daily dose of any preparation is preferable in terms of compliance and convenience, whilst valid, does not convince me as being important compared to possibly the more serious disadvantages of high serum peaks. Nevertheless, whilst holding this view, it is intriguing to contemplate the possibility emerging from this Congress that the maximum effects of lithium, at least on carbohydrate metabolism, seem to be produced by changing lithium concentration rather than the actual concentration itself. It was suggested therefore that intermittent dosage with lithium might be the treatment of choice. Such a suggestion will repay investigation as will also further studies on the minimum lithium level required to maintain a prophylactic effect. After these general comments, I now wish to describe some work carried out in out Unit. Little has been said in the earlier chapters concerning the well-recognized effect of lithium on thyroid function and it therefore seems desirable that I should try to remedy this.

THE EFFECT OF LITHIUM ON THYROID FUNCTION

With the increased use of lithium salts in the treatment of affective disorders, many investigators have reported lithium effects on thyroid function. These studies have indicated that females, especially those over 40, are more susceptible to lithium-induced hypothyroidism than males (1,2). Females over 40 however, whether treated with lithium or not, have a higher incidence of hypothyroidism. Nicholson *et al.* (3), for example, found three cases of unrecognised hypothyroidism in 98 unselected female psychiatric admissions, only one of whom was on lithium treatment; the incidence in female patients over 40 was 6%, excluding the lithium case.

Serum thyrotrophin (TSH) has been used as a sensitive indicator of hypothyroidism in patients receiving prophylactic lithium. Emerson *et al.* (4), reported raised TSH levels in 30% of 255 patients at some time during treatment and, at final testing, in 14% of patients who had been treated with lithium for an average period of 8 months. Linstedt *et al.* (5), have recently reported low T4 and raised TSH in 8 out of 53 patients (15%) who had received lithium at serum levels of 0.8-1.2 mmol/l for at least 2 years; all were females giving an incidence of 8/39 (20%) for female patients. Villeneuve *et al.* (6) reported hypothyroidism (low PBI and T4) in 14.7% of 149 cases on lithium treatment; for females the incidence was 23%. Transbøl *et al.* (7) have found raised TSH levels in 20/86 patients who had received lithium for an average of 80 months; 19/20 patients were females, all but one over 40, giving an incidence of hypothyroidism of 29% in females and 34% in females over 40.

We have recently determined thyroid function of 108 patients regularly attending our weekly clinic who have been maintained on lithium for an average period of 56 months. The thyroid tests were carried out by C. Chapman and C.J. Hayter of the Department of Nuclear Medicine, Leeds General Infirmary. Plasma thyroxine (T4) and tri-iodothyronine (T3) were measured using pre-precipitated double antibody developed in the Department of Nuclear Medicine and ^{125}I-labelled T4 and T3, both of high specific activity, obtained from the Radiochemical Centre, Amersham, Bucks. TSH was determined by a modification of the method of Odell *et al.* (8) as described by Chapman, Hutton & Hayter (9). Thyroid hormone distribution index THDI which indicates the distribution of thyroid hormones between the free and protein-bound fractions in plasma was measured as described by Macdonald, Chapman & Franklin (10). Serum T3 and T4 have been determined in each patient 2-10 times (mean 3.5) over a period of 8 months. When either or both of these were low, serum TSH was also measured. 7 of the 108 patients had been receiving 1-thyroxine as well as lithium for an average period of 40 months (range 9-54) because of previously detected persistent hypothyroidism (11). The age, sex, (M = male F = female) time on lithium, dosage and serum levels of this group of patients is given in Table 43.1.

Table 43.1. Characteristics of patients receiving thyroxine

	No.	Age (years)		Time on lithium (months)		Dosage (mg Li_2CO_3)		12 h serum lithium (mmol/l)	
		Mean	Range	Mean	Range	Mean	Range	Mean	Range
M	3	75.3	72-81	82.3	57-75	467	400-500	0.60	0.35-0.87
F	4	64.0	53-76	66.5	48-96	700	600-800	0.852	0.56-1.16

Of the remaining 101 patients, 64 had at least one low T3 and/or T4 result during the serial study. Normal ranges for the laboratory were 60-140 and 1.6-3.0 ng/ml for T4 and T3 respectively. 34 of these 64 patients had only one low result. 30 gave low values on 2-5 occasions. 12 were below the normal range on every occasion tested. Age, sex and treatment data for the euthyroid patients and for the group with at least one low thyroid result are shown in Table 43.2.

Table 43.2. Patient characteristics

	No.	Age		Time on lithium		Dosage (mg)		12 h serum level	
		Mean	Range	Mean	Range	Mean	Range	Mean	Range
A) Eurthyroid patients									
M	11	52.0	39-69	58.6	24-100	800	400-1200	0.507	0.22-0.72
F	26	53.7	18-73	63.3	3-120	721	250-1200	0.567	0.30-0.95
B) Patients with at least one low thyroid test									
M	19	52.7	20-71	61.8	3-115	941	500-1600	0.674	0.32-0.97
F	45	53.5	18-80	46.0	4-120	891	400-2000	0.707	0,35-1.12

It can be seen that the ages and times on lithium of all groups are very similar except that euthyroid females, contrary to expectation, have received lithium longer on average than females with hypothyroid values. The mean serum lithium levels of both euthyroid males and females however are significantly lower ($p < 0.001$) than their counterparts who show some indication of hypothyroidism.

The mean values and ranges of total T4, total T3 and the mean ± SEM of the free thyroxine index (FTI) in the euthyroid males and females and the rest of the patients are given in Table 43.3. THDI was within the normal range for the laboratory (1.2-2.0) in all except 2 patients.

Table 43.3.

	Total T4		Total T3		FTI	
	Mean	Range	Mean	Range	Mean	SEM
Euthyroid males	85.1	62-135	2.22	1.7-3.2	1.84	0.11
Euthyroid females	90.3	61-134	2.26	1.7-3.1	1.74	0.06
Males with 1 or >1 low test value	74.3	53-108	1.74	0.9-2.7	1.05	0.02
Females with 1 or >1 low test value	72.2	31-145	1.75	0.8-2.6	0.97	0.03

Despite the high incidence of abnormalities, albeit of a transient nature in some patients, it is surprising that only four patients (all females over 40) had TSH values above the normal range for the laboratory. Taking a raised TSH as the best laboratory criterion of primary hypothyroidism, the incidence of this condition in our patients on lithium, including 7 previously detected by other laboratory tests is 11/108 (10%), compared with 15%, 14% and 23%, respectively reported by Lindstedt *et al.* (5), Villeneuve *et al.* (6) and Transbøl *et al.* (7). Considering female patients unrelated to age, we have found hypothyroidism in 10.6% whereas incidences of 20%, 23% and 29% have been reported by the other groups. For females over 40, our figure is 12.5% (8/64) whilst Transbøl *et al.* (7) reported hypothyroidism in 34%. It may be that the lower incidence of hypothyroidism in our lithium-treated patients, despite the length of the average time of treatment, is related to the lower average levels of serum lithium we maintain without diminution of prophylactic effect. Some support for this suggestion is provided by the lower average dosages and serum levels of lithium found in our euthyroid patients compared to those of patients with at least occasionally low circulating thyroid hormones.

From the viewpoint of patient management, two considerations emerge: 1) the possibility of reducing the incidence of lithium-induced hypothyroidism by maintaining lower, but still effective, prophylactic blood levels, and 2) reinforcement of the view we put forward in 1972 and subsequently supported by other workers, such as Rosser (12), Transbøl *et al.* (7), Lindstedt *et al.* (5), of the importance of routine screening of thyroid function before starting and during lithium treatment. Opinions vary as to the frequency of monitoring required but, if facilities are readily available, there is much to be said for screening thyroid function not only before beginning lithium treatment but also on each visit once the blood lithium level been stabilised and certainly at 3- or 6-monthly intervals during treatment. Rosser (12) has drawn attention to the less common situation where treatment with lithium is complicated by thyrotoxicosis. Whilst the symptoms and signs of hypothyroidism can be mistaken for the early stage of a depressive relapse, the clinical signs of thyrotoxicosis may be confused with the side effects of lithium. If lithium is withdrawn as a consequence of this, the thyrotoxicity may be accentuated as a rebound phenomenon. In our hospital, we have seen two cases of thyrotoxicity in lithium-treated patients similar to those described by Rosser (12). Thus it is desirable that proper management of lithium treatment should include some schedule of monitoring thyroid function in addition to blood lithium.

Turning to the mechanisms underlying the effect of lithium on the thyroid gland: in laboratory studies, lithium has been shown to block the stimulating effect of TSH (13), to impair coupling of iodotyrosines (14,15) and to interfere with release of hormone from the gland by disrupting microtubules (17). However, in a patient with a normal thyroid gland, compensatory increase in the secretion of TSH from the pituitary results in a normal rate of thyroid hormone production though often with a lower serum PBI (11) and thyroxine concentration. In our survey, lithium-patients have again been shown to have T3 and T4 concentrations skewed towards the bottom of, and in some cases, below the range of values found in euthyroid, untreated, groups of similar age and sex distribution (Figures 43.1 and 43.2).

The report of Fyrö *et al.* (1) that serum thyroxine concentration may revert to its original level after long-term treatment with lithium is not supported in our patient population. A lower range of serum concentrations of T4, T3 and protein bound iodide (PBI) can therefore be expected in a patient receiving lithium. In the absence of clinically overt signs of hypothyroidism, such a finding requires no action. Hypothryroidism can occur in various forms ranging in severity from patients with decreased serum thyroid hormones, very high levels of TSH associated with overt clinical symptoms, through milder forms with low T3 and T4, raised TSH levels but only unspecific symptoms, to subclinical states with low T3 and T4, no obvious symptoms and no increase in TSH levels. It is remarkable that, in our cross-sectional study, only a few cases of raised TSH levels were found despite the widespread incidence of transient and even persistently low circulating levels of T3 and T4. How can this be

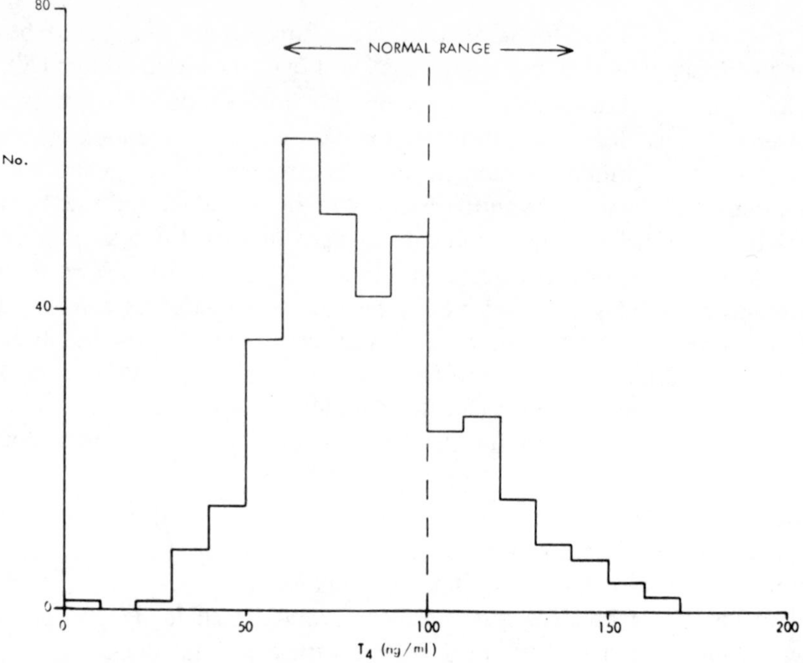

Figure 43.1. Distribution of T4 values amongst lithium-treated patients showing a skew towards the bottom range of, and sometimes below, the range of values noted in matched euthyroid untreated subjects

explained? Could it be that lithium in addition to its direct effect on thyroid hormone production, might also affect the pituitary-thyroid axis so that the expected response in TSH secretion is not forthcoming? Alternatively, the more sensitive and sophisticated laboratory tests of thyroid function used today may reveal hitherto unsuspected, subtle changes in the reserve capacity of the thyroid gland. There is little information available on serial changes in serum T3 and T4 in normal euthyroid individuals; these may be larger than anticipated from studies using less sensitive techniques.

Only one of the four patients discovered with persistently low serum thyroid hormones and markedly raised TSH levels in our study showed clinical signs and symptoms of hypothyroidism. There may be some discrepancy between the severity and persistence of hypothyroidism revealed by these laboratory tests and their clinical effect on the patient.

ALDOSTERONE-RENIN RELATIONSHIPS IN BIPOLAR MANIC-DEPRESSIVE PSYCHOSIS

On the first day of initiating lithium treatment, a sodium diuresis occurs

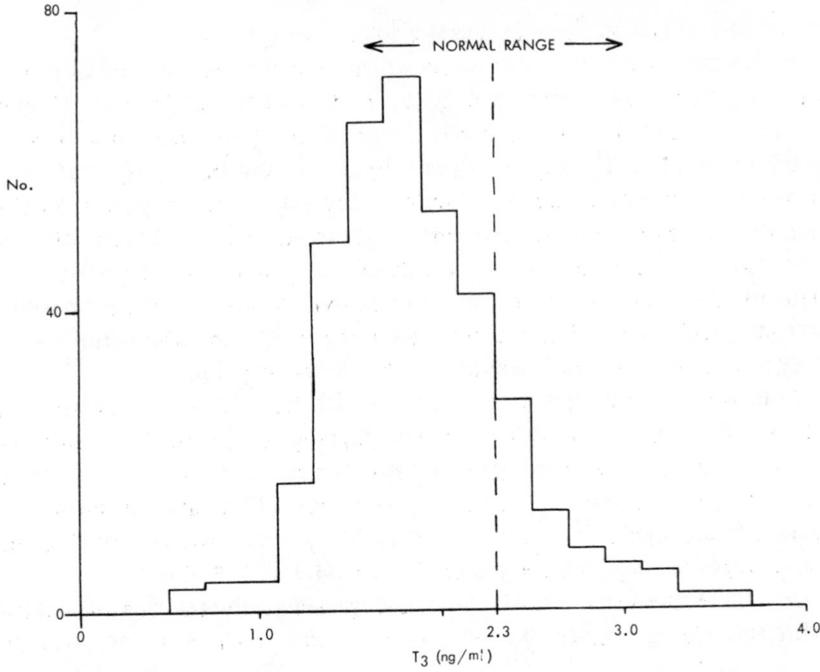

Figure 43.2. Distribution of T3 values amongst lithium-treated patients. Like the T4 values, these show a skew towards the lower end of, and below, the range of values noted in euthyroid untreated subjects

followed on subsequent days by a reduction in the urinary sodium excretion (on constant daily sodium intake) as lithium treatment continues (18). These changes in sodium metabolism result from an initial decrease in aldosterone production (19,20), followed by an increase during the first few weeks of treatment. Long-term effects of lithium upon the renin-aldosterone system have not been investigated until recently when Transbøl reported that, compared with control subjects, plasma levels of aldosterone and renin were increased in 17 manic-depressive patients on long-term lithium treatment (21). These effects of lithium on the aldosterone-renin system in affective disorders make it relevant to describe some of the work we have been carrying out in recent years on aldosterone renin relationships. It is possible to speculate on the possibility that this work could provide clues to construct another model to explain how lithium may exert its therapeutic and prophylactic effect. This work has been carried out by our Unit in collaboration with Drs M.J. Levell of the Division of Steroid Endocrinology and M.R. Lee of the Department of Medicine, University of Leeds. My colleagues, Drs R. McDonald, M.N.E. Allsopp, S.P. Tyrer, T.C. Jerram and M.J. O'Brien, have also been involved at different times in these various investigations.

A number of experimental results from animals and man indicate that factors other than plasma potassium and sodium, angiotensin II and ACTH act directly on the zona glomulerosa to influence aldosterone production (22). To explain these results it has been suggested that unknown stimulators and/or inhibitors may act at various points on the biosynthetic pathway of aldosterone. From experiments on sheep (23) and dog (24), a factor has been postulated, originating in the CNS and dependant on sodium concentration there, which directly influences aldosterone production. Thus the renin-angiotensin system, whilst important, may not be the only one involved in aldosterone secretion.

Following earlier work by ourselves and others (25-27) which showed abnormalities in the control of sodium metabolism in bipolar manic depressive patients, we investigated aldosterone production in such patients (28,29). It was shown that the aldosterone production rate fell during the switch from mania to depression, reaching a very low level during the early stages of the depressed phase (Figures 43.3 and 43.4).

A fall in the extra-cellular fluid and plasma volumes was associated with this change rather than the expected rise. Further support for an

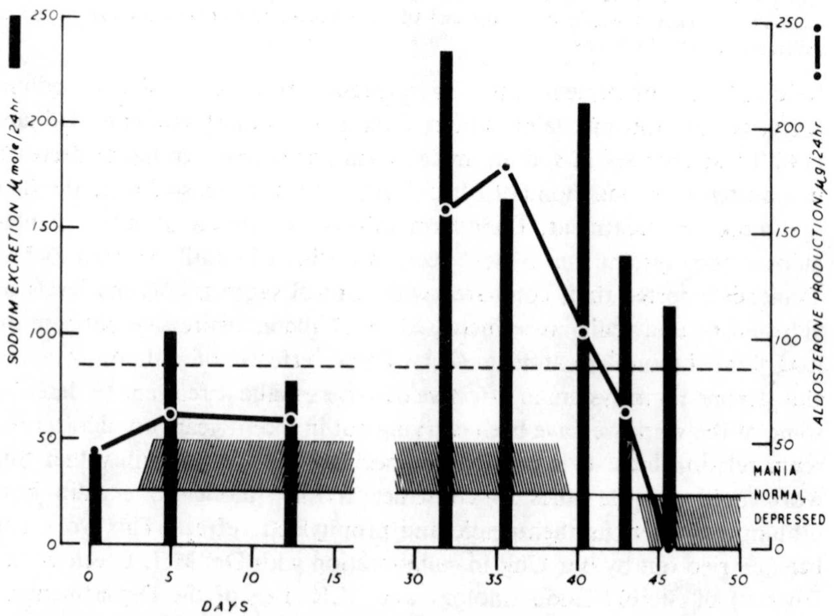

Figure 43.3. Sodium excretion and aldosterone production rates in bipolar manic depressive patients, related to prevailing mood state

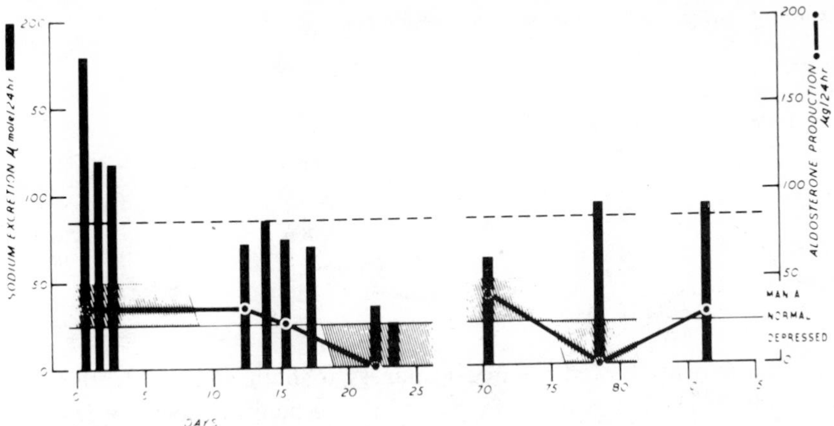

Figure 43.4. Sodium excretion and aldosterone production rates in different mood states

abnormality in the regulatory mechanisms for aldosterone in patients with manic depressive psychosis came from studies of a 40-year-old woman whose typical pattern of affective change was a 72-h cycle. The cycle involved depression on day 1 and the morning of day 2 followed by a rapid transition to mania (usually after a short sleep) which persisted for the remainder of that day and throughout the following day (day 3). For simplicity the three days are described as depressed, switch and manic days, respectively. Her urinary aldosterone excretion was studied over two 72-h cycles in a metabolic ward on a sodium intake of 90 mmol/24 h. Any deficiences of intake during her depression were made good by slow sodium tablets. The slow sodium was then increased to give a sodium intake of 270 mmol/day which was maintained until balance and constant weight had been achieved when a further 72-hour cycle was studied. The patient was then given diuretics and the sodium intake lowered until balance and constant weight were achieved on 15-20 mmol/24 h intake. The aldosterone excretion pattern was then investigated over another cycle.

The aldosterone excretion results for the various periods are shown in Table 43.4.

The excretions of aldosterone during sodium loading are not significantly different from those on the normal sodium intake. On the low sodium intake the daily aldosterone excretions were greater but only by a modest amount, not the 20-30 fold increase expected on such a low intake. Indeed, non-manic days the aldosterone excretion increased by only about 60% and even on manic days the increase was only of the order of 150%.

Table 43 4. Urinary aldosterone excretion (micro g/24 h)

Patient MG (female)	Normal sodium	High sodium	Low sodium
M	6.0	7.1	19.0
D	6.9	8.6	10.0
S	10.7	7:5	18.6

M = Manic D = Depressed S = Switch

Thus the patient showed blunted responses to both sodium deprivation and loading. The abnormality in regulatory mechanisms does not lead to abnormal values for aldosterone however, most reported values of aldosterone production (29) and excretion (19,20) in manic depressive patients being within the ranges found in healthy people.

The development of a radioimmunological assay for plasma renin activity has enabled us in recent years to examine the role of renin in the postulated defect of aldosterone regulation. Renin levels were found to be very high during the period of low aldosterone production observed in the switch from mania to depression.

A further study (30) of four manic depressive patients in a metabolic ward on constant daily sodium intake over two months has produced more evidence of aldosterone-renin abnormalities. Plasma renin activity (recumbent and upright), sodium and potassium were determined twice weekly together with packed cell volumes in each patient. Aldosterone production rate was measured on two occasions. Three of the patients showed at least one episode each of mania and depression during the study whilst the fourth patient, who was receiving prophylactic lithium throughout, showed one ten-day depressive period but was otherwise normal.

The group showed a high resting renin activity compared with controls (Table 43.5) and a blunted renin response to postural change (Table 43.6) compared with controls.

The distribution of individual renin activities found in manic depressive patients is shown in Figure 43.5. The patient on lithium carbonate, although normotensive, had a particularly high plasma renin activity in the range associated with extreme sodium deprivation whereas her aldosterone production was normal. Inappropriate aldosterone production rates for the renin activity found were also demonstrated.The aberrant relationship between renin and aldosterone is further illustrated in Table 43.7

Table 43 5. Recumbent plasma renin activity (ng/ml/h) in four manic-depressive patients and five control subjects

Patient	No. of measurements	Mean ± SEM
AB	27	2.18 ± 0.31
MG	30	2.84 ± 0.16
MWi	28	2.50 ± 0.25
MWa*	21	5.71 ± 0.89
Controls	5	1.53 ± 0.32

*Taking lithium carbonate

Table 43 6. Recumbent and ambulant plasma renin activities in controls and manic depressive patients (ng/ml/h) Mean ± SEM (n)

	Recumbent	Upright	Mean % increase
Controls (5)	1.53 ± 0.32	5.13 ± 1.27	235
Patient AB	2.18 ± 0.31 (27)	4.93 ± 1.21 (9)	126
MG	2.84 ± 0.16 (30)	4.03 ± 0.42 (11)	42
MWi	2.50 ± 0.25 (28)	2.94 ± 0.56 (10)	18
MWa*	5.71 ± 0.89 (21)	13.40 ± 2.47 (5)	134

*Patient on prophylactic lithium carbonate

Table 43 7. Aldosterone, renin and urinary sodium changes in four manic depressive patients receiving constant sodium intake

		Changes		
Patient	Mood	APR (mmol/24 h)	PRA (ng/ml/h)	Urine sodium (mmol/24 h)
AB	N D	+53	-2.50	-9
MG	D D	+31	-0.99	+35
MWi	N M	-119	+3.87	+28
MWa*	N N	+20	-2.35	-18

APR = Aldosterone production rate
PRA = Plasma renin activity

N = Normal
D = Depressed
M = Manic

*Patient receiving lithium carbonate

In patients AB and MWi., substantial differences of renin activity occurred between the 2 days when aldosterone production rates were measured and should have led to corresponding change in aldosterone production. Although substantial changes did occur it was in the wrong

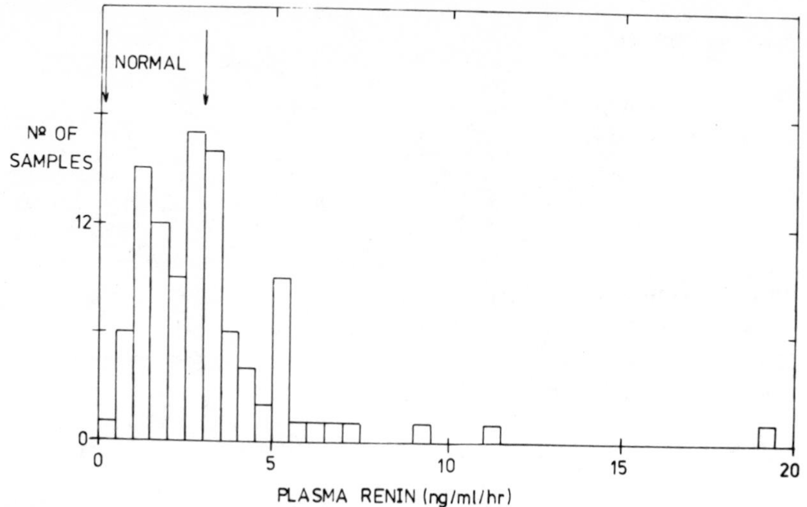

Figure 43.5. Distribution of individual renin activies found in depressive patients as compared with the range of normal values

direction in each case. MG and MWa also showed large changes in renin activity but no significant changes in aldosterone production rate.

A study carried out more recently in the Unit has given still further evidence of abnormalities of the renin-aldosterone system in manic depressive patients. Six patients under metabolic balance conditions were given an extra 200 mmol of oral potassium per day for 3 days. This produced the expected increases in plasma potassium and renin activity but no corresponding increase in plasma aldosterone occurred as would have been expected from current views of normal aldosterone control mechanisms.

Considering the results of all these investigations, there is strong cumulative evidence of a paradoxical relationship between renin and aldosterone in manic depressive psychosis. The results obtained could be explained by postulating that an inhibitor of aldosterone production is present during certain phases of a manic depressive illness. Some direct support for this concept is provided by results obtained with an ACTH-stimulated *in vitro* system of aldosterone production obtained from rat adrenal capsules. The effect of adding sera from manic depressive patients to this system was compared with that of sera from normal subjects and from hospital patients suffering from physical diseases (Figure 43.6). Only in certain of the manic depressive sera was a factor present which inhibited aldosterone production very markedly. There was a variable correlation between mood and inhibitor level — the highest degree of inhibitor

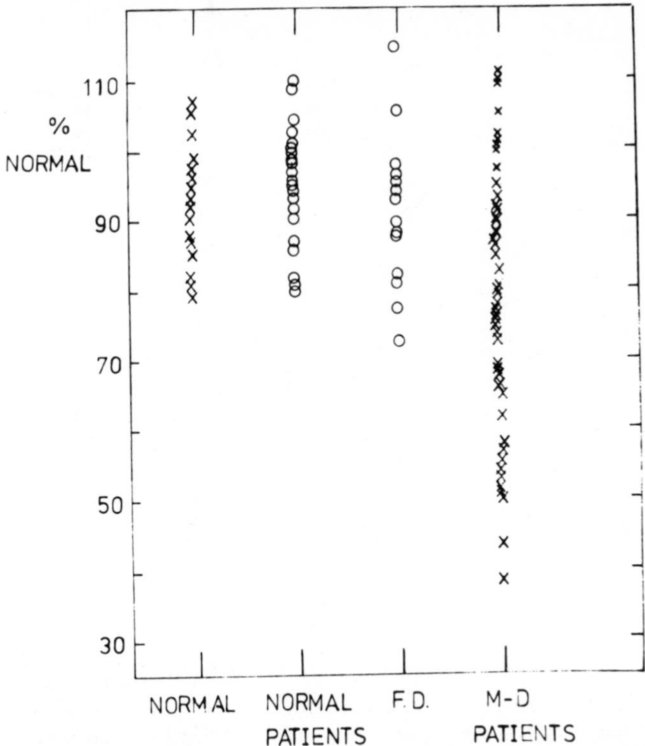

Figure 43.6. Aldosterone production in an *in vitro* system obtained from rat adrenal capsules, as affected by the addition of sera from different groups of subjects, including normal individuals, manic depressive patients, and patients with physical diseases

occurred in early depression and early mania in some patients (Figure 43.7), but was not associated with abnormal mood state in others (Figure 43.8). This patient AB showed the presence of inhibitor following change from mania to normal mood.

It is of interest that in the potassium loading of six patients which raised the plasma potassium and renin but failed to produce a corresponding immediate increase in aldosterone level, there was demonstrated an increase in inhibitor level as determined by the *in vitro* system. Some preliminary work to characterise and purify the inhibitory factor has been carried out by Dr O'Brien. On running normal plasma of Sephadex G-25, the elution profile showed two peaks, one stimulating and the other inhibiting the activity of the *in vitro* system (Figure 43.9). The inhibitory peak, after collection, ran on Sephadex G-50 as a single bond again near to the void volume.

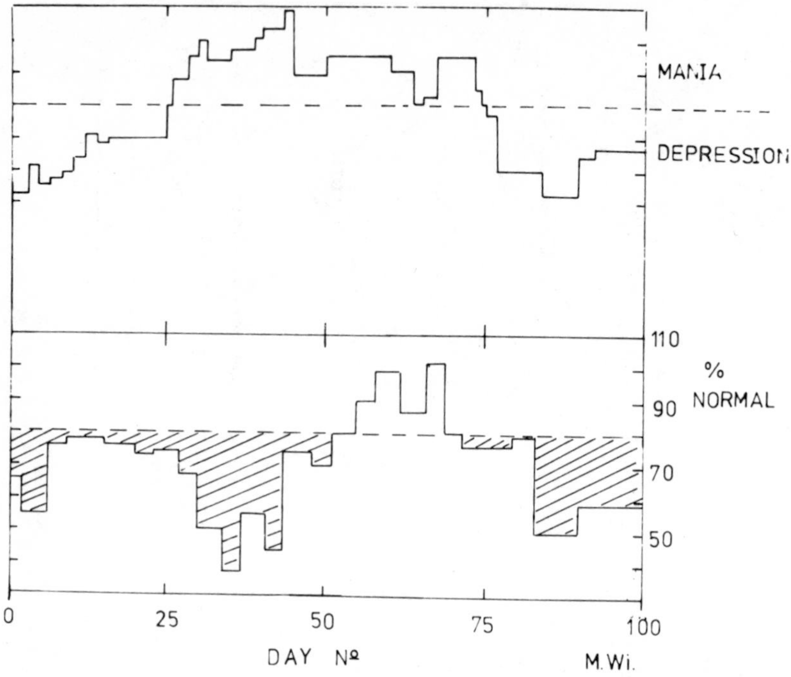

Figure 43.7. Inhibition of *in vitro* aldosterone by a serum factor which seems, in some patients, to fluctuate in its activity in a manner roughly correlated with mood state

Comparing elution profiles of normal and manic depressive sera on Sephadex G-50 (Figure 43.10) has given results for the manic depressive sera ranging from a picture similar to normal serum to a greatly-reduced or absent stimulatory peak in some sera, as shown at the bottom of Figure 43.10. The stimulator of the *in vitro* aldosterone system runs at a position indicating a molecular weight of about 1 000. It has not yet been identified but is not angiotensin II which does not stimulate rat adrenal cells to produce aldosterone. Work continues to clarify the situation.

CONCLUDING REMARKS

In conclusion, at the end of a conference devoted entirely to lithium it is right to ask the question 'Where do we go from here?' Research is fortunately an individual activity so each investigator will make his own choice about what to do and how to do it in terms of his own facilities and expertise. I will content myself with suggesting a few possibilities which might be fruitful.

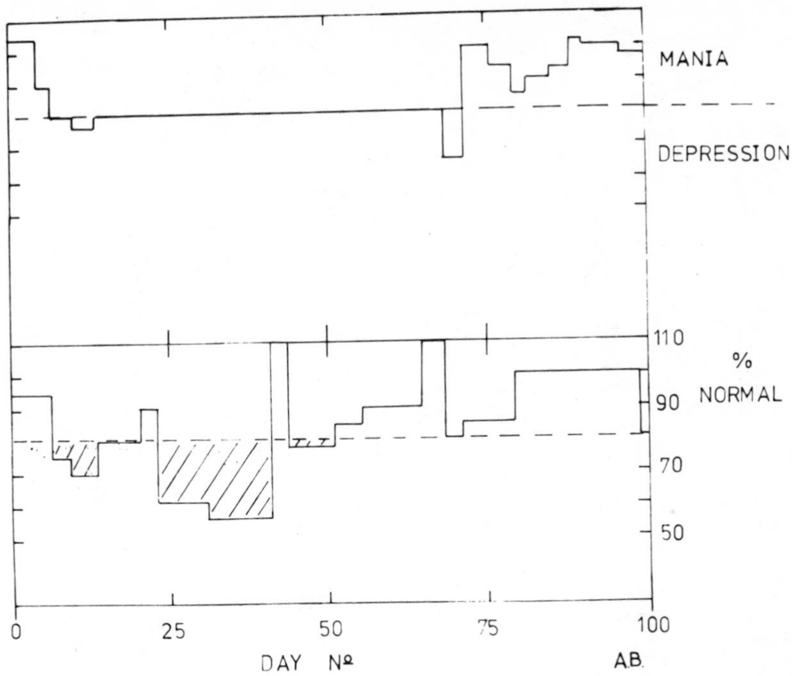

Figure 43.8. Lack of correlation in a patient between mood state and aldosterone production inhibiting effect of a serum-borne factor

1. As indicated earlier, further investigations of the long-term effects of lithium on the kidney is urgent so that extension of lithium therapy is not hindered by what may be merely a failure to control the treatment adequately.

2. Further work is required to determine the minimum blood levels of lithium which will produce maximum prophylactic effect. Unwanted side effects will be less the smaller the exposure of the organism.

3. Research to discriminate responders to lithium from non-responders is clearly important. Non-responders as a group will repay investigation in which the reasons for lack of response are sought.

4. The widespread nature of *in vitro* lithium effects will certainly continue to provide a fertile field. Provided these studies are related back to the patient at some stage, they should be of considerable value.

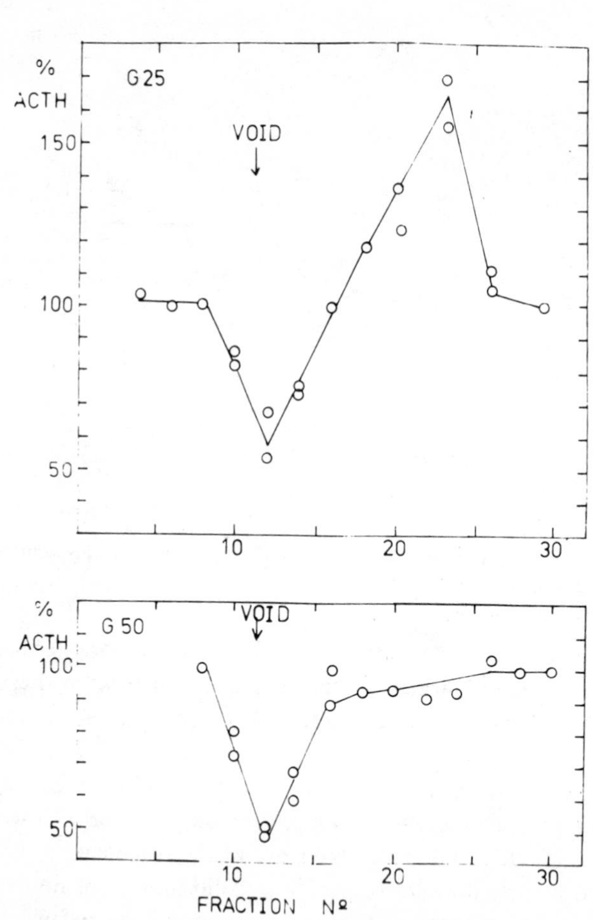

Figure 43.9. Elution profile of normal plasma on Sephadex G-25, showing two peaks, one stimulating and the other inhibiting *in vitro* aldosterone production. the lower profile shows the result of elution on Sephadex G-50 of the collected inhibitory peak

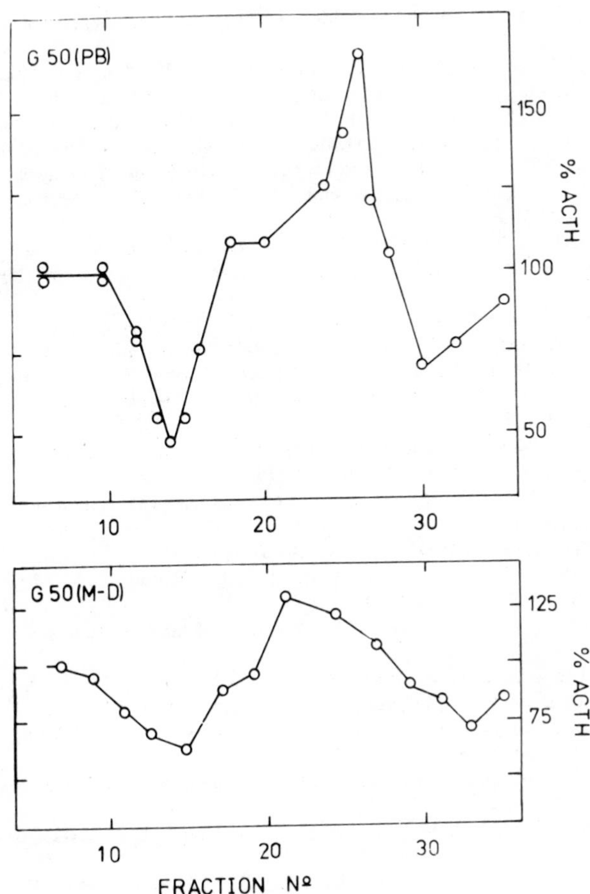

Figure 43.10. Elution profiles of sera from manic depressive subjects. These range in form from a picture similar to normal serum (top profile) to one in which the stimulatory peak is either reduced or completely absent (lower profile)

References

1. Fyrö, B., Petterson, U. and Sedvall, G. (1973). *Acta Psychiat. Scand.*, **49**, 230
2. Crowe, M.J., Lloyd, G.G., Bloch, S. and Rosser, R.M. (1973). *Psychol. Med.*, **3**, 337
3. Nicholson, G., Liebling, L.I. and Hall, R.A. (1976). *Br. J. Psychiat.*, **129**, 236
4. Emerson, C.H., Dyson, W.L. and Utiger, R.D. (1973). *J. Clin. Endocrinol. Metab.* **36**, 338
5. Lindstedt, G., Nilsson, L-A., Walinder, J., Skott, A. and Öhman, R. (1977). *Br. J. Psychiat.*, **130**, 452
6. Villeneuve, A., Gautier, J., Jus, A. and Perron, D. (1973). *Lancet*, **ii**, 502
7. Transbøl, I., Christiansen, C. and Baastrup, P.C. (1977). (Personal communication)
8. Odell, W.D., Wilber, J.F. and Paul, W.E. (1965). *J. Clin. Endocrinol.*, **25**, 1179
9. Chapman, C., Hutton, W.N. and Hayter, C.J. (1974). *Clin. Sci. Mol. Med.* **46**, 651
10. Macdonald, R.G., Chapman, C. and Franklin, H. (1976). *Br. J. Anaesth.*, **48**, 225
11. Hullin, R.P., McDonald, R. and Allsopp, M.N.E. (1975). *Br. J. Psychiat.*, **126**, 281
12. Rosser, R. (1976). *Br. J. Psychiat.*, **128**, 61
13. Lazarus, J.H. and Bennie, E.H. (1972) *Acta Endocrinol.*, **70**, 226
14. Berens, S.C., Bernstein, R.S., Robbins, J. and Wolff, J. (1970). *J. Clin. Invest.*, **49**, 1357
15. Männistö, P.T., Leppäluoto, J. and Virkkunen, P. (1973). *Acta Endocrinol.*, **74**, 492
16. Williams, J.A., Berens, S.C. and Wolff, J. (1971) *Endocrinology*, **88**, 1385
17. Bhattacharyya, B. and Wolff, J. (1976). *Biochem. Biophys. Res. Commun.*, **73**, 383
18. Hullin, R.P., Swinscoe, J.C., McDonald, R. and Dransfield, G.A. (1968). *Br. J. Psychiat.*, **114**, 1561
19. Murphy, D.L., Goodwin. F.K. and Bunney, W.E. (1969). *Lancet*, **ii**, 458
20. Aronoff, M.S., Evens, R.G. and Durell, J. (1971). *J. Psychiat. Res.*, **8**, 139
21. Transbøl, I., Christiansen, C., Baastrup, P.C., Nielsen, M.D. and Giese, J. (1977). (Personal communication)
22. Muller, J. (1971). *Regulation of Aldosterone Biosynthesis*
23. Abraham, S.F., Blair-West, J.R., Coghlan, J.P. Denton, D.A. Mouw, D.W. and Scoggins, B.A. (1973). *IRCS*, **1**, 22
24. McCoa, R.E., McCoa, C.S., Ott, C.E., Young, D.B. and Guyton, A.C. (1973). *IRCS*, **1**, 21
25. Coppen, A. and Shaw, D.M. (1963). *Br. Med. J.*, **2**, 1439
26. Coppen, A., Shaw, D.M. Malleson, A. and Costain, R. (1966) *Br. Med. J.*, **1**, 71
27. Hullin, R.P., Bailey, A.D., McDonald, R., Dransfield, G.A. and Milne, H.B. (1967). *Br. J. Psychiat.*, **113**, 584
28. Levell, M.J., Allsopp, M.N.E., Stitch, S.R. and Hullin, R.P. (1971). *J. Endocrinol.*, **51**, ix
29. Allsopp, M.N.E., Levell, M.J., Stitch, S.R. and Hullin, R.P. (1972). *Br. J. Psychiat.* **120**, 399
30. Hullin, R.P., Jerram, T.C., Lee, M.R., Levell, M.J, and Tyrer, S.P. (1977). *Br. J. Psychiat.*, **130** (in press)

Index